CARDIAC ARRHYTHMIAS

CARDIAC ARRHYTHMIAS

DIAGNOSIS AND TREATMENT

second edition

edited by

NOBLE O. FOWLER M.D.

Professor of Medicine, Department of Internal Medicine;
Director, Division of Cardiology, University of Cincinnati
College of Medicine, Cincinnati, Ohio

With 11 contributors

**First edition published under the title
Treatment of Cardiac Arrhythmias**

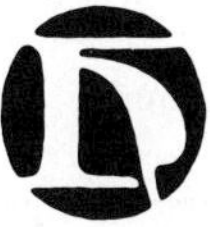

Medical Department
Harper & Row, Publishers
Hagerstown, Maryland
New York, San Francisco, London

Cover and text designed by Alice J. Sellers

77–78–79–80–81–82–10–9–8–7–6–5–4–3–2–1

CARDIAC ARRHYTHMIAS: Diagnosis and Treatment, Second Edition. Copyright © 1977 by Harper & Row, Publishers, Inc. All rights reserved. No part of this book may be used or reproduced in any manner whatsoever without written permission except in the case of brief quotations embodied in critical articles and reviews. Printed in the United States of America. For information address Medical Department, Harper & Row, Publishers, Inc., 2350 Virginia Avenue, Hagerstown, Maryland 21740.

Library of Congress Cataloging in Publication Data
Main entry under title:
Cardiac arrhythmias; diagnosis and treatment.
   Includes bibliographies and index.
   1. Arrhythmia.   2. Arrhythmia—Chemotherapy.
I. Fowler, Noble O. [DNLM: 1. Arrhythmia—
Therapy. WG330 T784]
RC685.A65C273   1977   616.1'28   76-40906
ISBN 0-06-140826-3

Contents

Contributors

Te-Chuan Chou, M.D.
Chapters 5, 9
Professor of Medicine, Division of Cardiology, University of Cincinnati College of Medicine, Cincinnati, Ohio

Gene F. Conway, M.D.
Chapter 12
Professor of Medicine, Department of Internal Medicine, University of Cincinnati College of Medicine, Cincinnati, Ohio

Leonard S. Dreifus, M.D.
Chapter 13
Professor of Medicine, Jefferson Medical College of Thomas Jefferson University; Chief, Cardiovascular Department, Lankenau Hospital, Philadelphia, Pennsylvania

Noble O. Fowler, M.D.
Chapters 1, 3, 6, 7, 8
Professor of Medicine, Department of Internal Medicine; Director, Division of Cardiology, University of Cincinnati College of Medicine, Cincinnati, Ohio

Donald C. Harrison, M.D.
Chapter 11
William G. Irwin Professor and Chief, Department of Cardiology, Stanford University School of Medicine, Stanford, California

John C. Holmes, M.D.
Chapter 14
Professor of Medicine, Department of Internal Medicine; Director, Cardiac Catheterization Laboratory, University of Cincinnati Medical Center, Cincinnati, Ohio

Mark E. Josephson, M.D.
Chapter 10
Assistant Professor of Medicine and Director, Medical Intensive Care Unit, Department of Medicine, University of Pennsylvania; Director, Clinical Electrophysiology Laboratories, Cardiovascular Section, Hospital of the University of Pennsylvania, Philadelphia, Pennsylvania

John A. Kastor, M.D.
Chapter 10
Associate Professor of Medicine, Department of Medicine, University of Pennsylvania School of Medicine; Associate Chief, Cardiovascular Section, Hospital of the University of Pennsylvania, Philadelphia, Pennsylvania

David McCall, M.D., Ph.D.
Chapter 2
Associate Professor of Medicine, Department of Internal Medicine; Director, Coronary Care Unit, University of Cincinnati Medical Center, Cincinnati, Ohio

Donald W. Romhilt, M.D.
Chapter 4
Associate Professor of Medicine, Department of Medicine, University of Cincinnati College of Medicine, Cincinnati, Ohio

Jonathan D. Satinsky, M.D.
Chapter 13
Associate Professor, Department of Medicine, Jefferson Medical College of Thomas Jefferson University; Associate Professor, Department of Cardiology, Lankenau Hospital, Philadelphia, Pennsylvania

Roger A. Winkle, M.D.
Chapter 11
Assistant Professor of Medicine, Cardiology Division, Stanford University Medical Center, Stanford, California

Foreword

Since the first edition of this book was published in 1970, significant new information has been developed which may be applied to the management of cardiac arrhythmias. While not many FDA-approved new drugs have appeared, certain important issues have become resolved. On the other hand, not only do some old questions remain unanswered, but a number of new questions have been posed.

Our understanding of the mechanism of action of antiarrhythmic drugs has been greatly improved. Despite this fact, the selection of antiarrhythmic agents is still largely empiric. Nevertheless, it is useful to remember that conduction within the ventricles is decreased by one group of antiarrhythmic agents (such as quinidine or procainamide) but is improved by another group (such as dilantin and lidocaine) (1). This information may be useful when an agent in one group is not effective in the management of a tachyarrhythmia. It would then appear to be more logical to use an agent from the other group.

Lidocaine, procainamide and other drugs given parenterally are very effective in the treatment of ventricular arrhythmias following acute cardiac infarction. However, it has become clear that the long-term management of ventricular premature beats is difficult, is often attended by drug-induced complications, and usually is of uncertain benefit. Most asymptomatic people with normal hearts probably should not receive drugs for management of premature cardiac contractions. When evaluated several weeks following myocardial infarction, patients who have premature ventricular contractions which exceed five per minute, are multifocal, or occur in salvos, appear to have an increased mortality rate during subsequent months. This same group of patients, however, usually has evidence of cardiac enlargement or left ventricular dysfunction. Controlled clinical trials are needed to determine whether or not antiarrhythmic drugs can reduce the prevalence of sudden death in such patients. It is unproven that coronary artery bypass surgery will be helpful in preventing fatal ventricular arrhythmias in this group of patients.

There have been significant advances in the surgical management of Wolff-Parkinson-White syndrome. Seely, Wallace and associates at Duke University have now treated over 30 patients successfully. Not only has the anatomy of AV nodal bypass tracts become more clearly defined, but also it now appears that effective surgical management is available for nearly all patients who fail to respond to drug management.

Coronary Care Unit observations indicate that a few patients with acute coronary insufficiency and associated ventricular tachyarrhythmias may not respond to drugs but may respond to coronary bypass surgery. An important issue with regard to the management of patients with acute myocardial infarction relates to the treatment of sinus bradycardia, which is extremely common in the first hour or two of infarction and may be observed in the majority of patients with acute inferior infarction if they are seen within the first few hours. Although Goldstein and his associates found that atropine may increase the prevalence of fatal ventricular arrhythmias in experimental infarction (3), this does not usually seem to be the case in humans with acute myocardial infarction and sinus bradycardia. In human infarction, when the heart rate is below 50 per minute and there is evidence of inadequate circulation, intravenous atropine is usually beneficial (5), probably in dosage of at least 0.5–1.0 mg to obviate the possibility of a muscarinic effect of low doses (2).

The indications for electrical DC cardioversion in patients with atrial fibrillation have been further defined. It now appears that this treatment is not indicated in the majority of patients with chronic atrial fibrillation because of the high rate of relapse.

Work is proceeding in the evaluation of new antiarrhythmic agents, such as Norpace

(4), and of oxyprenalol, tolamolol (4) and other beta adrenergic blocking agents. As yet, none of these is approved for general use. Practolol, a promising agent, has been withdrawn because of its tendency to cause cataracts. An effective agent which may be given orally for the long-term treatment of ventricular premature beats and which is free of the toxic effects of quinidine and procainamide is badly needed.

In the management of complete heart block, certain issues seem clarified; others remain uncertain. The value of, and indications for, temporary ventricular electronic pacing in patients with acute cardiac infarction who develop complete AV block are still unclear. The majority of patients with inferior infarction and complete AV block and a supraventricular pacemaker do not appear to require cardiac pacing, although it is usually employed. Patients who develop complete AV block as a complication of anterior infarction require AV pacing as a rule. However, because of their high mortality rate and extensive cardiac damage, it is difficult to show an improvement in survival rate. Cardiac pacing is indicated in most patients who have symptoms related to a persistently slow ventricular rate. In some centers, failure of the sinus pacemaker or "sick sinus syndrome" has emerged as a more common cause of syncope related to bradycardia than is AV block. Patients who have complete AV block with an idioventricular pacemaker should have electronic pacing because of their poor prognosis even though asymptomatic. At this time, asymptomatic patients who have chronic heart disease with evidence of bifascicular block such as right bundle branch block and left anterior hemiblock are not candidates for cardiac pacing since only a small percentage have been shown to progress to complete AV block. This is different from the situation that exists when this conduction disturbance appears in the course of acute infarction, where temporary pacing is probably indicated.

N. O. F.

References

1. Bassett AL, Hoffman BF: Antiarrhythmic drugs. Electrophysiological actions. Ann Rev Pharmacol 11:143, 1971
2. Das G, Talmers FN, Weissler AM: New observations on the effects of atropine on the sinoatrial and atrioventricular nodes in man. Am J Cardiol 36:281, 1975
3. Goldstein RE, Karish RB, Smith ER et al: Influence of atropine and of vagally mediated bradycardia on the occurrence of ventricular arrhythmias following acute coronary occlusion in closed-chest dogs. Circulation 47:1180, 1973
4. Lown B, Temte, JV, Reich P et al: Basis for recurring ventricular fibrillation in the absence of coronary heart disease and its management. New Engl J Med 294:623, 1976
5. Warren JV, Lewis RP: Beneficial effects of atropine in the pre-hospital phase of coronary care. Am J Cardiol 37:68, 1976

Preface

The second edition of CARDIAC ARRHYTHMIAS continues, like the first, to present concise descriptions of current diagnostic methods and current therapies applicable to cardiac arrhythmias commonly encountered in clinical practice. Since proper treatment depends upon correct identification of the arrhythmia, a detailed discussion of the diagnosis, including illustrations, particularly electrocardiograms, where appropriate, precedes the description of treatment. Where more than one treatment regimen is in common use, they are presented in the order of best performance. At the end of each chapter appears a carefully selected list of references to the current literature.

This second edition retains the basic structure of the first, with the addition of a new chapter by Dr. David McCall discussing the pharmacology of antiarrhythmic drugs. Considerable new information concerning the surgical treatment of Wolff-Parkinson-White syndrome is included in Dr. Chou's Chapter 5. Drs. Kastor and Josephson have written a new chapter on the difficult therapeutic decisions in the treatment of atrioventricular block with emphasis on the value of His bundle recordings in reaching a decision in some patients. Drs. Winkle and Harrison have updated the chapter on the use of beta adrenergic blocking agents in the treatment and prevention of cardiac arrhythmias; in addition to the previous information concerning propranolol, they have added much information concerning more recently developed beta blocking drugs. Dr. Donald Romhilt, in a new chapter on the treatment of premature cardiac contractions, emphasizes the difficulty in many instances in deciding on long-term treatment, especially in the absence of heart disease.

Considerable information made available since the first edition about the apparently increasing problems of the sick sinus syndrome is detailed in Chapter 3. Atrial and AV junctional tachycardias are described in a chapter by Dr. Chou; the management of atrial fibrilation and atrial flutter are described in separate chapters. There is now additional information about the long-term results of DC electrical shock in the management of supraventricular arrhythmias. The treatment of ventricular tachycardia is described and brought up-to-date in a separate chapter. Dr. Chou also presents much new information about digitalis-induced arrhythmias, especially with regard to improved diagnostic methods, correlation with serum digoxin levels, and about improved methods of treatment with drugs and cardiac pacing.

Dr. Conway has updated his excellent chapter on the prevention and treatment of cardiac arrhythmias complicating acute myocardial infarction and has emphasized the difficulty in decisions concerning the management of chronic arrhythmias following myocardial infarction. Drs. Dreifus and Satinsky present valuable information concerning the limitations of DC shock in the management of arrhythmias now that we have more experience with that therapeutic tool. Dr. John Holmes has updated his extremely important chapter on cardiac resuscitation.

This book should be of value to physicians specializing in internal medicine and to physicians who engage in family practice or in the general practice of medicine. It will be of interest also to nurses, especially those who work in coronary care and intensive care units, and to paramedical personnel who work in cardiac resuscitation units and emergency care units and life squads. Medical students and residents in training in internal medicine in hospitals will also find this information useful.

N. O. F.

CARDIAC ARRHYTHMIAS

1 | Modern Treatment of Cardiac Arrhythmias: A Perspective

NOBLE O. FOWLER

The first action that should be taken upon detection of a disorder of the heartbeat is to determine the setting in which the arrhythmia occurs. As is rapidly apparent when life is threatened by ventricular fibrillation or extremely rapid paroxysmal tachycardia, one may have to proceed with resuscitative measures, electric shock, or intravenous drugs without a detailed inquiry into the background of the disorder. Yet even in such an emergency, one would avoid electric shock if ventricular tachycardia were caused by digitalis intoxication.

ETIOLOGY OF ARRHYTHMIAS

Table 1–1 indicates some of the etiologic backgrounds of disorders of the heartbeat. Patients with apparently normal hearts may suffer from a variety of disturbances of the cardiac mechanism. Premature cardiac contractions are often unrelated to organic heart disease. They may be precipitated by fatigue, anxiety, overwork, caffeine-containing beverages, tobacco, alcohol, respiratory infections, or sympathomimetic drugs. In such patients treatment consists of a change in the pattern of living and perhaps in sedation. Brief paroxysms of atrial fibrillation may occur in persons with normal hearts, and perhaps 5–10% of patients with paroxysmal ventricular tachycardia have no clinical evidence of organic heart disease.

The myocardial diseases, including myocarditis, may be responsible for premature beats, paroxysmal tachyarrhythmias, and atrioventricular block of all degrees. Acute myocardial infarction is associated with some disorder of the heart beat in over 90% of instances. In infarction prophylaxis must be considered as well as treatment. Cardiac monitoring is needed for the first week or so to detect the patterns of ventricular premature beats, which are warning signs of ventricular tachycardia or fibrillation. Monitoring would also detect the actual occurrence of these disorders and other disturbances of the cardiac mechanism. Paroxysmal tachyarrhythmia in a young person may be a clue to such congenital diseases as the Wolff–Parkinson–White (W–P–W) syndrome or Ebstein's anomaly, or corrected transposition of the great vessels.

Atrial fibrillation and less often atrial flutter, complicate the course of severe mitral valve disease in a large percentage of instances. In such patients correction of the arrhythmia may be difficult unless the valvular deformity is al-

1

Table 1–1. ETIOLOGY OF CARDIAC ARRHYTHMIAS

Disorder	
Normal heart	Fatigue, caffeine, tobacco, alcohol, sympathomimetic drugs, respiratory infection
Myocardiopathy and myocarditis	Extrasystoles, AV block, atrial fibrillation, paroxysmal tachycardias
Coronary artery disease	Acute infarction
Congenital heart disease	Ebstein's anomaly, atrial septal defect, Wolff–Parkinson–White syndrome, short PR interval with normal QRS, corrected transposition of the great arteries
Rheumatic mitral disease	Atrial fibrillation and flutter
Digitalis intoxication	Extrasystoles, junctional rhythm, AV block; PAT with AV block; ventricular tachycardia
Electrolyte imbalance	Especially hypokaliemia, hyperkaliemia
Disturbances of ventilation and acid-base balance, especially hypoxia and hypocapnea with respiratory alkalosis	Atrial and ventricular tachyarrhythmias
Mitral click-murmur syndrome	Ventricular and atrial tachyarrhythmias
Congenital QT interval prolongation, deafness	Ventricular tachyarrhythmias

leviated surgically. Thyrotoxicosis may precipitate atrial flutter or fibrillation. The arrhythmia may be difficult or impossible to control or revert without treating the hyperthyroidism. A variety of paroxysmal arrhythmias including ventricular tachycardia or fibrillation may be caused by pheochromocytoma. When nodal (junctional) rhythms, ventricular tachycardia, or premature ventricular beats are caused by digitalis intoxication, the withdrawal of digitalis is essential to successful management. When digitalis intoxication has evoked a tachyarrhythmia the administration of potassium may be useful. The use of electric countershock should probably be avoided, since it may provoke ventricular fibrillation in this setting. Other drugs, such as quinidine, may be responsible for premature ventricular contractions or even for syncope or death caused by ventricular fibrillation (2). Electrolyte imbalance, especially potassium deficiency, may cause premature cardiac contractions or junctional rhythms. Hyperkaliemia may be responsible for atrial arrest, cardiac slowing, and syncope. Infusions of glucose and insulin, calcium salts, or sodium bicarbonate are useful in the emergency management of the latter. Especially in patients admitted to intensive care units and undergoing assisted respiration, disturbances of ventilation or acid-base balance may precipitate atrial and ventricular tachyarrhythmias. Hypoxia or respiratory alkalosis may be responsible for this condition (1).

REVERTING THE ARRHYTHMIA

In addition to determining the existence and background of cardiac or other disease which may be responsible for an arrhythmia, the physician must also determine whether the arrhythmia should be reverted to a sinus mechanism, and whether there are unjustifiable risks in permitting the arrhythmia to continue without treatment. Premature cardiac contractions may be harmless and may produce no symptoms; on the other hand, even though benign, they may cause disturbing palpitation. At the other extreme, when premature beats are frequent or multifocal they may warn of impending paroxysmal ventricular tachycardia or ventricular or atrial fibrillation. Atrial fibrillation or flutter, especially when associated with a rapid ventricular rate, may significantly impair cardiac function leading to heart failure and pulmonary edema. The latter is especially dangerous in mitral stenosis.

Atrial fibrillation increases the danger of systemic or pulmonary embolism and may result in disturbing palpitation. Yet in some patients, permanent reversion to a sinus mechanism is difficult or impossible and the only practical therapy is to slow the ventricular rate with digitalis, and perhaps to use supplemental anticoagulant therapy. Ventricular tachycardia may lead to shock or pulmonary edema, or to death from cardiac arrest. It is a special risk because of its frequent association with severe organic heart disease, the loss of atrial kick to ventricular filling, and the abnormal site of initial ventricular activation. Complete atrioventricular block is attended by the risk of syncope or sudden death caused by cardiac slowing, standstill or ventricular fibrillation, in addition to heart failure or renal failure.

REFERENCES

1. Ayres SM, Grace WJ: Inappropriate ventilation and hypoxemia as causes of cardiac arrhythmias. Am J Med 46:495, 1969
2. Selzer A, Wray HW: Quinidine syncope. Paroxysmal ventricular fibrillation occurring during treatment of chronic atrial arrhythmias. Circulation 30:17, 1964

2 | Pharmacology of Antiarrhythmic Drugs

DAVID MCCALL

The general principles to be followed in the management of cardiac arrhythmias are well defined in a recent publication by Winkle and his colleagues (68). These principles include an exact characterization of arrhythmias and the definition and treatment of underlying heart disease, if present. If the arrhythmias are suitable for pharmacologic suppression, precise therapeutic goals should be set documenting the efficacy of the drugs. Although in their article (68) these principles are directed mainly towards the therapy of ventricular arrhythmias, they are equally applicable to atrial arrhythmias.

Selection of the appropriate antiarrhythmic agent is based upon a knowledge of the possible underlying arrhythmogenic mechanisms combined with a knowledge of the electrophysiologic actions and pharmacokinetics of the available drugs. It is necessary to consider the electrophysiologic properties of an antiarrhythmic drug combined with a knowledge of its rates and modes of excretion, metabolic pathways and an understanding of the degree of plasma protein binding of that agent. The decision to pharmacologically suppress cardiac arrhythmias may be a decision involving a very short time span, such as suppression of arrhythmias associated with an acute myocardial infarction or myocarditis. However, it may be a decision subjecting the patient to pharmacologic intervention for the remainder of his life. In the latter setting it becomes extremely important to select an agent which will achieve satisfactory suppression of the arrhythmia combined with a minimal incidence of adverse side effects.

In any situation the presence of a cardiac arrhythmia is a reflection of altered underlying cellular electrophysiology. All of the antiarrhythmic drugs have effects on both normal and abnormal cardiac electrophysiology. A review of these topics is necessary to provide a better understanding of the mechanisms of the action of antiarrhythmic drugs. During the past decade considerable evidence has accumulated as to the basic electrophysiologic changes underlying many cardiac arrhythmias. These electrophysiologic changes have been the subject of more extensive and detailed reviews (18, 33, 39, 62, 64), and only a brief revision is within the scope of this chapter.

The first of these mechanisms to be considered is that of enhanced automaticity. This term is used to describe an increased rate of spontaneous discharge from subsidiary or ectopic pacemaker tissue situated either in the atrium, junctional tissue, Purkinje system or ventricular myocardium. Electrophysiologic studies have indicated that the most important determinant pacemaker activity is the slope of the slow intrinsic diastolic depolarization phase of pacemaker tissue. Enhanced automaticity is associated with an increase in the diastolic depolarization rate during this phase, which in turn may be associated with various underlying conditions. Increased rate of spontaneous diastolic depolarization has been observed in ischemic or hypoxic myocardium, in ventricular dilatation, such as occurs in heart failure, in hypokalemia, and exposure to endogenous or exogenous catecholamine activity. Enhanced automaticity is the probable mechanism underlying atrial, junctional and ventricular parasystolic rhythms. Arrhythmias based on enhanced automaticity are therefore by definition considered tachyarrhythmias. On the other hand suppression of automaticity will result in a bradyarrhythmia. Sinus bradycardia, for example, is due to decreased automaticity within the sinoatrial node mediated via acetyl choline released by vagal stimulation, ischemia of the pacemaker tissue or depletion of endogenous catecholamines. Altered automaticity may lead to both tachy and bradyarrhythmias, the more significant, however, being the tachyarrhythmias due to enhanced diastolic depolarization of latent pacemaker tissue.

The second important mechanism to be considered is that of decreased conductivity of the electric impulse within the cardiac tissue, resulting in impaired impulse transmission and decremental conduction. Decreased conduction velocity of the electric impulse and decremental conduction are capable of producing either unidirectional or bidirectional block, the former being largely responsible for the development of reentrant arrhythmias. Reentrant activity is used to describe a situation of continuous impulse propagation at a conduction rate slow enough to permit recovery from the refractoriness of the initiating focus before the circuit is complete. In this situation the slowly propagated impulse returns to the initiating point at a time when its effective refractory period is over and therefore is susceptible to restimulation, thereby reinitiating the circuit. Unidirectional block or decremental conduction through a localized area of myocardium is a necessary prerequisite for reentry since the initial response must fail to excite some area of tissue which is thereby capable of supporting a reentrant response.

Although reentrant arrhythmias may arise in any part of the myocardium, certain regions appear to be more vulnerable than others. In the atrium the distribution of specialized conduction networks provides the appropriate pathways for the development of the suspected circuit reentrant arrhythmia, presenting as atrial flutter. More recently reentrant pathways within the atrioventricular node have been associated with the occurrence of paroxysmal atrial tachycardia. The tachyarrhythmia appears to be sustained by reentry within the atrioventricular node itself. The peripheral ventricular conducting system, including Purkinje fibers and myocardial tissue, is probably more commonly implicated, resulting in reentrant ventricular premature beats. These premature beats will occur most often as coupled beats, usually with a fixed coupling interval. Sustained reentry in this setting may very easily result in ventricular tachycardia. Total suppression of conductivity, indicating bidirectional block, if strategically located within the conducting system, will produce the rhythms of heart block. This may be partial or complete or may reflect a block within one of the more peripheral areas of the conducting system, such as occurs in left or right bundle branch block, or in one of the individual fascicles comprising the left bundle system.

A third major electrophysiologic mechanism of arrhythmogenesis is that of temporal dispersion of action potential duration. This refers to a disparity in the duration of the individual action potentials of neighboring myocardial fibers following simultaneous activation. This process may be associated with focal reexcitation, but is basically different from reentrant activity since it does not require a complete circular pathway, nor does it require unidirectional block. The situation in this instance is that of the presence of fibers which have already repolarized, and hence are beyond their effective refractory period. These repolarized fibers are in close proximity to fibers which remain depolarized for much longer. This sets up a local potential difference between adjacent fibers, which may be sufficient to exceed the threshold for restimulation of the repolarized fibers. These fibers are then restimulated and a focal reexcitation process initiated. This asynchronous recovery of the membrane potential is generally associated clinically with closely coupled premature beats, although some controversy still exists as to the prominence of this reexcitation mechanism. Several factors are known to contribute to nonuniformity of action potential duration. These include digitalis toxicity, localized ischemia, hypokalemia and excess of various antiarrhythmic agents.

Although theoretically it is simple to conceptualize of these three basic mechanisms producing different types of cardiac arrhythmias, in practice any combination of these mechanisms may well be operative. Pharmacologic therapy therefore has to be directed towards the correction of the underlying electrophysiologic mechanism thought most likely in any given situation.

Antiarrhythmic agents produce profound electrophysiologic changes in cardiac tissue. On the basis of their electrophysiologic effects, antiarrhythmics have been classified into two major groups by Bassett and Hoffman (5). The more important of these electrophysiologic actions are summarized in Table 2–1. The drugs of group 1, including quinidine, procainamide, and propranolol, produce somewhat different electrophysiologic effects from those drugs of group 2, including lidocaine and diphenylhydantoin. All drugs listed

Table 2–1. ELECTROPHYSIOLOGIC ACTIONS OF ANTIARRHYTHMIC DRUGS

Electrophysiologic properties	Group I		Group II Lidocaine Diphenyl hydantoin
	Quinidine Procainamide	Propanolol	
Automaticity	↓	↓	↓
Excitability	↓	↓	—
Membrane responsiveness	↓	↓	— or ↑
Effective refractory period (ERP)	↑	↓	↓
Action potential duration (APD)	↑	↓	↓
ERP relative to APD	↑	↑	↑

↑ Increased   ↓ Decreased   — Unchanged

in Table 2–1 decrease automaticity by slowing the rate of diastolic depolarization in subsidiary pacemaker tissue. Quinidine and procainamide increase both action potential duration and effective refractory period, while diphenylhydantoin and lidocaine produce a decrease in both of those parameters. Propranolol, although included with group 1 drugs, differs from the other two drugs in this group in that it causes a decrease in action potential duration and effective refractory period similar to that seen with drugs of group 2. It is of interest that all of the drugs possess the property of increasing effective refractory period duration relative to total action potential duration. Since this effect is common to all antiarrhythmic agents listed and since all are effective in most clinical situations, it may be that this particular property represents the most important electrophysiologic requirement of an antiarrhythmic drug. At the present time it is impossible to select any one of the electrophysiologic characteristics which, in any given situation, will be arrhythmia suppressing. A combined consideration of the electrophysiologic basis of arrhythmias and a knowledge of the electrophysiologic actions of the antiarrhythmic drugs must act as a guide in the selection of an appropriate suppressive agent.

In addition to an understanding of the electrophysiologic effects of the antiarrhythmic drugs, the selection, dosage, and frequency of administration of any particular drug must be based on an understanding of the pharmacokinetic properties of that agent. Although the properties of the individual agents will be discussed with respect to the individual drugs, an outline of the general principles of antiarrhythmic drug administration should be considered at this point. For more extensive treatment of this subject the review of articles by Winkle and his colleagues (68) and Moss and Patton (51) are recommended to the reader.

Since both the therapeutic efficacy and the incidence of adverse side effects of most of the commonly used antiarrhythmic agents show a relationship to plasma drug level, it is important that plasma drug levels be monitored regularly. Knowledge of the kinetic characteristics of the individual drug must be employed in choosing the appropriate dose and frequency of administration. Pharmacologic principles dictate that antiarrhythmic drugs be given on a rigid time schedule, which in most cases, will include the necessity of the patient taking the drug at some time during the night. It is the experience (68) that most patients taking antiarrhythmic drugs do not take them on a regular dose schedule and therefore do not have the benefit of continuously therapeutic blood levels. Administration of an antiarrhythmic agent to a patient, whether by repeated regular oral dosage or by continuous intravenous infusion, requires a basic understanding of the rate of excretion of the drug, the amount of plasma protein binding expected, and the rate of metabolism, together with the various metabolic pathways involved. It is also important to consider the compartment or compartments throughout which the drug is distributed and the manner in which it is distributed, since this will affect the ultimate concentration of the agent at its desired therapeutic target organ. To consider all of these parameters in a scientifically accurate way would necessitate the use of complex mathematic formulas, which in most cases is beyond the scope of practical clinical care of the patient.

A somewhat more simplified approach, could be summarized as the "plateau principle" (31). This concept, summarizing the kinetics of drug accumulation in the body, incorporates pharmacodynamics of distribution, binding, degradation, and excretion. It is fundamental to the understanding of steady state, constant rate infusions and to the dosing interval of intermittently administered agents. The concept does incorporate some assumptions as to the kinetics of absorption and elimination, but in the light of present knowledge these assumptions can be reasonably incorporated into our clinical therapeutic regimes. The concept defines that the establishment of a stable serum level of the drug is determined primarily by the rate of excretion, or elimination, from the body, which also determines the so-called biologic halftime of the agent. During a constant rate of drug infusion it was found (31) that plasma levels increased steadily and reached 90% of the desired plateau blood level after approximately three half-times had elapsed. The implications of this are clear, for example, in the case of lidocaine. Lidocaine has a half-time of about 100 minutes (61), and would require about 5–6 hours of constant infusion before a steady therapeutic blood level is reached. When contemplating continuous infusions it is apparent that a steady plasma level cannot be rapidly obtained, except by the administration of large initial loading doses given at the time of initiation of the continuous infusion. This is now the usually recommended procedure. In addition (31) if one shifts from one steady state of infusion to another in an attempt to increase the plasma drug level, it will again take approximately three half-times to reach 90% of the anticipated new plateau steady state. For this reason it is also recommended that when the infusion rate is increased in an attempt to elevate the plasma level of an agent, a further bolus injection be given at the time of the increase.

The principles outlined above for continuous infusion of antiarrhythmic agents can also be used to determine the appropriate dosing interval of intermittently administered oral drugs. Since the overall principle in the administration of antiarrhythmic therapy is to achieve constant serum levels as nearly as possible, one should accept fluctuations of effective drug concentrations of no greater than 50% in any given 24 hour interval. Since a decrease of 50% in the serum level requires a time interval equal to the half-time of excretion or biologic half-time of the drug, it follows that the dosing interval of any agent should approximately equal the known biologic half-time of that agent. The actual concentration of an agent in the blood, is a reflection not only of the rate of excretion and dosing interval, but also of the amount given together with other variables indicated above, such as plasma protein binding and variable compartmental distribution. It is therefore imperative that blood levels of the drug should be obtained during the initial phases of stabilization on an agent so that a guide as to the frequency and amount of drug administration to any given patient can be obtained. The rate of excretion of a drug or its rate of metabolic conversion may be significantly altered by various disease states. For this reason it is not possible to set down hard and fast rules as to the amount and frequency of administration of any given drug and in the following descriptions of the individual agents only broad, general guidelines are suggested.

With regard to the continuous intravenous infusion of antiarrhythmic drugs one further point merits some discussion. It is the opinion of the author that whenever this route of administration is selected, serious consideration should be given to the use of a continuous infusion pump. This offers several distinct advantages over conventional intravenous drip infusion. First, the use of an infusion pump allows much more accurate control of the infusion rate. The second consideration is one of safety. An infusion pump offers much more protection against inadvertent increases in infusion rate, which may occur for a variety of reasons with the more usual drip infusions. One further consideration of some importance is the volume of fluid required, as a vehicle, to administer any given quantity of the drug. Since all infusion pumps generate pressure very low overall flow rates (as low as 3–5 cc/hour) are required to maintain the patency of indwelling venous cannulas, of fine bore, for prolonged periods of time. Such is not the case with drip infusions, where flow rates as low as this would inevitably lead to cessation of the infusion due to local thrombosis within a very short time. Using an infusion pump it is therefore possible, by increasing the concentration of the drug in the solution, to administer maximal doses of an agent without subjecting the patient to an unnecessary volume load. This is clearly an advantage in situations where one wishes to rigidly control a patient's fluid balance, such as following an acute myocardial infarction or in the presence of congestive heart failure. For these reasons it is felt that, whenever possible, an infusion pump should be used for the continuous intravenous administration of medications. The type of pump used is largely a matter of the individual physician's preference, but both syringe pumps and tubing pumps (for example, Sigmamotor pumps) are equally suited to this use.

As can be seen from Table 2–1, the antiarrhythmic drugs can conveniently be divided into two groups and consideration of the individual agent will follow these groupings as closely as possible, commencing with consideration of the drugs in group 1.

QUINIDINE

Quinidine represents the prototype antiarrhythmic drug of the Group 1 category, and has been in active clinical use for many years. Electrophysiologically the drug has both direct and indirect actions on the heart. The direct actions predominantly reflect decreased automaticity of pacemaker cells. This is true not only of the normally functioning pacemaker tissue of the sino-atrial node, but is also seen, perhaps to an even greater extent, in latent pacemakers under situations of enhanced automaticity. The rate of spontaneous diastolic depolarization is slowed in the presence of quinidine and it is postulated that this and the other electrophysiologic effects of the drug are related to its effects on membrane ion exchange (53). Quinidine also decreases the rate of rise of phase O, the initial rapid depolarization phase of the action potential, and since this is one of the prime determinants of rate of conduction of the subsequent impulse, it decreases the conduction velocity of the impulse in atrial, Purkinje and ventricular tissues. In atrial muscle and Purkinje fibers, quinidine prolongs the effective refractory period without altering the total action potential duration (64). In ventricular tissue quinidine prolongs both the action potential duration and the effective refractory period, simultaneously increasing the ratio of effective refractory period to total action potential duration (5). The drug also decreases atrial and ventricular excitability (64), producing a situation in which the electric impulse necessary to initiate activation is significantly increased. Membrane responsiveness is depressed, thereby decreasing the likelihood of a propagated impulse at low levels of membrane potential.

The direct action of quinidine on the atrioventricular node is to decrease conduction velocity in normal nodal tissue (64). However, it should be noted that quinidine does have some vagolytic effect, which may accelerate conductivity through this tissue.

In addition to these effects quinidine has some antiadrenergic and vagolytic effects, the latter occasionally being manifest by an increase in sinus rate at ordinary therapeutic doses. With small to moderate dosage schedules quinidine has only a minimal depressant effect on cardiac contractility; however, an increase in the QT interval on the electrocardiogram is usually noted, and on rare occasions some QRS prolongation may be seen.

Various oral quinidine preparations are available, including quinidine sulfate and quinidine gluconate. Quinidine gluconate is also available for intramuscular and intravenous administration. Quinidine sulfate is rapidly and completely absorbed from the gastrointestinal tract, the onset of action noted within 30 minutes, and a peak effect achieved in 2–3 hours. Thereafter, the effect decreases with a half-time of some 5–6 hours. Following absorption quinidine is widely distributed in the body but demonstrates a high affinity for protein binding. The tissue to plasma protein binding ratio is approximately 20:1 with 70% of the plasma-bound quinidine being related to the albumin fraction.

Ninety percent of an administered dose of quinidine is metabolized in the liver and the other 10% is excreted, unchanged, in the urine. Urinary excretion is enhanced in an acid urine since the compound itself represents a weak base. Combined hepatic metabolism and renal excretion of the drug results in a biologic half-time in the body of some 4–6 hours (32). This means that with either oral quinidine sulfate or parenteral administrations of the gluconate, the frequency of quinidine administration necessary to maintain plasma levels is in the range of 4–6 hours. Administered more frequently, the drug may accumulate and produce undesirable side effects. In congestive heart failure and renal failure elimination of quinidine may be significantly slowed and the dose interval will have to be increased beyond the normal 4–6 hours to prevent toxic accumulation. Therapeutic blood levels of quinidine are generally accepted to be in the range of 4–6 mg/liter (36).

The principal indications for the use of quinidine include the suppression of atrial, junctional, and ventricular premature contractions and tachyarrhythmias. The drug is also a valuable agent to be used in prophylaxis against occurrence or recurrence of these arrhythmias. Quinidine, although rarely used in this context today, may be used for the conversion of atrial flutter to sinus rhythm; in this respect caution must be exercised (25). Since quinidine reduces intraatrial conduction velocity, it may result in the slowing of atrial flutter to around 200/min prior to conversion to sinus rhythm. At this slower rate, particularly when one considers the vagolytic effect of the drug on the atrioventricular node, this combination may allow an increase in AV conduction resulting in an increase in ventricular rate to undesirable levels. This possibility requires that any patient be fully digitalized before using quinidine in this setting. Since quinidine is one of the few antiarrhythmic agents which prolong atrial refractory time, it is particularly valuable in the management of atrial arrhythmias and has also been used to prevent recurrences of atrial arrhythmias following electric cardioversion. Quinidine may also be used to terminate the reentrant paroxysmal atrial tachycardia of the Wolff–Parkinson–White syndrome. Following acute myocardial infarction quinidine significantly reduces the incidence of premature ventricular contractions (13). Quinidine is also of value in controlling digitalis-induced ventricular arrhythmias. With the advent of safer agents for the parenteral treatment of ventricular tachycardia, quinidine is rarely used parenterally since this is associated with a very high incidence of significant complications.

Contraindications to the use of quinidine include heart block of either the AV nodal or trifasicular type and a history of previous significant adverse or idiosyncratic reactions to the drug.

Unfortunately adverse drug reactions with quinidine are frequent. Lown (48) reports side effects significant enough to require discontinuation of therapy in 30% of his patients receiving the drug. Common side effects include nausea or vomiting, diarrhea, cramping abdominal pain, and headaches. These side effects may occur at ordinary therapeutic doses. At higher dose levels hypoprothrombinemic hemorrhage may occur due to quinidine-induced depression of prothrombin formation and caution has to be exercised with patients receiving concomitant anticoagulant therapy. The drug has been known to produce ventricular tachycardia and ventricular fibrillation even at ordinary therapeutic dosage (21). Sudden arrhythmic death has been estimated by Lown (48) to occur in 0.5% of patients taking the drug. It is postulated that these ventricular arrhythmias induced by quinidine are resultant upon decreased conduction velocity and consequent reentrant mechanisms. Ventricular tachyarrhythmias occurring at regular therapeutic dosages may be considered to represent specific hypersensitivity reaction to the drug. The effects of toxic overdosage of quinidine include the syndrome of cinchonism, hypotension, and significant electrocardiographic abnormalities. Heart block may occur, as may intraatrial block and bundle branch block. In a susceptible individual idiosyncratic reactions occur. In addition to skin rash, angioneurotic edema, thrombocytopenia, hemolytic anemia, and agranulocytosis, these reactions may include any of the previously described adverse reactions usually associated with excessive dosage of the agent.

PROCAINAMIDE

From the electrophysiologic standpoint procainamide behaves in a manner identical to quinidine (5) and requires no further description at this point.

Procainamide, as the hydrochloride salt, is available in both oral and parenteral preparations. When given orally the drug is rapidly absorbed from the gastrointestinal tract, peak serum levels occurring within 1 hour following administration of the drug. With intramuscular injection a therapeutic level is obtained within 5 minutes, with a peak level in 15–30 minutes. Given intravenously maximum antiarrhythmic activity is seen within a very few minutes. Once absorbed, procainamide is distributed widely in all body tissues, but shows some tendency to become concentrated in the kidney, liver, spleen, lungs, heart, and skeletal muscle. It is weakly bound to plasma proteins, with only 15% of the plasma concentration being protein bound (25), resulting in prompt excretion of the drug. This results in the very short biologic half-time of approximately 3 hours compared to 6 hours in the case of quinidine. Almost 60% of an administered dose of the drug is excreted unchanged in the urine (48), with only 5–10% being metabolized to paraaminosalicylic acid in the liver. Although under normal circumstances there is extremely rapid elimination of procainamide from the body, renal excretion is delayed in patients with either congestive heart failure or renal failure (49). The commonly recommended therapeutic blood level of procainamide is in the range of 4–6 mg/liter (8, 44), although one authority recommends levels as high as 10–20 mg/liter (8). Given orally for prophylaxis of ventricular arrhythmias following acute myocardial infarction, a 1 g loading dose of the drug followed by a maintenance of 250–500 mg every 3 hours will maintain a plasma concentration between 4–8 mg/liter. Procainamide may also be given intravenously as a bolus. Although safer than quinidine in this respect, it should be given cautiously at an infusion rate of not greater than 50 mg/min up to a maximum dose of 1.0 g. It may also be given by continuous intravenous infusion at the rate of 4–8 mg/min in the prophylaxis and management of ventricular arrhythmias following acute myocardial infarction.

The principal indications for use of procainamide are the suppression of premature ventricular contractions and ventricular tachycardia. In the latter situation it has been proven to be very efficacious (44). Following acute myocardial infarction, procainamide given either orally or by continuous intravenous infusion decreases the frequency of ventricular premature contractions. It has also been shown to provide significantly greater protection against ventricular fibrillation than either lidocaine or diphenylhydantoin (66).

Intravenously, procainamide is effective in terminating established ventricular tachycardia; but to some extent it has been superseded in this respect by lidocaine, or by direct current cardioversion. The drug is also of value in the treatment of digitalis-induced arrhythmias. Although effective in some situations, attempts to use procainamide to control atrial arrhythmias have proved, generally, to be rather disappointing.

As is the case with quinidine, unpleasant side effects constitute a significant problem with procainamide. The most frequent of those are gastrointestinal, including anorexia, nausea, vomiting, and diarrhea. However, flushing, weakness, giddiness, and occasional hallucinations have also been reported with considerable frequency (32). Drug fevers and drug rashes may occur, and 50% of patients receiving long term procainamide therapy have a positive antinuclear antibody test, with a clinical lupuslike syndrome occurring in at least 20% (16). Other tissue antibodies which have been noted are positive latex and Coombs tests. In one prospective study to detect the efficiacy of prophylactic antiarrhythmic therapy in acute myocardial infarctions, 500 mg every 8 hours of procainamide was associated with adverse reaction in as many as 58% of the patients (48). The allergic reactions to procainamide, including the drug fever and drug rash, usually clear within a short period of time after cessation of therapy. In some cases a positive antinuclear antibody test has persisted for months, or even years. With excessive or toxic doses profound hypotension and shock may occur due to decreased peripheral vascular resistance or depressed ventricular contractility, or a combination of both (8). On the surface electrocardiogram there may be an apparent increase in QRS duration or evidence of AV block. Ventricular ectopic beats, ventricular tachycardia, and ventricular fibrillation have been reported with procainamide. These represent, as they do in the case of quinidine, either toxic overdosage or an idiosyncratic reaction (43).

In order to achieve continual therapeutic levels the drug has to be given at regular 3 to 4 hour intervals. In most individuals this will constitute a significant disturbance from their daily routine. Since it will almost certainly include 2 doses during normal sleeping hours, there will be considerable upset of normal sleep pattern. To many patients this will present an unacceptable intrusion on their life style.

The third drug of this group is propranolol, which has electrophysiologic properties very similar to those of both quinidine and procainamide, differing from them only in that it does not prolong action potential duration. Propranolol together with other β adrenergic antagonists are considered in a later section of this book.

Drugs belonging to the second electrophysiologic category include lidocaine and diphenylhydantoin.

LIDOCAINE

Electrophysiologically, lidocaine has been the subject of considerable study (5), and although it is generally considered to have markedly different effects from those drugs in group 1, there is some controversy on this point (59). The effects of lidocaine differ depending on the concentration used and according to the extracellular potassium concentration (59). Lidocaine generally decreases automaticity by reducing the rate of spontaneous depolarization in both normal and enhanced ectopic pacemaker tissue (22). On the other hand, conduction velocity in cardiac muscle, atrioventricular node, or Purkinje system is unaffected by lidocaine in normal concentrations (22). The effective refractory period (ERP) and total action potential duration (APD) in Purkinje fibers are shortened, but the ratio ERP/APD is increased, as it is with other antiarrhythmic drugs. Minimal effects on ventricular muscle have been recorded (10). Membrane responsiveness, as indicated by the rate of rise of initial depolarization of the action potential particularly in Purkinje fibers (5), is either unaffected or increased by lidocaine. Thus, lidocaine tends to increase antegrade conduction velocity of a propagated electric impulse; by this mechanism it may abolish decremental conduction and unidirectional block in the distal Purkinje system, thereby abolishing reentrant tachyarrhythmias. Because of the effect of lidocaine on action potential duration, particularly in the Purkinje system, temporal dispersion of action potential duration in adjacent fibers will be minimized and localized reexcitation reduced accordingly. Lidocaine is generally considered (5) to have little or no effect on ventricular excitability, although it has been reported (35) that excitability is decreased, causing an elevation in the magnitude of electric stimulation required to initiate depolarization during diastole. The electrophysiologic effects described above are thought to occur at ordinary therapeutic concentrations, but at higher concentrations of lidocaine the effective refractory period in ventricular fibers is prolonged (22) and there is a concomitant decrease in membrane responsiveness. Since the concentrations of lidocaine necessary to produce these latter effects are not encountered clinically, their relevance to the antiarrhythmic action of the drug is minimal.

From the pharmacologic standpoint lidocaine is effective only when given parenterally, preferably by intravenous injection. It is of note, however, that a new, oral lidocainelike agent has been shown to possess significant antiarrhythmic activity in both experimental animals (15) and man (67, 69). Given intravenously lidocaine begins to act within a very few minutes. Following administration lidocaine is largely metabolized in the liver by processes of deamination and deethylation, and only approximately 10% of the drug is excreted, unchanged, in the urine. Metabolic processes, however, are rapid, resulting in a halftime of lidocaine disappearance from the serum following cessation of intravenous medication of about 1½ hours. The clinical implications of this, regarding both initiation of lidocaine infusion and changing to a new infusion rate, are discussed under general pharmacodynamic principles.

In order to achieve adequate therapeutic blood levels lidocaine should be administered as a bolus injection of 50–100 mg intravenously, followed immediately by a constant infusion of 2–4 mg/min (28). Failure to administer the initial dose injection will result in a lapse of some 6 hours before adequate therapeutic blood levels are obtained. This same procedure must be carried out when a change of infusion rate in an upward direction is contemplated, since without a bolus injection there would be unnecessary lapse of time before the subsequent new blood level was attained. It has also been shown (6) that 300 mg of lidocaine, given intramuscularly in adult subjects, is effective in suppressing ventricular premature contractions for at least 45 minutes, with peak plasma levels of some 2.5 mg/liter being obtained 30 minutes after the injection. Analysis of blood lidocaine levels is a technically difficult procedure and is not commonly used for control of therapy. Therapeutic plasma levels of lidocaine are considered to lie within the range 2–5 mg/liter, with serious toxic effects occurring when levels of 10 mg/liter are reached (28). Care should be exercised in the administration of lidocaine to patients with congestive heart failure or liver disease. In both of these conditions, because of impaired hepatic detoxification of the drug a prolonged lidocaine half-time may occur, and values up to 8 hours have been obtained. In this situation, obviously there could be a significant cumulative effect, with early appearance of toxic symptomatology. The infusion rate must be appropriately decreased in these conditions.

It is generally considered, in contradistinction to both quinidine and procainamide, that lidocaine in therapeutic doses has minimal hemodynamic effects in both normal subjects and in patients with heart disease. Intravenous administration of up to 50 mg of lidocaine has been shown to produce no significant depression of cardiac output, left ventricular end-diastolic pressure, or left ventricular dp/dt. In large doses (26) depression of ventricular contractility and hypotension may occur. Little or no change in the surface electrocardiogram occurs during the administration of ordinary dosage of lidocaine.

The principal indication for the use of lidocaine lies in the prevention and suppression of ventricular tachyarrhythmias, particularly in settings in which it is desired to use an agent with minimal hemodynamic or myocardial depressant effects. In this context lidocaine has become the preferred agent for the treatment of ventricular arrhythmias complicating acute myocardial infarction. Numerous clinical studies have documented its efficacy in this respect (42, 47, 48). Lidocaine is particularly effective in suppressing premature ventricular contractions, and for both terminating and preventing repetitive ventricular arrhythmias such as ventricular tachycardia. The drug, is relatively ineffective in treating and suppressing atrial arrhythmias. Successful therapy of atrial arrhythmias was observed in less than 20% of treated patients (42). Although it is generally considered that lidocaine has little or no effect on atrioventricular conduction time, the agent is contraindicated in heart block since it may suppress life-sustaining ventricular or junctional escape rhythms. At ordinary therapeutic doses the drug is capable of producing sinus arrest due to depressed automaticity of the sinoatrial node tissue.

Despite the very widespread and universal use of lidocaine, the reported incidence of side effects of the drug is very small and almost exclusively representative of toxic reactions due to overdosage. These might have resulted from continuous infusion rates of greater than 4 mg/min, or administration of the drug to patients with advanced liver disease. The most prominent and most alarming side effects or toxic reactions to lidocaine are those involving the central nervous system. These may be manifest by muscular twitching, visual disturbances, tinnitus, paresthesias, dizziness, drowsiness, or dysarthria. The patient may complain of an intense feeling of apprehension, or may alternatively appear to be extremely euphoric. The patient may enter a state of profound obtundation, and if lidocaine is continued in this situation, respiratory center depression and convulsions may ensue (58). Excessively large doses may produce cardiovascular depression, with evidence of decreased contractility, reduction of peripheral vascular resistance, hypotension and shock. Ectopic beats may occur, but more commonly there is a bradyarrhythmia, usually sinus bradycardia consequent upon the drug's suppression of sinoatrial automaticity. Idiosyncratic reactions to the drug are rare and no significant or sustained toxic reactions have been reported following the administration of a single therapeutic intravenous injection of the drug.

DIPHENYLHYDANTOIN

Although in use for many years as an antiepileptic agent, it was not until the 1950s that this drug was introduced as a possible antiarrhythmic agent. It was initially reported (34) to be effective in the treatment of cardiac arrhythmias following experimental myocardial infarction in dogs. Thereafter several reports as to its efficacy in man were published.

Electrophysiologically diphenylhydantoin suppresses automaticity in the manner similar to that of other antiarrhythmic agents by depressing spontaneous diastolic depolarization. Reports as to its effect in atrial tissue indicate that the drug may either enhance or depress membrane responsiveness in this tissue and that the magnitude of its effects in this respect are dependent on a number of variables (41). In the Purkinje system its electrophysiologic effects are similar to those of lidocaine in therapeutic doses, causing a shortening of both APD and ERP. The drug, both in Purkinje fibers and in ventricular myocardium, increases the rate of initial depolarization of the action potential and thereby increases the conduction velocity of a propagated impulse. In this respect its effect on reentrant tachyarrhythmias is similar to that of lidocaine, decreasing the likelihood of decremental conduction and unidirectional block. It should be emphasized, (5) that the electrophysiologic effects of diphenylhydantoin are somewhat inconsistent and unpredictable. The effect of diphenylhydantoin on atrioventricular conduction may show improvement or at least no suppression of atrioventicular conduction velocity (12), but the maximum rate of ventricular response to atrial beats may well be diminished (37). The electrophysiologic effects of diphenylhydantoin may be reflected on surface electrocardiograms (11), where it may decrease the PR interval and QT intervals, while heart rate and QRS duration remain normal.

Diphenylhydantoin, as an antiarrhythmic agent, may be given either orally or by intravenous injection. When given orally the drug is slowly absorbed from the gastrointestinal tract, peak blood levels not being obtained until some 8–12 hours after ingestion of the drug. Once absorbed the drug is concentrated mainly in liver, kidney, brain, adipose tissue, and muscle (61). The drug is principally detoxified in the liver and excreted in the bile, which contains only 2% of the unaltered compound. Approximately 90% of diphenylhydantoin in the blood is plasma-protein-bound, resulting in a long plasma halflife of approximately 24 hours. This is subject to alteration and plasma protein binding is considerably reduced by coexistent chronic renal disease. In this situation there is enhanced urinary excretion of the drug. Similarly in patients receiving barbiturates there is enhanced hepatic metabolism of diphenylhydantoin, resulting in a shortening of the plasma half-life. On the other hand in patients with chronic liver disease, the half-life is prolonged and such patients are particularly prone to develop toxic reactions.

It is generally considered (11) that the therapeutic, antiarrhythmic effects of diphenylhydantoin are noted at blood levels between 10–20 mg/liter, while toxic effects are seen when serum levels exceed the upper figure. For rapid achievement of therapeutic blood levels, it is suggested (11) that 50–100 mg of the drug be given intravenously every 5 minutes until the arrhythmia is abolished or until a total of 1000 mg are given. For effective oral administration these same investigators (11) recommend an oral loading dose of 1000 mg the first day, 500 mg the second and third days, and a maintenance dose of 300–400 mg/day. Other investigators have recommended more conservative schedules, with an initial intravenous injection of only 5–10 mg/kg of body weight slowly over a 15 minute period (24). Because of the long plasma half-life (11), unless loading doses are given, a maintenance regimen of 300–400 mg/day results in an established plateau level only after 3–5 days. When administered intravenously diphenylhydantoin is associated with some depression in myocardial contractility and reduction in peripheral vascular resistance (55). This was reflected in an increase in left ventricular end-diastolic pressure (45), decreased cardiac output and a fall in left ventricular dp/dt (50). These effects, are usually transient and do not last more than 30 minutes.

It is now considered that the main indication for the use of diphenylhydantoin is in the treatment of digitalis-induced arrhythmias. Indeed the drug has proven efficacious in the treatment of only a small group of arrhythmias. It has been used successfully in treating both supraventricular and ventricular arrhythmias induced by digitalis and is considered by many to be the drug of choice in this situation, since it is unlikely to depress atrioventricular conduction further (19). It has also been advocated that diphenylhydantoin will improve the toxic to therapeutic ratio of digitalis and that the drug provides prophylaxis against digitalis toxicity (38). Other situations in which diphenylhydantoin has been successfully used include the immediate postoperative state and following cardioversion. The usefulness of the drug in controlling myocardial infarction related arrhythmias is somewhat controversial (60). A study designed to assess the effect of the drug in preventing recurrences of ventricular tachycardia in patients with coronary disease showed that the drug was uniformly ineffective in this area (60). Dilantin is rarely effective in atrial flutter or other supraventricular arrhythmias unrelated to digitalis intoxication. At present clinical experience has indicated that although diphenylhydantoin may be a useful adjunct to other antiarrhythmic therapy in certain situa-

stuffiness, diarrhea, nausea, and fatigue. There may be disturbance of micturition and, occasionally, painful parotid swelling has been reported. The most prominent life-threatening reaction is very marked hypotension, which may occur even in the supine position and is due to marked peripheral vasodilatation. The drug may occasionally produce sinus bradycardia. Hypersensitivity and idiosyncratic reactions can be anticipated with higher doses, and the drug is contraindicated in the presence of pheochromocytoma. Hypotension should be treated by the recumbent position, appropriate vasopressor therapy and volume loading. Patients receiving bretylium are extremely sensitive to sympathomimetic drugs, particularly epinephrine and amphetamine, which should be given only as a last resort. Isoproterenol does not produce peripheral vasoconstriction and is not an effective antagonist to bretylium.

ATROPINE

For the treatment of arrhythmias atropine is used only for bradyarrhythmias, since the drug effectively abolishes the action of acetylcholine on the heart. From the electrophysiologic standpoint one action of atropine is important. Since it abolishes the effect of acetylcholine, it selectively creates an increase in the rate of spontaneous depolarization in pacemaker cells. This results in an increase in the intrinsic rate of pacemaker tissue above the level of the atrioventricular node. The effect is to increase the rate of the sinoatrial and atrioventricular junctional pacemakers. In addition conduction velocity through the AV node increases, since under most circumstances this is under some degree of vagal control. Atropine therefore increases the resting heart rate, tends to abolish bradyarrhythmias, and accelerates atrioventricular conduction. Atropine shortens the PR interval of the surface electrocardiogram during sinus rhythm, and digitalis-induced heart block may in part be abolished. It should be noted (20) that in very small doses atropine may, in fact, cause a paradoxical effect, with slowing of the heart rate and increase in atrioventricular conduction time. Therefore care should be taken that atropine is administered in an adequate anticholinergic amount.

Following intravenous administration atropine has a peak effect in 30–90 seconds, thereafter disappearing rapidly from the blood. It is distributed widely throughout the body tissues. Fifty percent or more of the administered dose of atropine is metabolized, presumably in the liver, and the remainder is excreted unchanged in the urine. The pharmacologic half-life of atropine is very short, approximately 2–3 hours.

Atropine has widespread anticholinergic actions which to some extent are dose-dependent (32). At low dosages there is inhibition of secretion of the salivary, bronchial, and sweat glands; whereas at moderate dosages sinus tachycardia, pupillary dilatation, and inhibition of accomodation may occur. At higher dosages bladder dysfunction may be present and gastrointestinal motility is depressed. Central nervous system stimulation occurs as a manifestation of atropine overdosage.

Atropine produces few hemodynamic changes other than by its effect on heart rate. This alone, may effect a significant improvement in hemodynamics when hypotension or a low cardiac output is caused by bradyarrhythmia. With a normal resting heart rate, atropine produces little change in blood pressure, cardiac output or total peripheral resistance. In the management of bradyarrhythmias atropine should be given intravenously in an initial dose of 1 mg. This dose may be repeated in 15–30 minutes if required. In the prophylaxis of bradyarrhythmias atropine may be administered subcutaneously in a similar dosage every 4–6 hours.

The most important clinical use of atropine is in the treatment and abolition of bradyarrhythmias. The drug has been shown to be effective in treating supraventricular bradyarrhythmias accompanying acute myocardial infarction (1) and in AV conduction disturbances associated with acute inferior wall myocardial damage (70). Atropine may also prove useful in managing digitalis-induced sinoatrial bradycardia and atrioventricular block. In this respect atropine has been more effective in terminating the conduction disturbances accompanying acute digitalis overdosage, for example, in a suicide attempt. Adverse side effects of atropine include dryness of the mouth, loss of visual accommodation, constipation, micturition disturbances and minor aberrations of mental function, particularly at higher dose levels. Elderly patients are more prone to develop adverse reactions to atropine, although they frequently demonstrate a less than optimal therapeutic response. Precipitation of glaucoma represents a significant side effect. Prior to administration of atropine a history of symptoms suggestive of glaucoma should be sought in each patient. The adverse side effects of atropine usually disappear promptly upon termination of therapy with the drug.

DIGITALIS

No discussion of antiarrhythmic agents would be complete without a mention of the antiarrhythmic properties of the cardiac glycosides. Although generally considered mainly as positive inotropic agents for use in the therapy of congestive heart failure, the digitalis glycosides have very useful antiarrhythmic properties, predominantly allowing adequate control of supraventricular tachyarrhythmias. The cardiac glycosides produce both direct and indirect electrophysiologic effects on the heart. The direct actions on the heart result from the inhibitory effect of the drug on active transport of sodium and potassium by the cell membrane sodium-potassium-activated ATPase (30). The indirect actions of the drugs are due to a centrally mediated increase in vagal tone.

In many ways the direct and indirect actions are antagonistic; thus somewhat varying electrophysiologic effects have been ascribed to the drugs (40). The indirect actions, via vagal release of acetylcholine, result in a decreased rate of phase 4 depolarization in sinoatrial tissue and in the pacemaker cells of the junctional region. This action will also prolong the effective refractory period of the atrioventricular node and result in a decreased conduction through the node, which may give rise to varying degrees of atrioventricular block.

On the other hand, the direct action, particularly in toxic amounts, will enhance the intrinsic automaticity of tissues in the atrioventricular junction, His–Purkinje System and ventricular myocardium. Digitalis increases the excitability of His–Purkinje fibers and although the action potential duration is prolonged, the effective refractory period is usually shortened. Prolongation of the action potential duration may not be uniform, leading to some temporal dispersion of the action potentials. Since the effective refractory period is shortened, localized reentrant pathways may be initiated. The direct electrophysiologic effects of the glycosides reflect changes in membrane permeability to sodium and potassium, consequent upon inhibition of active transport of those ions, and are the effects largely responsible for the common digitalis-induced arrhythmias.

A wide variety of digitalis preparations are available. The difference between them largely represents differences in rates of absorption and excretion. For a more complete discussion of these individual compounds the reader is referred to reference (32). In the present discussion only digoxin will be considered, since it represents the most commonly used digitalis preparation at the present time. Digoxin is well absorbed from the gastrointestinal tract to the extent of approximately 80% of the administered dosage. Oral absorption, however, is decreased in various malabsorption syndromes and may well vary from preparation to preparation (46). Following oral administration the peak action of digoxin is achieved within 2–2½ hours, whereas following intravenous administration the peak action is seen within 30 minutes. Digoxin is partially bound to plasma proteins, approximately 20% of the circulating amount of the drug being protein bound. The drug is widely distributed throughout various body tissues with the highest concentrations being found in the gastrointestinal tract, liver, and kidney; somewhat lower concentrations are found in the heart, lungs, and spleen. The myocardium itself has no selective affinity for digitalis. Since the primary site of action is the sodium potassium ATPase of the cell membrane, it attaches to these sites throughout all body tissues. Approximately 30–40% of an administered dose of digoxin is excreted unchanged in the urine and 10% is metabolized in the liver. Renal excretion of digoxin is influenced to some extent by plasma protein binding. It is much more significantly influenced by the presence of renal disease, in that patients with an elevated blood urea nitrogen (BUN) or serum creatinine tend to excrete a proportionally smaller percentage of the administered dose per day. The effective plasma halftime for digoxin is approximately 1.6 days and therapy should generally be monitored by obtaining plasma digoxin levels. Therapeutically the plasma level should lie within the range of 1–2 ng/ml. Since excretion is markedly altered in patients with impairment of renal function, the usual daily dosage of 0.125–0.5 mg/day should be tailored to the individual and followed by frequent measurements of the serum digoxin level.

The most frequent antiarrhythmic use of the cardiac glycosides is to control and convert supraventricular tacharrhythmias. Digoxin is effective in controlling a rapid ventricular response to atrial flutter and atrial fibrillation primarily via its indirect action on atrioventricular conduction. In the presence of atrial fibrillation or atrial flutter digoxin frequently results in a slowing or control of the ventricular response. If the rhythm is of recent onset, the drug may effect a conversion to sinus rhythm by virtue of a stabilizing influence on abnormal atrial mechanisms. In general terms higher doses of digoxin are required to control the ventricular response in atrial flutter than in atrial fibrillation, but the exact mechanism for this phenomenon is uncertain. Digoxin has also been shown to be effective in reducing the frequency of attacks of paroxysmal atrial tachycardia and for terminating acute attacks once they occur. It is impossible to lay down hard and fast dosage schedules for digoxin to be used in the treatment of acute supraventricular tachyarrhythmias. In general terms the drug should be given as outlined in the appropriate chapters of this text, until the therapeutic end point is achieved or until evidence of digitalis toxicity supervenes. In this respect the recent availability of serum digoxin levels has been of considerable benefit. Generally, the serum digoxin level 5–6 hours after the last oral dose should not exceed 2 ng/ml. Occasionally this level may need to be exceeded in order to achieve a satisfactorily controlled ventricular response, particularly in the presence of atrial flutter.

Adverse reactions to digitalis glycosides are common (32) and only a brief description of the more common syndromes will be presented. Most frequent initial side effects which may occur at ordinary therapeutic dosage include headaches, gastrointestinal upset, and visual disturbances. The most alarming aspect of digitalis toxicity is the production of cardiac arrhythmias. Almost any arrhythmia may result from digitalis toxicity, but by far the most frequent are premature ventricular contractions which usually occur with a fixed coupling interval and often with bigeminy. More significant ventricular tacharrhythmias, including sustained ventricular tachycardia and ventricular fibrillation, may occur as may various accelerated junctional and supraventricular tachycardias. In addition to the tachyarrhythmias a variety of bradyarrhythmias may result from suppression of the atrioventricular or sinus nodes. First degree atrioventricular block is common and second degree block, usually of the Wenckebach type, may occur and even progress to complete heart block. Sinus node suppression resulting in sinus bradycardia or sinus arrest may be associated with junctional or ventricular escape rhythms, due to the enhanced automaticity of the intrinsic pacemakers of those regions. The occurrence of tachyarrhythmias, particularly supraventricular tachyarrhythmias during the course of digitalis therapy may give rise to a significant diagnostic dilemma. Clinically it is often uncertain as to whether this represents insufficient digitalization, or whether it represents a manifestation of digitalis toxicity. The availability of serum digoxin levels in the last few years has considerably aided in this problem, but in only a relatively few institutions can these be obtained with any degree of rapidity. When faced with this particular situation, unless there are significant hemodynamic sequels to the arrhythmia, it is often considered better to regard the situation as one of digitalis toxicity and hold any further therapy until the serum digoxin level is available.

SELECTION OF AN ANTIARRHYTHMIC AGENT: GENERAL CONSIDERATIONS

Although a variety of agents are available for the management of arrhythmias, it is clear that there is no single ideal antiarrhythmic drug. Although the drugs discussed, if carefully selected for the appropriate arrhythmia, are clinically effective, all are associated with a high incidence of significant side effects. At the present time no new antiarrhythmic agents are available for general use in the United States, although preliminary reports from Europe have shown encouraging results, with some recent additions to this field. These include a new quinidinelike agent, Norpace. Verapamil and newer β-blocking agents such as Oxprenolol and Sotalol are likely to prove useful. Some of these agents, including Norpace, Verapamil, and Oxprenolol, have been granted investigational new drug status by the Food and Drug Administration. The early reports of the clinical trials of the new oral lidocainelike agent, Astra W–36095–HCl, are encouraging, but at this time insufficient experience has been gained to fully assess its efficacy.

It is apparent that there are many similarities between the presently available agents, although some important differences do exist. The selection of any particular agent to control an arrhythmia must take into account a consideration of the pharmacologic actions of the drugs together with a consideration of the possible underlying arrhythmogenic mechanism and a detailed knowledge of the pharmacokinetics of the available agents. This latter is of particular importance when one is contemplating long-term therapy and is also of considerable importance in attaining and maintaining a high degree of patient compliance. Since it is imperative (68) that relatively constant blood levels of an antiarrhythmic agent be maintained throughout a 24 hour span, the frequency of administration of the drugs, depending on the halftime of elimination of the agent, must be rigidly controlled. For example relatively stable quinidine levels can be achieved only by a regular 6 hour schedule, which usually requires that the patient awake from his normal sleep for one dose. Greater inconvenience to the patient results from the administration of oral procainamide, which should be given every 4 hours. The higher degree of inconvenience probably will result in a lesser degree of patient compliance. In addition to the inconvenience dictated by the obligatory therapeutic regimens of the antiarrhythmic agents, one has also to consider the relative incidence of adverse side effects. Unfortunately at this time there is no effective antiarrhythmic agent which has no, or only minimal, side effects. Quinidine and procainamide are probably the two most commonly used antiarrhythmic drugs at this time. Long term therapy with oral procainamide is associated with an alarmingly high incidence of positive Lupus Erythematosus Cell (LE) tests and a significant incidence of a frank lupus syndrome. On the other hand quinidine is by no means an innocuous agent, with some 30% of patients showing significant side effects which necessitate discontinuation of therapy. Selection of the appropriate antiarrhythmic agent must therefore be made on very carefully considered grounds. The economic consideration of cost effectiveness, which in certain circumstances may become an important determinant in the selection of any specific drug (52), must also be weighed.

From Table 2–1 it is apparent that there are several similarities between the electrophysiologic effects of the various antiarrhythmic agents. Each of the agents listed is commonly used for suppression of ventricular arrhythmias, suppresses automaticity in latent pacemakers and prolongs the effective refractory period of Purkinje fibers and ventricular myocardium. This latter effect means that the earliest premature beats will occur at a more negative membrane potential, resulting in a more rapid rate of rise of the resultant action potential and hence a more rapid conduction of any propagated impulse. This may enhance conduction in the Purkinje system and ventricular myocardium, and possibly eliminate reentrant arrhythmias generated in part by depressed conduction velocity. Several differences between the drugs, however, do exist. The drugs of Group 1, including propranolol, depress membrane responsiveness and depress the conduction velocity of an electric impulse in the Purkinje system and ventricular myocardium. The drugs in group 2 have an exactly opposite effect when used in therapeutic concentrations. Both of these actions, however, may result in an overall beneficial effect, particularly in consideration of a reentrant arrhythmia. The drugs of group 1, probably by virtue of their depressant effect, convert an area of unidirectional block into an area of bidirectional block, thereby breaking the circus movement responsible for the reentrant arrhythmia. On the other hand the drugs of group 2, by enhancing antegrade conduction through the depressed area, favor the establishment of normal conduction and thereby eliminate the reentrant mechanism. Both groups of agents may correct the arrhythmogenic mechanism of temporal dispersion of action potential duration; group 1 agents by prolonging overall action potential duration, and group 2 agents by shortening the action potential duration in those tissues with the initially prolonged action potential duration. Unfortunately the surface electrocardiogram from which the decision to use an antiarrhythmic agent is usually made provides little or no evidence as to the underlying electrophysiologic mechanism. The selection of an appropriate agent from either of the two groups therefore remains, at this time, largely a matter of trial and error.

Clear indications for use of one or other of the agents listed above exist in only a few situations. Examples of these include the use and selection of a digitalis preparation for control of the ventricular response in atrial fibrillation and atrial flutter and for treatment of supraventricular tachycardia. In other situations selection of the initial antiarrhythmic agent should be based on the general principles outlined above and, in greater detail, by Winkle and his colleagues (68). The first selected agent should be given in fully therapeutic amounts, utilizing blood levels of the drug to determine the proper dose frequency. The dosage of the drug should be gradually increased until it is likely that a maximal therapeutic dose level has been obtained. The effective therapeutic range of most antiarrhythmic agents is quite narrow and failure to achieve this range may result in inefficacy of the preparation, whereas slightly exceeding this range may result in significant toxic side effects. When the optimal dosage of one agent has proved to be ineffective, selection of an agent with different electrophysiologic properties should be made. For example when an agent of the group 1 category of drugs has failed to control a particular arrhythmia, it would appear logical to try the effect of one of the drugs of group 2, since it will apply a different electrophysiologic mechanism to the underlying arrhythmogenic process. As with the original drug selection this drug should also be given in maximum therapeutic dosages; both the dose and frequency of administration should be closely controlled by following plasma levels of the agent. Only when an agent has been given so that optimal blood levels are obtained, can a persistent arrhythmia be considered refractory to that particular agent. When the optimal dosage of one or more agents administered singly has proved ineffective, the combination of two or more agents should be tried. Additional agents should be such that they complement the electrophysiologic properties of the initial drug. Thus there is little advantage in combining quinidine with procainamide, since the basic antiarrhythmic properties of the two drugs are identical. Instead a combination of an agent from one of the electrophysiologic groups with that of one from the other group should be tried, since the antiarrhythmic activity of these combinations is often complementary.

By following this logical sequence and by paying close attention to blood levels of the drugs, optimal dosage regimen can be established that offer the best change for satisfactory therapeutic control of an arrhythmia.

REFERENCES

1. Adgey AAJ, Geddes JS, Mulholland HC et al.: Incidence, significance, and management of early bradyarrhythmias complicating acute myocardial infarction. Lancet 2: 1097, 1968
2. Allen JD, Zaida SA, Shanks RG, Pantridge JF: The effects of bretylium on experimental cardiac dysrhythmias. Am J Cardiol 29:641, 1972
3. Aviado AM, Dil AH: The effects of a new sympathetic blocking drug (Bretylium) on cardiovascular control. J Pharmacol Exp Ther 129:328, 1960
4. Bacaner M: Bretylium tosylate for suppression of induced ventricular fibrillation. Am J Cardiol 17:528, 1966
5. Bassett AL, Hoffman BF: Antiarrhythmic drugs: electrophysiological actions. Annu Rev Pharmacol 11:143, 1971
6. Bellet S, Roman L. Kotis JB et al.: Intramuscular lidocaine in the therapy of ventricular arrhythmias. Am J Cardiol 27:291, 1971
7. Bernstein JG, Koch–Weser J: Effectiveness of bretylium tosylate against refractory ventricular arrhythmias. Circulation 45:1024, 1972
8. Bigger JT, Heissenbuttel RH: The use of procaine amide and lidocaine in the treatment of cardiac arrhythmias. Prog Cardiovasc Dis 11:515, 1969
9. Bigger JT, Jaffe CC: The effect of Bretylium Tosylate on the electrophysiologic properties of ventricular muscle and Purkinje fibers. Am J Cardiol 27:82, 1971
10. Bigger JT, Mandel WJ: Effect of lidocaine on the electrophysiological properties of ventricular muscle and Purkinje fibers. J Clin Invest 49:63, 1970
11. Bigger JT, Schmide DH, Kutt H: Relationship between plasma level of diphenylhydantoin sodium and its cardiac antiarrhythmic effects. Circulation 38:363, 1968
12. Bigger JT, Steiner C, Burris JO: The effect of diphenylhydantoin on atrioventricular conduction in man. Clin Res 15:196, 1967

13. Bloomfield SS, Romhilt DW, Chou TC, Fowler NO: Quinidine for prophylaxis of arrhythmias in acute myocardial infarctions. N Engl J Med 285:979, 1971
14. Cohen HC, Gozo EG, Langendorf R et al.: Response of resistant ventricular tachycardia to bretylium. Circulation 47:331, 1973
15. Coltart DJ, Berndt TB, Kernoff R, Harrison DC: Antiarrhythmic and circulatory effects of Astra W36095. A new lidocaine-like agent. Am J Cardiol 34:35, 1974
16. Condemi JJ, Blomgren SE, Vaughan JH: The procainamide-induced lupus syndrome. Bull Rheum Dis 20:604, 1970
17. Cooper JA, Frieden J: Bretylium tosylate. Am Heart J 82:703, 1971
18. Cranefield PF, Wit AL, Hoffman BF: Genesis of cardiac arrhythmias. Circulation 47:190, 1973
19. Damato AH: Diphenylhydantion: pharmacological and clinical use. Prog Cardiovasc Dis 12:1, 1969
20. Das G, Talmers FN, Weissler AM: New observations on the effects of atropine on the sinoatrial and atrioventricular nodes in man. Am J Cardiol 36:281, 1975
21. Davies P. Leak D, Oram S: Quinidine-induced syncope. Br Med J 2:517, 1965
22. Davis LD, Temte JV: Electrophysiological actions of lidocaine on canine ventricular muscle and Purkinje fibers. Circ Res 24:639, 1969
23. Day HW, Bacaner M: Use of bretylium tosylate in the management of acute myocardial infarction. Am J Cardiol 27:177, 1971
24. Dreifus LS, Rabbino MD, Watanabe Y: Newer agents in the treatment of cardiac arrhythmias. Med Clin North Am 48:371, 1964
25. Friedberg CK: Disease of the Heart, 3rd ed. Philadelphia, WB Saunders, 1966
26. Frieden J: Lidocaine as an antiarrhythmic agent. Am Heart J 70:713, 1965
27. Furchgott RF: Receptors for sympathomimetic amines. In Vane JR, Wolstenholme GEW, O'Connor M (eds): Adrenergic Mechanisms. Boston, Little, Brown, 1960, pp 246–252
28. Gianelly RE, von der Groeben JO, Spivack AP et al.: Effect of lidocaine on ventricular arrhythmias in patients with coronary heart disease. N Engl J Med 277:1215, 1967
29. Gillis RA, Clancy MM, Anderson RJ: Deleterious effects of bretylium in cats with digitalis-induced ventricular tachycardia. Circulation 47:974, 1973
30. Glynn IM: The action of cardiac glycosides on ion movement. Pharmacol Rev 16:381, 1964
31. Goldstein A, Aronow L, Kalman S: Principles of Drug Reaction. New York, Harper & Row, 1968, p 292
32. Goodman LS, Gilman A: The Pharmacological Basis of Therapeutics, 4th ed. New York, MacMillan, 1970
33. Han J: The concepts of reentrant activity responsible for ectopic rhythms. Am J Cardiol 28:253, 1971
34. Harris AS, Kokernot RH: Effects of diphenylhydantoin sodium (Dilantin Sodium) and phenobarbital sodium on ectopic ventricular tachycardia in acute myocardial infarction. Am J Physiol 163:505, 1950
35. Harrison DC, Sprouse JH, Morrow AG: The antiarrhythmic properties of lidocaine and procainamide. Circulation 28:486, 1963
36. Heissenbuttel RH, Bigger JT: The effect of oral quinidine on intraventricular conduction in man: correlation of plasma quinidine with changes in QRS duration. Am Heart J 80:453, 1970
37. Helfant RH, Lau SH, Cohen SI et al.: Effects of diphenylhydantoin on atrioventricular conduction in man. Circulation 36:686, 1967
38. Helfant RH, Scherlag BJ, Damato AN: Protection from digitalis toxicity with prophylactic use of diphenylhydantoin sodium. Circulation 36:119, 1967
39. Hoffman BF: The genesis of cardiac arrhythmias. Prog Cardiovasc Dis 8:319, 1966
40. Hoffman BF, Singer DH: Effects of digitalis on electrical activity of cardiac fibers. Prog Cardiovasc Dis 7:226, 1964
41. Jensen RA, Katzung BG: Electrophysiological actions of diphenylhydantoin on rabbit atria. Circ Res 26:17, 1970
42. Jewitt DE, Kishon Y, Thomas M: Lignocaine in the management of arrhythmias after acute myocardial infarction. Lancet 1:266, 1968
43. Kayden HJ, Brodie BB, Steele JM: Procaine amide. Circulation 15:118, 1957

44. Koch–Weser J, Klein S, Foo–Canto LL et al.: Antiarrhythmic prophylaxis with procainamide in acute myocardial infarction. N Engl J Med 281:1253, 1969
45. Lieberson AD, Schumacher RR, Childress RH et al.: Effects of diphenylhydantoin on left ventricular function in patients with heart disease. Circulation 36:692, 1969
46. Lindenbaum J, Mellow MH, Blackstone MD, Butler VP: Variation in biologic availability of digoxin from four preparations. N Engl J Med 285:1344, 1971
47. Lown B, Vassaux C: Lidocaine in acute myocardial infarction. Am Heart J 76:586, 1968
48. Lown B, Wolf M: Approaches to sudden death from coronary heart disease. Circulation 44:130, 1971
49. Mark LC, Kayden HJ, Steele JM et al.: The physiologic disposition and cardiac effects of procaine amide. J Pharmacol Exp Ther 102:5, 1951
50. Mixter CG, Moran JM, Austen WG: Cardiac and peripheral vascular effects of diphenylhydantoin sodium. Am J Cardiol 17:332, 1966
51. Moss AJ, Patton RD: Antiarrhythmic Agents. Springfield, Ill, CC Thomas, 1973 p 23
52. Moss AJ, Patton RD: Antiarrhythmic Agents. Springfield, Ill, CC Thomas, 1973 p 109
53. Pamintuan JC, Dreifus LS, Watanabe Y: Comparative mechanisms of antiarrhythmic agents. Am J Cardiol 26:512, 1970
54. Papp JGY, Vaughan–Williams EM: The effect of bretylium on intracellular cardiac action potentials in relation to its anti-arrhythmic activity and local anaesthetic activity. Br J Pharmacol 37:380, 1969
55. Pari PS: The effect of diphenylhydantoin sodium (Dilantin) on myocardial contractility and hemodynamics. Am Heart J 82:62, 1971
56. Romhilt DW, Bloomfield SS, Lipicky RJ et al.: Evaluation of bretylium tosylate for the treatment of premature premature ventricular contractions. Circulation 45:800, 1972
57. Sanna G, Arcidiacono R: Chemical ventricular defibrillation of the human heart with bretylium tosylate. Am J Cardiol 32:982, 1973
58. Selden K, Sasahara AA: Central nervous system toxicity induced by lidocaine. JAMA 202:908, 1967
59. Singh BN, Vaughan–Williams EM: Effect of altering potassium concentration on the action of lidocaine and diphenylhydantoin on rabbit atrial and ventricular muscle. Circ Res 29:286, 1971
60. Stone N, Klein MD, Lown B: Diphenylhydantoin in the prevention of recurring ventricular tachycardia. Circulation 43:420, 1971
61. Svensmark O, Scheller PJ, Buchtal F: 5,5-diphenylhydantoin (Dilantin) blood levels after oral or intravenous dosage in man. Acta Pharmacol Toxical (Kbh) 16:331, 1960
62. Thomson PD, Rowland M, Melmon KL: The influence of heart failure, liver disease and renal failure on the disposition of lidocaine in man. Am Heart J 82:417, 1971
63. Vassalle M: Automaticity and automatic rhythms. Am J Cardiol 28:245, 1971
64. Wallace AG, Cline RE, Sealy WC et al.: Electrophysiologic effects of quinidine. Circ Res 19:960, 1966
65. Watanabe Y, Dreifus LS: Newer concepts in the genesis of cardiac arrhythmias. Am Heart J 76:114, 1968
66. Weisse AB, Moschos CB, Passannante AJ et al.: Relative effectiveness of three antiarrhythmic agents in the treatment of ventricular arrhythmias in experimental acute myocardial ischemia. Am Heart J 81:503, 1971
67. Winkle RA, Fitzgerald JW, Meffin PJ et al.: A new oral lidocaine-like antiarrhythmic drug, W36095: antiarrhythmic efficacy in man. Circulation 52(supp II): 74, 1975
68. Winkle RA, Glantz SA, Harrison DC: Pharmacologic therapy of ventricular arrhythmias. Am J Cardiol 36:629, 1975
69. Woosley RL, McDevitt DG, Smith RF et al.: Antiarrhythmic and pharmacokinetic properties of 2-ammo-2″, 6′–proprionoxylidide HCl (W–36095–HCl, Astra) in man. Circulation 52 (supp II):75, 1975
70. Zipes DP: The clinical significance of bradycardic rhythms in acute myocardial infarction. Am J Cardiol 24:814, 1969

3 | Sinus Bradycardia, Sick Sinus Syndrome and Sinus Tachycardia

NOBLE O. FOWLER

The term sinus bradycardia indicates that both atrial and ventricular rates are below 60/min with the normal sequence of sinus node-atrio-ventricular activation. As a rule resting heart rates between 50–60/min are not ominous, and are often associated with health rather than disease (24). Sinus bradycardia is more likely to be significant when the heart rate is 40–50/minute, although resting heart rates in this range are not uncommon in athletes. When the heart rate is below 40/min, symptoms are likely to be present (24). These symptoms may include light-headedness, dizziness, fatigue, or syncope.

The term *sick sinus syndrome* has gained popularity as a label for patients who have symptoms related to failure of the normal sequence of sinus node activation and impulse conduction to the atrium (8,9). In such patients disease of the sinus node and/or atrium may be manifest in one of several ways:

1. Sinus bradycardia
2. Sinus bradycardia with periods of atrial tachyarrhythmia, such as atrial flutter, paroxysmal atrial tachycardia (brady-tachy syndrome) (Fig. 3–1)
3. AV junctional escape rhythm with or without sinus bradycardia or arrest
4. Sinus node arrest
5. Sinoatrial block (Fig. 3–2)

It is estimated that 70% of patients with symptoms related to sinus bradycardia also have periods of atrial tachyarrhythmia. In some centers sick sinus syndrome is now being recognized more often than AV block as a cause of syncope requiring electronic pacemaker implantation.

SINOATRIAL BRADYCARDIA AND SICK SINUS SYNDROME

Sinus bradycardia may be found in a variety of settings. The individual may be healthy, there may be a disease primarily outside the heart, or there may be heart disease. The causes of sinus bradycardia may be classified as follows:

1. Normal individuals. Young adults, especially athletes, old age (2)
2. Neurohumoral mechanisms.
   a. Vagal stimulation. Carotid sinus syncope, esophageal diverticulum, increased intracranial pressure, vasodepressor syncope (6)

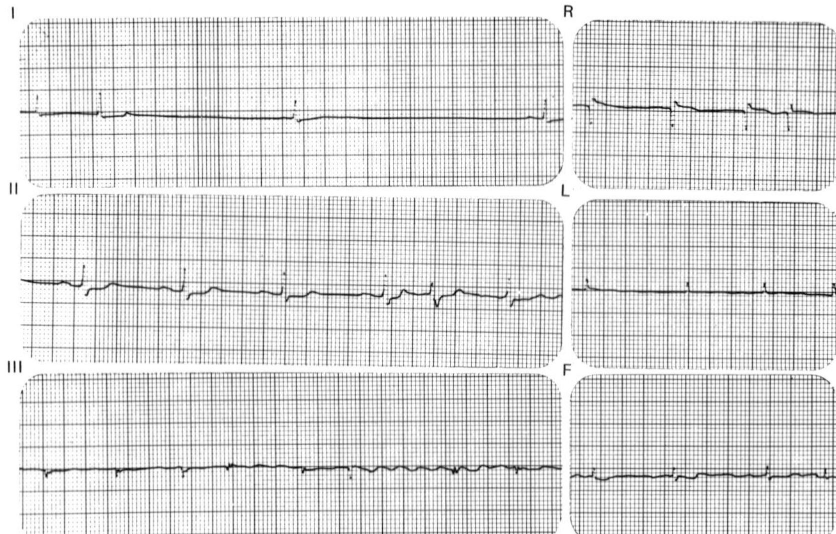

Fig. 3–1.   **Sinus bradycardia (Lead I) and atrial fibrillation (Lead III) in the same electrocardiogram of an octogenerian with sick sinus syndrome. Syncope had occurred while he was driving an automobile. (From Fowler N O; Cardiac Diagnosis and Treatment, 2nd ed Hagerstown, Harper & Row, 1976)**

Fig. 3–2.   **Sinoatrial block, probably caused by digitalis. Following the first and the second P-QRS-T complexes of the electrocardiogram, a cardiac cycle is missing. The interval between P_2 and P_3 is exactly twice the normal PP interval and there is no blocked premature P wave, so that an undetected blocked premature atrial systole is unlikely. A similar phenomenon occurs following the third and the fourth beats.**

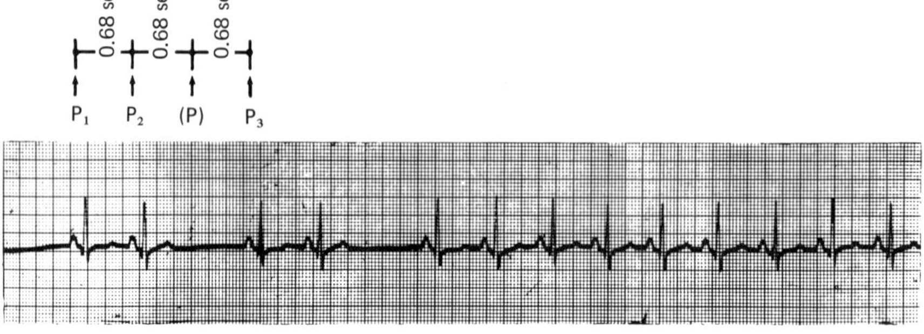

    b. Catecholamine depletion or β-sympathetic blockade, reserpine (3) or propranolol therapy (5)

3. Metabolic disorders. Hypothyroidism (14), hypothermia

4. Drug and electrolyte effects. Digitalis (21) or quinidine administration (17), hyperkaliemia (25), Lidocaine toxicity

5. Disease of the atrium or sinoatrial node.

    a. Acute or chronic coronary artery disease (24)

    b. Inflammations, myocarditis

    c. Invasive disease, neoplasms and myocardiopathy, including facio-scapulo-humeral muscular dystrophy and amyloidosis
    d. Familial sinus bradycardia
6. Following surgical repair of congenital heart disease, especially transposition of the great arteries and tetralogy of Fallot (15)

Sinus bradycardia must be distinguished from other causes of a slow ventricular rate, especially when the ventricular rate is near 40/min. The other common cause of such rates is complete AV block, and occasionally lesser degrees of AV block. With complete AV block one usually finds intermittent cannon *a* waves in the neck veins, varying intensity of the first heart sound, and the heart rate changes little if at all with exercise. With sinus bradycardia the heart rate usually increases with exercise, cannon *a* waves are absent, and the first heart sound is constant. When sinus bradycardia is caused by disease of the sino-atrial node, the response of the heart rate to exercise may be subnormal. The electrocardiogram serves to make the precise diagnosis of the bradycardia (Fig. 3–3), if made when bradycardia is present, but often shows a normal mechanism since the bradyarrhythmia is often paroxysmal (12).

DIAGNOSIS

A common problem is that the patient has symptoms of paroxysmal syncope or dizziness without obvious cause and the cardiac rhythm is normal at the time of the examination. In this case electrocardiographic monitoring of the cardiac rhythm in hospital for several days may be useful in disclosing a paroxysmal arrhythmia. In ambulatory patients a portable electromagnetic tape apparatus may be utilized to obtain 10–24 hour records of the electrocardiogram (dynamic electrocardiography). Other methods are less satisfactory. One may study the electrocardiogram during exercise (stress electrocardiography) for evidence of exercise related impairment of the sinoatrial mechanism. One may study the sinoatrial recovery time following electronic stimulation of the right atrium at a rate of 130/min for 3 min. The sinus node should begin pacing the atrium within one second after electronic pacing is discontinued (Fig. 3–4). Unfortunately this test fails to show an abnormal delay in sinus node recovery in many patients with sick sinus syndrome (22).

TREATMENT

Whether or not sinus bradycardia requires treatment depends upon the cause and upon whether or not there are symptoms. Heart rates in the fifties are common in healthy young adults at rest, and heart rates in the forties and even in the upper thirties may be found in resting athletes (16). When sinus bradycardia is related to myxedema or increased intracranial pressure, the treatment is that of the underlying disease. When drugs such as digitalis, propranolol,

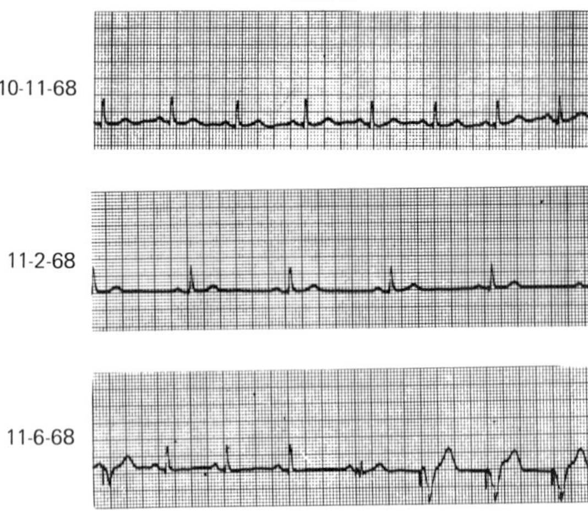

Fig. 3–3. Electrocardiogram, 51-year-old male, of 10/11/68 reveals normal sinus mechanism; heart rate was 72/min. Electrocardiogram of 11/2/68 reveals sinus bradycardia with heart rate of 50/min. Record of 11/6/68 shows that some QRS complexes are activated from the atrium, and others at a rate of 75/min by pervenous demand ventricular pacemaker.

Fig. 3–4. Induction of bradycardia following right atrial pacing at a rate of 143/min in a patient with sick sinus syndrome (top ECG strip). "S" indicates electronic pacing stimulus artefact. There is prolonged sinus node depression after rapid atrial pacing at 143/min, with a very slow junctional escape rhythm. In order to restore adequate circulation, atrial electronic pacing was reinstituted, this time at a rate of 86/min (bottom ECG strip). (Courtesy by Robert J. Adolph, M.D.)

R.W. 83 ♂
1-25-71
RA pacing 143/min

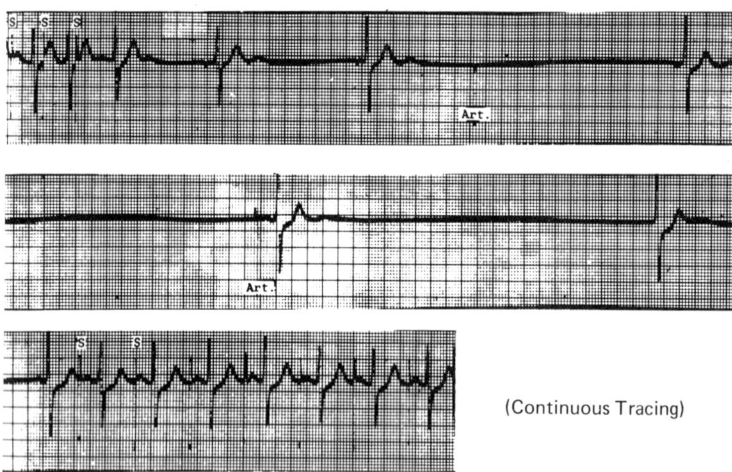

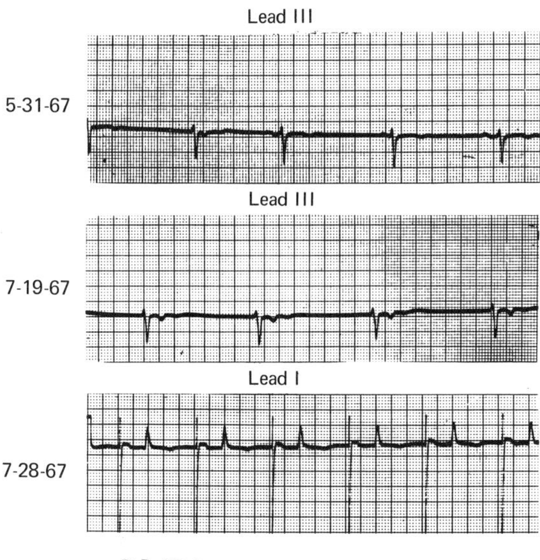

Fig. 3–5. **Electrocardiogram, 75-year-old male, 5/31/67 shows sinus bradycardia, with periods of sinus arrest and junctional escape rhythm. Second QRS complex is followed by evidence of retrograde activation of atria. On 7/19/67 there is AV junctional rhythm, type III. On 7/28/67 atria are paced electronically by pervenous atrial stimulation at a rate of 60/min. The PR interval is prolonged, being 0.28 sec. [From Fowler, Fenton, and Conway (12).]**

other β-adrenergic blocking agents, or reserpine are responsible, one may need to reduce the dosage of the drug or withdraw it. Especially in elderly patients one may find sinus bradycardia without obvious cause, often with an inadequate increase in heart rate in response to exercise. At times there is sinus arrest with an escape nodal rhythm. In such patients treatment may not be indicated if there are no symptoms. Such symptoms as fatigue, exertional dyspnea, dizziness, or syncope suggest that a pervenous demand ventricular pacemaker is indicated (Fig. 3–3). Chronic right atrial pacing may also be employed for this purpose (18) (Fig. 3–5) but is usually considered less desirable for several reasons. Chronic right atrial pacing, when carried out pervenously, tends to be less stable than right ventricular pacing but may be attempted via the right atrial appendage or coronary sinus. Since patients with sick sinus syndrome are often elderly, thoracotomy for chronic right atrial pacing is likely to be undesirable. Another reason for the lack of appeal of chronic right atrial pacing is the frequent occurrence of AV block in patients with sick sinus syndrome. Thus right ventricular pacing, despite the loss of atrial systole as an aid for ventricular filling, is more likely to ensure a stable ventricular mechanism. When the patient has a large heart or heart failure, sequential AV pacing to maintain the atrial aid to ventricular filling should be considered (10). When sinus bradycardia is a chronic symptomatic disorder, and especially when there is syncope, drugs such as atropine or isoproterenol are unlikely to provide continuous relief.

Sinus bradycardia is said to occur in approximately 20% of patients with acute myocardial infarction (24). It is said to occur in 61% of patients seen within the first hour of acute inferior infarction (1). The event may be spontaneous, or result from the administration of morphine or from the extreme pain. Heart rates of 50–60/min are usually of little clinical significance and other than observation by cardiac monitoring, no special treatment is required. In acute myocardial infarction sinus bradycardia with a heart rate of below 50 suggests that atropine, 1.0 mg intravenously, be given, especially if there is a fall of blood pressure or cardiac output. Up to 2 mg doses may be given at intervals of 3–4 hours (15). Alternatively one may use isoproterenol, 1 mg in 500 ml 5% dextrose, infused at 1–2 ml/min. Uncommonly, temporary pervenous atrial pacing at a rate of 70–80/min is needed. Usually such treatment is no longer required after the first week or so of infarction.

Kent and associates, using information from animal experiments, suggest that use of atropine may be hazardous in the sinus bradycardia of acute infarction and may tend to cause ventricular fibrillation in this setting (19). On the other hand, Chadda and associates found that intravenous atropine improved the blood pressure and cardiac output without evoking ventricular fibrillation when given to patients with acute cardiac infarction who had sinus bradycardia accompanied by a fall in blood pressure (4).

SINUS TACHYCARDIA

There are several physiologic mechanisms for the production of sinus tachycardia. Sympathetic stimulation may result from a fall in blood pressure affecting the baroreceptor mechanisms in the carotid sinus and aortic arch. The same mechanism also decreases parasympathetic discharge. Hypoxia or anxiety may stimulate adrenal and sympathetic catecholamine release. Elevation of right atrial pressure in heart failure may cause tachycardia by the Bainbridge reflex, although this reflex is in dispute. Elevation of body temperature increases the heart rate. Humoral substances, for example, thyroid hormone, may cause tachycardia by a direct effect upon the myocardium. Exercise produces tachycardia in several ways: sympathetic stimulation, catecholamine release, and by a third poorly understood mechanism which is operative even in the denervated heart after β-sympathetic blockade.

Clinical causes of sinus tachycardia may be listed as follows:

1. Anxiety
2. Fever
3. Exercise
4. Hyperthyroidism
5. Anemia
6. Hypoxia
7. Congestive heart failure

8. Idiopathic high cardiac output states
9. Pheochromocytoma
10. Related to drugs, e.g., ephedrine or epinephrine
11. Myocarditis
12. Shock
13. Pulmonary embolism

It may be observed in most instances that sinus tachycardia is not directly related to heart disease; hence, usually it is not to be treated with such cardiac drugs as digitalis or quinidine. In fact an attempt to decrease the heart rate with digitalis when heart failure is not the cause may lead to serious digitalis intoxication. The excessive use of digitalis may produce atrial or junctional tachycardia. When this is not recognized, further attempts to slow the heart with still more digitalis may evoke a more serious or fatal arrhythmia.

Sinus tachycardia in the adult is said to exist when there is a sinus mechanism with a heart rate above 100/min. In most clinical settings, the heart rate with sinus tachycardia lies between 100–150 beats/min; occasionally the rate is 170/min or faster. With maximal exercise, however, the heart rate may reach 190 ± 12/min in young adults (23). The maximal exercise heart rate decreases with advancing age (7).

DIAGNOSIS

As a rule the recognition of sinus tachycardia presents no problem when the heart rate is 100–150/min and the rhythm is regular. Usually there is demonstrable cause and the onset, unlike paroxysmal tachycardia, is gradual rather than sudden. With sinus tachycardia there is usually some variation in the heart rate from hour to hour, but a constant rate is usually found with paroxysmal tachycardia. When the heart rate is near 150/min the possibility of atrial flutter with 2:1 AV block or of atrial or AV junctional tachycardia may arise. The electrocardiogram usually enables one to make the distinction; it may be necessary to employ carotid sinus pressure during the recording. With sinus tachycardia there are usually normal P waves preceding each QRS complex; carotid sinus pressure either has no effect or causes a gradual slowing of the rate, with a gradual return to the previous rate upon release of pressure (Fig. 3–6). With atrial flutter there are usually visible saw-tooth flutter waves in Leads II and III and the atrial activity is visible in Lead V_1 (Fig. 3–7). At times carotid sinus pressure is needed to increase the AV block to disclose the flutter waves (Fig. 3–8). With atrial or AV junctional tachycardia, the P waves are usually not visible, often being superimposed upon the preceding T wave, or buried within the QRS complex. When P waves are visible with atrial tachycardia they tend to be of altered configuration and the PR interval is usually different from that seen in the same patient during normal sinus rhythm. In junctional tachycardia the P waves are negative in Leads II, III, and AVF. With atrial or junctional tachycardia, carotid sinus pressure either has no effect or converts the rhythm to a sinus mechanism (Fig. 3–9).

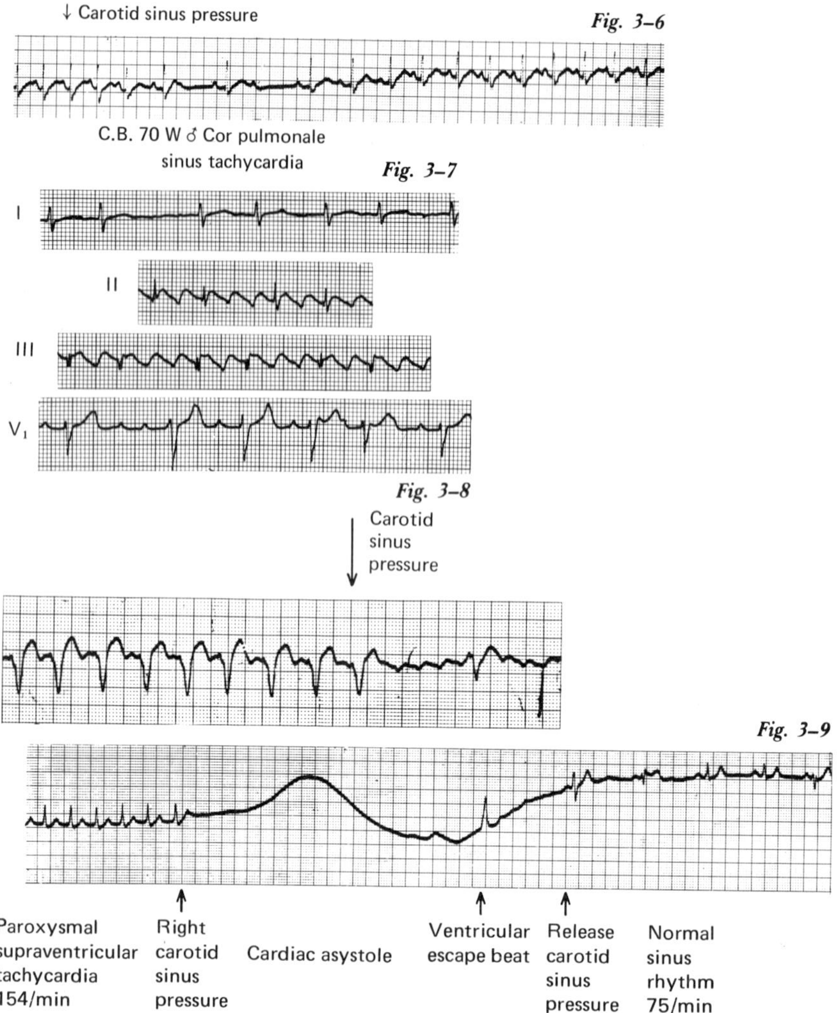

TREATMENT

The therapy of sinus tachycardia is to be directed toward the underlying cause, as indicated in the list previously given. Digitalis is not indicated unless there is underlying heart failure; the heart rate should not be used as a sole guide to therapy when there is a sinus mechanism accompanying heart failure. As a rule the tachycardia of heart failure is not great, and the heart rate seldom exceeds 100–120/min. Quinidine is not indicated in the management of sinus tachycardia. Propranolol (Inderal) is effective in the tachycardia of the idi-

◀ *Fig. 3–6.* **Sinus tachycardia with heart rate of 150 beats/min in 70-year-old male with cor pulmonale. Application of carotid sinus pressure (arrow) is followed by slowing of heart rate and failure of conduction of some atrial beats to ventricles. After carotid sinus pressure is released, heart rate gradually returns to original rate of 150 beats/min. The response is different from that in paroxysmal atrial tachycardia; in the latter there is either no change in heart rate or heart rate remains slow upon release of carotid sinus pressure indicating that rhythm has been converted to normal sinus rhythm. [From Fowler (11).]**

◀ *Fig. 3–7.* **Atrial flutter with varying AV block, showing characteristic saw-tooth pattern of flutter waves in Leads II and III. Flutter activity is poorly seen in Lead I. In Leads II and III there is constant activity of the base line with no isoelectric interval between the flutter waves. This is rather characteristic of atrial flutter. There is an atrial rate of 250/min with varying atrioventricular conduction so that ventricular rhythm is irregular. [From Fowler (11).]**

◀ *Fig. 3–8.* **Carotid sinus pressure unmasking atrial flutter in patient with atrial flutter and 2:1 atrioventricular block. In absence of carotid sinus pressure, atrial activity cannot be visualized with certainty. The ventricular rate is 120 beats/min with regular rhythm. The broad QRS complexes are caused by bundle branch block. With carotid sinus pressure the atrioventricular block is increased, and characteristic saw-tooth pattern of flutter waves is visualized. The atrial rate is 240 beats/min. [From Fowler (11).]**

◀ *Fig. 3–9.* **Supraventricular tachycardia with a heart rate of 154 beats/min, showing conversion to normal sinus rhythm by right carotid sinus pressure. Application of carotid sinus pressure is followed by sinus standstill and then a ventricular escape beat. Upon release of carotid sinus pressure there is normal sinus rhythm with occasional premature ventricular contractions. [From Fowler (11).]**

opathic high output states (13), but probably should not be used in other varieties of sinus tachycardia. It is contraindicated in the tachycardia of heart failure, since it tends to impair ventricular function. Propranolol may decrease the heart rate in thyrotoxicosis, but should be used with caution in this setting since it does not improve the increased oxygen consumption (20). In most patients the proper management of sinus tachycardia requires first a diagnosis of the cause, and then attention to the underlying anxiety, infection, shock, anemia, or metabolic abnormality.

REFERENCES

1. Adgey AAJ, Geddes JS, Mulholland HC et al.: Incidence, significance and management of early bradyarrhythmia complicating acute myocardial infarction. Lancet 2:1097, 1968
2. Agruss NS, Rosen EY, Adolph RJ et al.: Significance of chronic sinus bradycardia in elderly people. Circulation 46:925, 1972
3. Alper MH, Flacke W, Krayer O: Pharmacology of reserpine and its implications for anesthesia. Anesthesiology 24:524, 1963
4. Chadda KD, Lichstein E, Gupta PK et al.: Bradycardia-hypotension syndrome in acute myocardial infarction. Am J Med 59:158, 1975
5. Cohen LS, Braunwald E: Amelioration of angina pectoris in idiopathic hypertrophic subaortic stenosis with beta-adrenergic blockade. Circulation 35:847, 1967
6. Ebert RV: Syncope. Circulation 27:1148, 1963
7. Ellestead MH, Allen W, Wan CKW, Kempt GL: Maximal treadmill stress testing for cardiovascular evaluation. Circulation 39:517, 1969
8. Ferrer MI: Sick sinus syndrome. Circulation 27:635, 1973
9. Ferrer MI: The Sick Sinus Syndrome. Mt Kisco, NY, Futura, 1974

10. Fields J, Berkovits BV, Matloff JM: Surgical experience with temporary and permanent A–V sequential demand pacing. J Thorac Cardiovasc Surg 66:865, 1973
11. Fowler NO: Cardiac Diagnosis and Treatment, 2nd ed. Hagerstown, Harper & Row, 1976
12. Fowler NO, Fenton JC, Conway GF: Syncope caused by bradycardia without atrioventricular block. Am Heart J 80:303, 1970
13. Frohlich ED, Tarazi RC, Dustin HP: Hyperdynamic β-adrenergic circulatory state. Arch Intern Med 123:1, 1969
14. Graettinger JS, Muenster JJ, Checchia CS et al.: Correlation of clinical and hemodynamic studies in patients with hypothyroidism. J Clin Invest 37:502, 1958
15. Greenwood RD et al.: Sick sinus syndrome after surgery for congenital heart disease. Circulation 52:208, 1975
16. Hanson JS, Tabakin BS: Comparison of the circulatory response to upright exercise in 25 "normal" men and 9 distance runners. Br Heart J 27:211, 1965
17. James TN, Nadeau RA: Mechanism of action of quinidine on the sinus node studied by direct perfusion through its artery. Am Heart J 67:804, 1964
18. Kastor JA, DeSanctis RW, Harthorne JW, Schwartz GH: Transvenous atrial pacing in the treatment of refractory ventricular irritability. An Intern Med 66:939, 1967
19. Kent KM, Smith ER, Redwood DR et al.: Electrical stability of acutely ischemic myocardium: influences of heart rate and vagal stimulation. Circulation 47:291, 1973
20. Leonard JJ, deGroot WJ: Thyroid state and the cardiovascular system. Mod Concepts Cardiovasc Dis 38:23, 1969
21. Margolis JR et al.: Digitalis and the sick sinus syndrome. Circulation 52:162, 1975
22. Narula OS, Samet P, Javier RP: Significance of the sinus node recovery time. Circulation 45:140, 1972
23. Sheffield LT, Reeves TJ: Graded exercise in the diagnosis of angina pectoris. Mod Concepts Cardiovasc Dis 34:1, 1965
24. Shillingford J, Thomas M: Treatment of bradycardia and hypotension syndrome in patients with acute myocardial infarction. Am Heart J 75:843 1968
25. Surawicz B: Relation between electrocardiogram and electrolytes. Am Heart J 73:814, 1967

4 | Treatment of Premature Cardiac Contractions

DONALD W. ROMHILT

VENTRICULAR PREMATURE CONTRACTIONS

The treatment of premature ventricular contractions depends on the clinical setting in which they occur. Premature ventricular contractions occur in the following principal settings: acute myocardial infarction; with other syndromes of coronary artery disease including postmyocardial infarction and acute coronary insufficiency; with other varieties of organic heart disease, particularly the cardiomyopathies, mitral valve click-murmur syndrome, and prolonged QT interval syndrome; with digitalis toxicity; in subjects without evidence of organic heart disease. Patients who have premature ventricular contractions without evidence of organic heart disease usually do not require treatment with antiarrhythmic drugs.

ACUTE MYOCARDIAL INFARCTION

During the first few days after an acute myocardial infarction almost all patients have premature ventricular contractions. The frequency of premature ventricular contractions is highest in the first few hours after the infarction and gradually decreases during the next few days. Lown and coworkers (28) recognized certain features of premature ventricular contractions (serious ventricular arrhythmias) that commonly preceded ventricular fibrillation in patients with acute cardiac infarction. These were: occurrence at a rate of 5 or more/min, R on T phenomenon, (an early premature beat whose R wave by electrocardiogram falls on the T wave of the preceding normal beat) multifocal premature beats, consecutive premature ventricular beats in runs of two or more, and ventricular tachycardia. When premature ventricular contractions fulfilling these criteria occur, antiarrhythmic drugs should be administered to suppress these arrhythmias. When serious ventricular arrhythmias were treated with lidocaine, Lown et al (30) reported only a 2% incidence of primary cardiac arrest in 300 patients with acute myocardial infarction. If lidocaine proves to be ineffective, then procainamide should be given intravenously as a second choice.

The routine prophylactic administration of antiarrhythmic agents in all patients with acute myocardial infarction in the coronary care unit has been evaluated extensively. Most studies reported a significant decrease in premature ventricular contractions and serious ventricular arrhythmias without an effect on mortality when such agents as procainamide, quinidine or lidocaine were used prophylactically (7, 22, 27, 32). Since the majority of deaths secondary to acute myocardial infarction occur prior to hospitalization, Lown and Vassaux (29) recommend the administration of 200 mg of intramuscular lidocaine as soon as a myocardial infarction is suspected if the heart rate is over 70 beats/min. The effectiveness of immediate prophylactic administration of an antiarrhythmic agent to reduce mortality in patients with suspected myocardial infarction needs to be evaluated in a controlled clinical trial.

CHRONIC CORONARY ARTERY DISEASE

In cases of previous myocardial infarction several studies have reported an increased mortality and an increased frequency of sudden death in patients who have premature ventricular contractions or certain of the serious ventricular arrhythmias (11, 24, 33, 48). The lack of an antiarrhythmic agent that is suitable for long term oral administration in the United States has limited clinical studies designed to determine whether prophylactic administration of an antiarrhythmic agent will decrease mortality in postmyocardial infarction patients. In Sweden recent controlled clinical trials with alprenolol demonstrated a significant reduction in sudden deaths in postmyocardial infarction patients (1, 50). A large multicenter trial with practolol in postmyocardial infarction patients in England also demonstrated a significant reduction in sudden death. In addition overall mortality was reduced in patients with anterior wall myocardial infarction (34). However the trial had to be terminated because of the ocular complications associated with long-term practolol administration. Since in one study (1) the incidence of reinfarction was also significantly decreased, the mechanism of the beneficial effect of the β-adrenergic blocking drugs in decreasing mortality and sudden death may not be entirely related to their antiarrhythmic properties.

Patients discharged from a coronary care unit after an episode of acute coronary insufficiency or unstable angina have a mortality rate of 10%–15% in the year following discharge (25, 43). In acute coronary insufficiency, propranolol was reported to relieve pain promptly (13) and may also decrease the frequency of acute myocardial infarction (14). Additional studies will be needed to evaluate the effect of β-adrenergic blockers and other antiarrhythmic agents on mortality rate in patients who are discharged after an episode of acute coronary insufficiency.

At the present time it is possible that oral antiarrhythmic agents (either quinidine, procainamide, or propranolol) on a long-term basis may be beneficial in patients with coronary artery disease who demonstrate serious ventricular arrhythmias, if the side effects of the individual drug do not prohibit its use. Large multicenter trials are needed in the United States to determine if the long-term prophylactic administration of oral antiarrhythmic agents will decrease mortality in patients with the various subsets of chronic coronary artery disease.

OTHER VARIETIES OF ORGANIC HEART DISEASE

Certain other patients with organic heart disease appear to have a predilection for ventricular arrhythmias. Patients with the mitral valve click-murmur syndrome tend to have premature ventricular contractions, which are often precipitated by exercise. Propranolol will usually suppress the premature ventricular contractions in this syndrome. In patients with the congestive cardiomyopathies, at times an attempt is made to suppress the serious ventricular arrhythmias with quinidine or procainamide. Symptomatic patients with the prolonged QT interval syndrome and paroxysmal ventricular arrhythmias, with or without deafness, should be treated. Digitalis, propranolol, diphenylhydantoin, and bretylium were each reported to be effective in some instances (15, 20, 37, 44).

DIGITALIS TOXICITY

Patients with premature ventricular contractions secondary to digitalis toxicity should usually be observed and the digitalis stopped. If the premature ventricular contractions conform to the criteria for serious ventricular arrhythmias, the observation should be conducted in the coronary care unit. If specific therapy is required potassium chloride or lidocaine will usually suppress premature ventricular contractions secondary to digitalis toxicity. Premature ventricular contractions secondary to other drugs, including quinidine, procainamide, clofibrate, and phenothiazine derivatives or other agents (as in glue sniffing), will resolve when the drug or agent is discontinued.

WITHOUT ORGANIC HEART DISEASE

The problem of premature ventricular contractions in patients without apparent organic heart disease is even more difficult with respect to treatment. We generally avoid the use of antiarrhythmic drugs in individuals without evidence of organic heart disease. In the Tecumseh Study persons over the age of 30 with premature ventricular contractions on a routine electrocardiogram had a significant increase in sudden death (10). There was also a correlation between premature ventricular contractions and coronary artery disease in persons over age 30; thus the presence of the premature ventricular contractions may only be identifying the persons with coronary artery disease who are at a level of increased risk of sudden death from this disease. The problem is compounded further by the report of Hinkle and coworkers (17), which states that 62% of middle-aged American men had premature ventricular contractions during a 6 hour period. In this group, also, the presence of either premature ventricular contractions or more than 10 premature ventricular contractions per 1000 beats correlated with an increased risk of death, and also with the presence of underlying coronary artery disease. Rodstein *et al.* (38) studied individuals who were considered to have a normal life expectancy at the time of examination for life insurance. The presence of premature ventricular contractions, if fewer than 10/min, did not increase their mortality rate. However there was an increase in death rate in persons with complex premature ventricular contractions, or when the frequency increased to 10–30 min. In the individuals without heart disease premature ventricular contractions were frequently found to occur as a result of fatigue, anxiety, or overindulgence in coffee, tobacco, tea or alcohol. Removal of these causative agents often decreased or eliminated the premature ventricular contractions.

ATRIAL PREMATURE CONTRACTIONS

Premature atrial contractions (also nodal or junctional premature beats) are also frequent and occur in a variety of clinical settings. Premature atrial contractions were not found to be associated with an increased mortality or with an increased incidence of coronary artery disease (10, 17). In patients without evidence of organic heart disease they may occur in relation to fatigue, anxiety, or overindulgence in coffee, alcohol or tobacco and usually require no treatment. Removal of these agents will often decrease or eliminate the premature beats. Rarely, when the sensation of palpitations is annoying, sedation, digitalis or quinidine may be needed. In patients with organic heart disease, particularly those with atrial enlargement, premature atrial contractions may be premonitory for atrial tachyarrhythmias. Treatment of the underlying cardiac condition will often result in their elimination. Again digitalis or quinidine may be used for suppression, as needed.

DIGITALIS

Digitalis, if thought to cause premature contractions, should be discontinued temporarily. In the presence of organic heart disease digitalis often eliminates premature contractions, especially those of atrial origin. In patients with cardiomegaly and congestive heart failure digitalis may decrease premature ventricular contractions by improvement in cardiac function.

Digitalization may be carried out slowly over several days by the oral administration of digoxin 0.5 mg daily for 6 days (31), followed by a maintenance dose which usually ranges from 0.125–0.50 mg/day (average 0.375 mg) given as a single or divided dose. When rapid digitalization is required the loading dose method is used. Within a 24 hour period a total of 1.5–2.0 mg of digoxin may be administered orally in divided doses. The dosage of digoxin should be decreased in the elderly, in patients with renal disease, and frequently when pulmonary disease is present. Jelliffe published graphs and computer-assisted dosage regimens to guide the use of digitalis preparations in patients, and especially in patients with decreased renal function (18, 19). When one administers diuretics concurrently with digitalis oral potassium supplemement will usually be needed to prevent hypokalemia and possibly digitalis toxicity. The recent development of techniques to assay serum digitalis glycoside levels is very useful in the prevention and detection of toxicity. In patients with digitalis toxicity 87% had digoxin levels above 2.0 ng/ml, whereas 90% of patients without evidence of toxicity had levels less than 2.0 ng/ml. (45).

QUINIDINE

Quinidine sulfate decreases the rate of phase 4 depolarization of the action potential, increases the effective refractory period and action potential duration, and tends to abolish atrial and ventricular premature contractions. Despite its limitations quinidine is the most commonly used oral antiarrhythmic agent in the treatment of premature cardiac contractions. The usual oral dosage range is 0.2–0.4 g every 6 hours, although occasionally larger dosages will be needed to provide adequate serum levels. A loading dose regimen, with administration every 3 hours for 3 doses, may be used to achieve therapeutic levels more rapidly (7). The desired serum level is 4–6 mg/liter when measured one hour before the next dose, although antiarrhythmic effect begins around a level of 2.5 mg/liter (7). Acidification of the urine markedly enhances the excretion of quinidine, whereas alkalinization of the urine can be used to increase the serum level if needed (16). Serum levels should be determined after 2–3 days of drug administration.

The disadvantages of quinidine are a number of unpleasant side effects including nausea, vomiting, diarrhea, blurred vision, and tinnitus, and occur in 20–25% of patients during long-term administration. Although less common, more serious side effects are fever, thrombocytopenic purpura, hypotension, and ventricular tachycardia or fibrillation. Quinidine serum levels of 10 mg/liter or more are frequently toxic and associated with prolongation of the QRS interval, sinoatrial and atrioventricular nodal block, and ventricular tachycardia and fibrillation. Toxic levels tend to develop more readily in the elderly or in patients with congestive heart failure or renal insufficiency. Quinidine syncope due to ventricular fibrillation may occur at therapeutic serum levels.

PROCAINAMIDE (PRONESTYL)

Procainamide has the same electrophysiologic properties as quinidine and is effective in the treatment of atrial and ventricular premature contractions. The drug may be given orally or parenterally. Intravenous procainamide is usually administered as a bolus of 100 mg every 2–3 min up to a maximum dose of 1 g. The blood pressure and electrocardiogram should be monitored for arterial hypotension and widening of the QRS complex. If the premature contractions are suppressed by the bolus administration of procainamide, an intravenous drip of 1–5 mg/min can be used for continued suppression. Procainamide is nearly completely absorbed from the gastrointestinal tract. The oral or intramuscular dosage ranges from 250–500 mg every 3–4 hours.

Koch–Weser and Klein (21) found that it was necessary to give oral procainamide every 3 hours to maintain a relatively stable plasma concentration. The effective serum level usually ranges from 4–8 mg/liter, and toxic effects are common when the serum level exceeds 12 mg/liter (21).

The side effects of procainamide are anorexia, diarrhea, mental depression, and occasionally agranulocytosis. The most serious side effect is the causation of a lupuslike syndrome and positive antinuclear antibody studies which limit its usefulness for long-term administration. In a study (23) evaluating procainamide as a long term oral antiarrhythmic agent, 23% of patients had to discontinue the drug during the first 3 weeks because of early reactions; 100% of patients who took the drug for more than 1 year had a positive antinuclear antibody titer; at least 50% of the patients who took the drug more than 3 months developed a lupuslike syndrome. The syndrome was usually resolved within several days after stopping the drug (23).

XYLOCAINE (LIDOCAINE)

Lidocaine, available only for parenteral use, is effective in the suppression of premature ventricular contractions. Lidocaine decreases the rate of depolarization in phase 4 of the action potential; in contrast to quinidine and procainamide, it decreases the action potential duration and effective refractory period. Lidocaine is usually given by an intravenous bolus of 50–100 mg, which may be repeated once or twice. If the premature ventricular contractions are suppressed by the bolus of lidocaine, then a continuous infusion of 2–4 mg/min is initiated. Lidocaine is usually the first drug administered to patients with acute myocardial infarction when serious ventricular arrhythmias are recognized on the coronary care unit monitor. Lidocaine is also effective in the suppression of premature ventricular contractions secondary to digitalis toxicity. Lidocaine is rapidly metabolized by the liver and has a serum halflife of 20–30 min. The effective serum level ranges from 1.5–6.0 mg/liter (2). There are additional patients who will respond to intermittent high dosages of lidocaine, with serum levels approaching 10 mg/liter (2).

In patients with inadequate liver function, shock, congestive heart failure or hypovolemia, the dosage of lidocaine should be decreased and administered cautiously. The side effects of lidocaine include confusion, drowsiness, coma, central nervous system excitability manifested by convulsions, arterial hypotension, bradycardia or asystole, and respiratory arrest. Minor side effects are lightheadedness, tinnitus, muscle twitches, and visual disturbances. In our experience the problem of mental confusion is particularly common in patients with acute myocardial infarction who are in the coronary care unit and are receiving other analgesics and sedatives.

DIPHENYLHYDANTOIN (DILANTIN)

Diphenylhydantoin is used in the treatment of atrial and ventricular premature contractions, particularly those secondary to digitalis toxicity. Its electrophysiologic properties are similar to those of lidocaine. Intravenous diphenylhydantoin is given as 50–100 mg boluses every 5 min up to a total dose of 300 mg while the electrocardiogram is observed carefully. When given orally or intramuscularly, a loading dose of 1 g/day should be given for 1–2 days, followed by a maintenance dose of 100 mg 3 or 4 times a day (6). The effective serum level ranges from 10–18 mcg/ml (6). Oral diphenylhydantoin was not effective in the long-term suppression of recurrent ventricular tachycardia (46), and is usually the last choice for the suppression of premature ventricular contractions which are not secondary to digitalis toxicity.

The side effects of diphenylhydantoin are drowsiness, nystagmus, vertigo, nausea and vomiting, sinus bradycardia, and cardiac arrest. The side effects following long-term administration include megaloblastic anemia, lymphoma-like syndrome, gum hypertrophy, and lupuslike syndrome.

PROPRANOLOL (INDERAL)

Propranolol is the only β-adrenergic blocking agent currently approved for use in the United States, and may be effective in the treatment of atrial and ventricular premature contractions. Its antiarrhythmic properties are similar to those of quinidine. Intravenous propranolol is usually given as a 1 mg bolus every 2–3 min up to a total dose of 5–7 mg, with careful monitoring of the electrocardiogram for sinus bradycardia or sinus arrest and the blood pressure for arterial hypotension. This method is not ordinarily used for treatment of premature beats alone. Orally the total antiarrhythmic dose ranges from 40–160 mg/day in 4 divided doses. Occasionally larger doses will be effective. It is the second or third choice in either immediate or long-term suppression of premature cardiac contractions, but in certain situations such as the mitral valve click-murmur syndrome it is the first choice. Propranolol is usually contraindicated in patients with congestive heart failure, atrioventricular block or asthma. Side effects include dizziness, hypotension, sinus bradycardia, sinus arrest, cardiac arrest, hypoglycemia and precipitation of congestive heart failure.

NEW ANTIARRHYTHMIC AGENTS

There are a number of drugs that have been evaluated or are currently being evaluated for effectiveness as antiarrhythmic agents. The purpose of this section is to mention a few of them briefly. Bretylium tosylate, an adrenergic neuronal blocking agent, is effective in the suppression of ventricular tachyarrhythmias and premature ventricular contractions (3, 4, 39). It differs from other antiarrhythmic agents in that it increases cardiac automaticity and has a positive inotropic effect (5, 8, 52). The parenteral dosage usually ranges from 4–8 mg/kg. Oral absorption is erratic and the oral dosage is usually about twice the parenteral dose. Its primary side effect is hypotension, which is increased by assuming the upright posture. Nausea and vomiting may occur after intravenous administration. Bretylium tosylate should not be used to treat premature ventricular contractions secondary to digitalis toxicity.

Disopyramide phosphate (Norpace) has electrophysiologic properties similar to those of quinidine and is effective in the suppression of atrial and ventricular premature contractions (35, 49). It is well absorbed from the gastrointestinal tract and has a plasma half-life of 5–6 hours. Norpace appears to be as effective as quinidine, but may be better tolerated. Side effects are primarily due to its anticholinergic properties (dry mouth, difficulty with urination, constipation) and its negative inotropic properties.

Aprinidine (12, 47), Astra-W36095 (51, 53), and Mexiletine (9) are three new drugs similar to lidocaine and are effective in the suppression of ventricular arrhythmias. Each of the three drugs is absorbed well after oral administration and each has a prolonged half-life. Thus oral administration should be required no more often than 2–3 times per day. Each of the three also has central nervous system side effects similar to those of lidocaine.

QX-572 is another drug similar to lidocaine; however it is not absorbed orally. It can be given only parenterally; but it has a long duration of action, does not cause the central nervous system side effects of lidocaine, and is effective in ventricular arrhythmias refractory to lidocaine (41). It causes a mild tachycardia in all patients and hypotension in some (41).

There are many β-adrenergic blocking drugs currently under investigation for antiarrhythmic effectiveness. As previously mentioned alprenolol and practolol significantly reduced mortality in postmyocardial infarction patients (1, 34, 50). The ocular and mucocutaneous side effects (54) of practolol have resulted in its withdrawal from clinical use for the present. Additional β-adrenergic blocking drugs under study are oxprenolol, sotalol, acebutolol, and talamolol.

Perhexiline is an antianginal drug that possesses antiarrhythmic properties similar to those of quinidine (36). It was effective in the suppression of atrial and ventricular premature contractions (36). Perhexiline is well absorbed orally and has a prolonged half-life. Side effects include dizziness, insomnia, anorexia, nausea, and elevation of hepatic enzyme levels and other liver function studies.

Verapamil blocks the slow inward current of sodium and calcium in myocardial fibers. The major antiarrhythmic action of verapamil is related to its depression of the rate of phase 4 depolarization since it has little effect on the action potential and effective refractory period (40). This agent appears to be more effective in supraventricular arrhythmias and arrhythmias secondary to digitalis toxicity than in premature ventricular contractions (42). Side effects include hypotension, bradycardia, and asystole; verapamil should not be used in conjunction with β-adrenergic blocking drugs (26).

The new antiarrhythmic agents mentioned briefly in this section will continue to undergo evaluation for effectiveness in comparison with drugs in current use. There is a particular need for an oral agent without significant side effects that is effective in the long-term suppression of premature ventricular contractions and can be administered once or twice a day.

REFERENCES

1. Ahlmark G, Saetre H, Korsgren M: Reduction of sudden deaths after myocardial infarction. Lancet 2:1563, 1974
2. Alderman EL, Kerber RE, Harrison DC: Evaluation of lidocaine resistance in man using intermittent large-dose infusion techniques. Am J Cardiol 34:342, 1974
3. Bacaner MB: Treatment of ventricular fibrillation and other acute arrhythmias with bretylium tosylate. Am J Cardiol 21:530, 1968
4. Bernstein JG, Koch–Weser J: Effectiveness of bretylium tosylate against refractory ventricular arrhythmias. Circulation 45:1024, 1972
5. Bigger JT, Jaffe CC: The effect of bretylium tosylate on the electrophysiologic properties of ventricular muscle and Purkinje fibers. Am J Cardiol 27:82, 1971
6. Bigger JT, Schmidt DH, Kutt H: Relationship between the plasma level of diphenylhydantoin sodium and its cardiac antiarrhythmic effects. Circulation 38:363, 1968
7. Bloomfield SS, Romhilt DW, Chou TC, Fowler NO: Quinidine for prophylaxis of arrhythmias in acute myocardial infarction. N Engl J Med 285:979, 1971
8. Boura ALA, Green AF: The actions of bretylium: adrenergic neurone blocking and other effects. Br J Pharmacol 14:536, 1959
9. Campbell NPS, Kelly JG, Shanks RG, Chaturvedi NC, Strong JE, Pantridge JF: Mexiletine (Kö 1173) in the management of ventricular dysrhythmias. Lancet 2:404, 1973
10. Chiang BN, Perlman LV, Ostrander LD, Epstein FH: Relationship of premature systoles to coronary heart disease and sudden death in the Tecumseh epidemiologic study. Ann Intern Med 70:1159, 1969
11. Coronary Drug Project Research Group: Prognostic importance of premature beats following myocardial infarction. JAMA 223:1116, 1973
12. Fasola AF, Zipes DP, Noble RJ: Treatment of drug refractory ventricular arrhythmias with aprinidine. Circulation 52 Supp. (II): 75, 1975
13. Fischl SJ, Herman MV, Gorlin R: The intermediate coronary syndrome. N Engl J Med 288:-1193, 1973
14. Fox KM, Chopra MP, Portal RW, Aber CP: Long-term beta blockade: possible protection from myocardial infarction. Br Med J 1:117, 1975
15. Garza LA, Vick RL, Nora JJ, McNamara DG: Heritable Q–T prolongation without deafness. Circulation 41:39, 1970
16. Gerhardt RE, Knouss RF, Thyrum PT, Luchi RJ, Morris JJ: Quinidine excretion in aciduria and alkaluria. Ann Intern Med 71:927, 1969
17. Hinkle LE, Carver ST, Stevens M: The frequency of asymptomatic disturbances of cardiac rhythm and conduction in middle-aged men. Am J Cardiol 24:629, 1969
18. Jelliffe RW: An improved method of digoxin therapy. Ann Intern Med 69:703, 1968
19. Jelliffe RW, Buell J, Kalaba R: Reduction of digitalis toxicity by computer-assisted glycoside dosage regimens. Ann Intern Med 77:891, 1972
20. Jervell A, Thingstad R, Endsjö T: The surdo-cardiac syndrome (three new cases of congential deafness with syncopal attacks and QT prolongation on the electrocardiogram). Am Heart J 72:582, 1966
21. Koch–Weser J, Klein SW: Procainamide dosage schedules, plasma concentrations, and clinical effects. JAMA 215:1454, 1971
22. Koch–Weser J, Klein SW, Foo–Canto LL, Kastor JA, DeSanctis RW: Antiarrhythmic prophylaxis with procainamide in acute myocardial infarction. N Engl J Med 281:1253, 1969
23. Kosowsky BD, Taylor J, Lown B, Ritchie RF: Long-term use of procaine amide following acute myocardial infarction. Circulation 47:1204, 1973
24. Kotler MN, Tabatznik B, Mower MM, Tominaga S: Prognostic significance of ventricular ectopic beats with respect to sudden death in the late postinfarction period. Circulation 47:959, 1973
25. Krauss KR, Hutter AM, DeSanctis RW: Acute coronary insufficiency, course and follow-up. Circulation 45–46, Supp. (1):66, 1972
26. Krikler DM, Spurrell RAJ: Verapamil in the treatment of paroxysmal supraventricular tachycardia. Postgrad Med J 50:447, 1974

27. Lie KI, Wellens HJ, vanCapelle FJ, Durrer D: Lidocaine in the prevention of primary ventricular fibrillation. N Engl J Med 291:1324, 1974
28. Lown B, Fakhro AM, Hood WB, Thorn GW: The coronary care unit. JAMA 199:188, 1967
29. Lown B, Vassaux C: Lidocaine in acute myocardial infarction. Am Heart J 76:586, 1968
30. Lown B, Vassaux C, Hood WB, Fakhro AM, Kaplinsky E, Roberge G: Unresolved problems in coronary care. Am J Cardiol 20:494, 1967
31. Marcus FI, Burkhalter L, Cuccia C, Pavlovich J, Kapadia GG: Administration of tritiated digoxin with and without a loading dose. Circulation 34:865, 1966
32. Mogensen L: Ventricular tachyarrhythmias and lidocaine prophylaxis in acute myocardial infarction. Acta Med Scand [Suppl] 513:39, 1970
33. Moss AJ, DeCamilla J, Engstrom F, Hoffman W, Odoroff C, Davis H: The posthospital phase of myocardial infarction. Circulation 49:460, 1974
34. Multicentre International Study: Improvement in prognosis of myocardial infarction by long-term beta-adrenoreceptor blockade using practolol. Br Med J 3:735, 1975
35. Norpace symposium. Angiology 26 (Supp. 1) 65–164, 1975
36. Perhexiline symposium. Postgrad Med J 49 (Supp. 3) 1–32, 1973
37. Ratshin RA, Hunt D, Russell RO, Rackley CE: QT interval prolongation, paroxysmal ventricular arrhythmias, and convulsive syncope. Ann Intern Med 75:919, 1971
38. Rodstein M, Wolloch L, Gubner RS: Mortality study of the significance of extrasystoles in an insured population. Circulation 44:617, 1971
39. Romhilt DW, Bloomfield SS, Lipicky RJ, Welch RM, Fowler NO: Evaluation of bretylium tosylate for the treatment of premature ventricular contractions. Circulation 45:800, 1972
40. Rosen MR, Ilvento JP, Gelband H, Merker C: Effects of verapamil on electrophysiologic properties of canine cardiac Purkinje fibers. J Pharmacol Exp Ther 189:414, 1974
41. Ryden L, Hjalmarson A, Wasir H, Werkö L: Effects of a long-acting antiarrhythmic agent-QX-572-on therapy resistant ventricular tachyarrhythmias. Br Heart J 36:811, 1974
42. Schamroth L, Krikler DM, Garrett C: Immediate effects of intravenous verapamil in cardiac arrhythmias. Br Med J 1:660, 1972
43. Schroeder JS, Fitzgerald J, Harrison DC: Detection of the high-risk patient for sudden death. Adv Cardiol 15:25, 1975
44. Singer PA, Crampton RS, Bass NH: Familial QT prolongation syndrome. Arch Neurol 31:64, 1974
45. Smith TW, Haber E: Digoxin intoxication: the relationship of clinical presentation to serum digoxin concentration. J Clin Invest 49:2377, 1970
46. Stone N, Klein MD, Lown B: Diphenylhydantoin in the prevention of recurring ventricular tachycardia. Circulation 43:420, 1971
47. Van Durme JP, Bogaert MG, Rosseel MT: Therapeutic effectiveness and plasma levels of aprinidine, a new antidysrhythmic drug. Eur J Clin Pharmacol 7:343, 1974
48. Vismara LA, Amsterdam EA, Mason DT: Relation of ventricular arrhythmias in the late hospital phase of acute myocardial infarction to sudden death after hospital discharge. Am J Med 59:6, 1975
49. Vismara LA, Mason DT, Amsterdam EA: Disopyramide phosphate: clinical efficacy of a new oral antiarrhythmic drug. Clin Pharmacol Ther 16:330, 1974
50. Wilhelmsson C, Wilhelmsen L, Vedin JA, Tibblin G, Werkö L: Reduction of sudden deaths after myocardial infarction by treatment with alprenolol. Lancet 2:1157, 1974
51. Winkle RA, Fitzgerald JW, Meffin PJ, Bell PA, Harapat SR, Harrison DC: A new oral lidocaine-like antiarrhythmic drug. W36095: antiarrhythmic efficacy in man. Circulation 52 (Supp. II):74, 1975
52. Wit AL, Steiner C, Damato AN: Electrophysiologic effects of bretylium tosylate on single fibers of the canine specialized conducting system and ventricle. J Pharmacol Exp Ther 173:344, 1970
53. Woosley RL, McDevitt DG, Smith RF, Nies AS, Wilkinson GR, Oates JA: Antiarrhythmic and pharmacokinetic properties of 2-amino-2″, 6′–propionoxylidide HCl (W–36095–HCl, Astra) in man. Circulation 52 (Supp. II):75, 1975
54. Wright P: Untoward effects associated with practolol administration: oculomucocutaneous syndrome. Br Med J 1:595, 1975

5 | Atrial and AV Junctional Tachycardia

TE–CHUAN CHOU

PAROXYSMAL ATRIAL AND AV JUNCTIONAL TACHYCARDIA

In paroxysmal atrial tachycardia the abnormal impulse originates from an ectopic focus in the atrium. The tachycardia is characterized by its clocklike regularity, abrupt onset and termination. It occurs intermittently and may last for seconds, hours, or days. The heart rate generally ranges from 140–220/min, most commonly between 180–200/min. It is not an uncommon arrhythmia. Among atrial arrhythmias it is observed more often than atrial flutter, but less often than atrial premature beats and atrial fibrillation.

The term paroxysmal AV junctional tachycardia has replaced paroxysmal nodal tachycardia to indicate ectopic tachycardia originating from the atrioventricular node area (23). Recent electrophysiologic studies have failed to identify automatic fibers in AV node proper (12). The source of the so-called "nodal beats" has been shown to be above or below the N region of the node. For the same reason the designation of "upper, middle, and lower nodal" origin of the arrhythmia, based on the relationship of the P wave to the QRS complex, is without an anatomic foundation. Furthermore, the relationship of a retrograde P wave to the QRS complex is not only dependent on the proximity of the ectopic pacemaker to the atria and ventricles, but also on the relative speed of impulse conduction in either direction. For example, if the impulse originates in the bundle of His and there is considerable antegrade conduction delay, the retrograde atrial activation may precede rather than follow the ventricular activation.

The mode of onset and termination of paroxysmal AV junctional tachycardia and its rate and regularity are similar to those of paroxysmal atrial tachycardia. This is also true in regard to their etiology and clinical consequences. They are often lumped together as paroxysmal supraventricular tachycardia. Recent intracardiac electrocardiographic studies also suggest that both tachyarrhythmias may involve a similar electrophysiologic mechanism. A circus movement is probably present with the atrium and AV node involved in the reentry pathway (10).

Although paroxysmal atrial and AV junctional tachycardias may be seen in patients with rheumatic, arteriosclerotic, and hypertensive heart disease, the arrhythmias are well known for their frequent occurrence in healthy, often young individuals who have no evidence of heart disease. The cause of the arrhythmias in such patients is obscure. Occasionally the paroxysms seem to be related to emotional stress, mental or physical fatigue, excessive consumption of tobacco, coffee, alcoholic beverages, and disease of the digestive tract.

They are also the most common types of arrhythmias seen in patients with the Wolff–Parkinson–White syndrome; the mechanism involved in this condition will be discussed in a later section of this article.

The tachycardia, either atrial or AV junctional, may be quite alarming and disturbing to the patient but is usually well tolerated without serious hemodynamic consequences. A prolonged attack even in an otherwise healthy individual may cause overt congestive heart failure or shock due to a significant decrease in cardiac output. Angina may develop as the coronary blood flow is reduced. Cerebral ischemia may be manifested by dizziness and syncope. An interesting phenomenon described by Wood (30) is the occurrence in many patients of polyuria during paroxysmal supraventricular and ventricular tachycardias. Such polyuria has been uncommon in our own experience.

DIAGNOSIS

The diagnosis of paroxysmal atrial or AV junctional tachycardia is often suggested clinically by its characteristic mode of onset and termination, and its rate and regularity of the rhythm, especially if the patient has no other evidence of heart disease. A regular rhythm with a ventricular rate ranging from 140–220/min suggests one of the following mechanisms: sinus tachycardia, paroxysmal atrial tachycardia, paroxysmal junctional tachycardia, atrial flutter with 2:1 AV conduction, and paroxysmal ventricular tachycardia. If an electrocardiograph is not available during the episode, vagal stimulation such as carotid sinus massage may be helpful in the differentiation of these arrhythmias. In sinus tachycardia the rate will decrease gradually with carotid sinus stimulation and then gradually resume its previous level shortly after the pressure is released. In paroxysmal atrial or AV junctional tachycardia, the rhythm will either be unchanged or reverted abruptly to a normal sinus mechanism. In atrial flutter any change in the rhythm is usually the result of an increase in the degree of AV block and there will be a jerky slowing of the heart beat upon carotid massage, followed by a jerky return to its previous regular rhythm after the procedure is terminated. Paroxysmal ventricular tachycardia is not affected by the procedure.

ELECTROCARDIOGRAM

In the electrocardiogram the remarkable regularity of the rhythm is observed. In paroxysmal atrial tachycardia the P waves, when identifiable, are different in configuration from those observed in the same patient during sinus rhythm. The PR interval is within normal limits or prolonged. There is a QRS complex following each P wave, and the duration of the QRS complex is usually normal and its configuration resembles that observed during normal sinus rhythm. In some patients the QRS complex may be widened because of aberrant ventricular conduction or preexisting ventricular conduction defect. In paroxysmal AV junctional tachycardia the P waves are inverted in Leads II, III, and aVF, and the PR interval is less than 0.12 sec. The P waves may precede, coincide with, or succeed the QRS complexes.

Even with the electrocardiogram a definitive diagnosis of paroxysmal atrial or AV junctional tachycardia is often difficult. When the heart rate in sinus tachycardia exceeds 140/min it may resemble closely paroxysmal atrial tachycardia. In sinus tachycardia the P waves tend, in general, to be quite clear-cut, while those in paroxysmal atrial tachycardia are usually small and hard to identify. Sometimes it is useful to compare the heart rate at the beginning with that at the end of the tracing. Any change in the RR interval during the period would speak in favor of sinus tachycardia. Carotid sinus massage during the recording of the electrocardiogram may also be helpful as previously discussed. Because of the short interval between the beats, the P waves are often fused with the preceding T waves and become difficult to identify. Separation of this rhythm from other types of supraventricular tachycardia may be impossible from the conventional body surface leads. If the patient has previous intraventricular conduction defect, such as left or right bundle branch block, Wolff–Parkinson–White syndrome, or develops aberrant ventricular conduction because of the rapid heart rate, the arrhythmia may resemble closely paroxysmal ventricular tachycardia. Under these circumstances esophageal and intraatrial lead electrocardiograms have been found very useful to record P waves of larger magnitude and demonstrate the relationship between the atrial and ventricular activities. The esophageal electrocardiogram has been seldom used in recent years and has been replaced mainly by the intraatrial electrogram. The former suffers from lack of cooperation from many patients because of the discomfort involved in the procedure. A technically good tracing is difficult to obtain. Figure 5–1 illustrates an intraatrial electrocardiogram of a patient with paroxysmal AV junctional tachycardia. The P waves which are superimposed on the QRS complexes are easily identified by the intraatrial lead.

Fig. 5–1. **Paroxysmal nodal tachycardia. Lead II and the intraatrial lead were recorded simultaneously. Large P waves are demonstrated by the intraatrial electrogram, as the electrode is advanced from the superior vena cava (SVC) into the right atrium (RA). P waves cannot be identified from Lead II.**

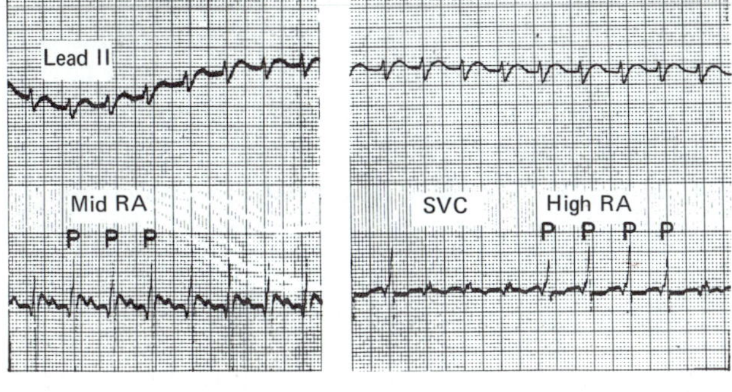

DISTINGUISHING SUPRAVENTRICULAR FROM VENTRICULAR TACHYCARDIA

Even if the atrial activities can be clearly demonstrated, the differential diagnosis between paroxysmal supraventricular tachycardia with *wide* QRS complexes and ventricular tachycardia is not always easy and may sometimes be impossible from the body surface leads alone. Certain observations are useful for the separation of the two types. If the onset of the arrhythmia is recorded, the presence of an ectopic and premature P wave at the beginning of the tachycardia strongly supports the supraventricular origin of the rhythm. If there is a P wave preceding each QRS complex and the PR interval is constant, the diagnosis of supraventricular tachycardia is quite certain. If the P wave follows the QRS complex and is inverted in Leads II, III, and aVF, the rhythm may be either AV junctional or ventricular in origin with retrograde capture of the atria. A short RP interval of 0.10 sec or less is in favor of junctional tachycardia. The availability of a previous tracing when the patient has normal sinus rhythm could be very helpful as it may demonstrate the preexisting bundle branch block or other ventricular conduction defects. If the wide QRS is the result of aberrant conduction secondary to the rapid heart rate, its configuration in Lead V_1 is often triphasic (an RSR' pattern) and the initial portion of the QRS complex usually resembles that when the conduction is normal. On the other hand, if the QRS complex has the same configuration as that of the premature ventricular contractions when the basic rhythm was sinus in origin, ventricular tachycardia is likely. It should be emphasized that the mere demonstration of independent atrial and ventricular rhythms is not necessarily indicative of ventricular tachycardia. A junctional tachycardia without retrograde capture of the atria may also result in the dissociation of the atrial and ventricular activities. However when ventricular captures or fusion beats are also present the tachycardia is, with rare exceptions, ventricular in origin.

In recent years the recording of His bundle electrogram offers a more definitive means for the differentiation of supraventricular tachycardia with wide QRS complex and ventricular tachycardia (8). In supraventricular tachycardia with aberrancy or intraventricular conduction defect a His bundle spike is present preceding each QRS complex. Such a spike is absent and obscured within each ventricular depolarization in ventricular tachycardia. Atrial pacing may also be helpful in the differential diagnosis. If the atrium is stimulated at a faster rate than that of the tachycardia and the ventricular captures have a narrower QRS, the presence of aberrancy can be excluded (5). However, under most circumstances in which this diagnostic problem occurs, these invasive procedures are not accessible or practical. The therapeutic approach has to depend on the surface electrocardiogram and clinical judgment.

RECORDING ELECTROCARDIOGRAM IN AMBULATORY PATIENTS

If the paroxysms are brief the tachycardia may terminate before the patient is seen by a physician or before an electrocardiogram can be recorded. Verification of the arrhythmia may be obtained by the use of the Holter monitor (dynamic electrocardiogram) (13). This portable magnetic tape recorder has the ability to record the electrocardiogram continuously for up to 24 hours in the ambulatory patient. The magnetic tape is then scanned rapidly at a speed 60 or 120 times faster than the actual recording time. Any significant finding may be transcribed to obtain a permanent record. Figure 5–2 illustrates the onset of an episode of paroxysmal atrial tachycardia in a middle-aged man who complained of frequent palpitation for many years. As the attacks were of very short duration, they were not documented by electrocardiography until such an apparatus was employed.

TREATMENT OF THE ACUTE EPISODE

During an acute attack the patient should be reassured as to the usually benign nature of the tachycardia. A sedative, such as phenobarbital 100 mg or secobarbital 100 mg, may be given by mouth. In many patients the tachycardia will revert spontaneously without further treatment.

VAGAL STIMULATION

Various types of vagal stimulation are perhaps the most useful maneuver for the termination of the tachycardia. A Valsalva maneuver may first be performed by instructing the patient to expire forcefully while holding his breath after a deep inspiration.* Occasionally the episode may be stopped by induced gagging or vomiting by irritating the throat. If any one of these simple procedures is found to be effective, the patient may be asked to use them in the event of future episodes.

Vagal stimulation by carotid sinus massage is the most useful procedure employed by the physician. The carotid sinus is located just below the angle of the jaw approximately at the level of the upper border of the thyroid cartilage. The wall of the carotid sinus is supplied by pressure receptors which carry the impulse to the vasomotor and cardioinhibitor centers in the brain

Fig. 5–2. Onset of paroxysmal atrial tachycardia as recorded by the Holter apparatus. Changes in the configuration of the QRS complexes after onset of tachycardia are due to aberrant ventricular conduction, which is most marked in first two beats.

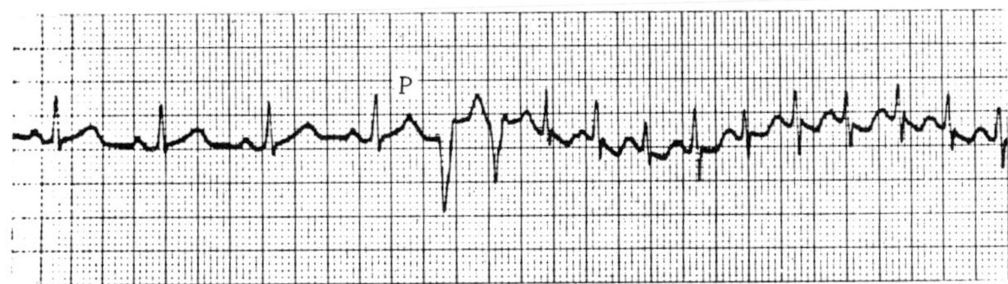

*With his breath held, the patient may immerse his face in a basin of cold water. The vagal effect of this "diving reflex" was successful in seven patients with paroxysmal atrial tachycardia. (Wildenthal K, Atkins JM, Leshin SJ, et al.: The diving reflex used to treat paroxysmal atrial tachycardia. Lancet 1:12, 1975)

stem. The procedure should be done with the patient in a supine position and his head extended and turned to the opposite side. The rhythm should be monitored with an electrocardiograph, if available, or the heart rate checked by listening to the heart simultaneously. The right carotid sinus is usually tried first because it is generally more effective. Pressure and massage are applied upon the carotid sinus posteriorly and medially against the vertebral spine. It is to be continued only a few seconds at a time. Simultaneous bilateral carotid sinus stimulation should never be done. The procedure is contraindicated in patients with a history of cerebrovascular disease. In certain individuals with a sensitive carotid sinus, pressure may result in prolonged bradycardia due to sinus arrest, complete heart block or even cardiac standstill. Other types of vagal stimulation, such as the cold pressor test or eyeball pressure are sometimes used in place of carotid sinus stimulation; however, they are generally not quite as effective and the latter method is unpleasant and may be hazardous (causing detached retina or other ocular injury).

PARASYMPATHOMIMETIC DRUGS

Neostigmine (Prostigmin) 0.5–1.0 mg may be given subcutaneously or intramuscularly. If this alone is unsuccessful, carotid sinus stimulation may be applied 15–20 minutes after the injection to potentiate the vagal effect. The drug is contraindicated in patients with history of bronchial asthma. Edrophonium chloride (Tensilon) 5–10 mg given intravenously has also been found moderately effective to terminate paroxysmal supraventricular tachycardia (11). It has a more rapid and shorter effect than Neostigmine.

PHENYLEPHRINE HYDROCHLORIDE

If the above described procedures are not successful the use of a pressor amine to stimulate the vagal reflex may be indicated. Phenylephrine hydrochloride (Neo-Synephrine) 0.5 mg is given rapidly intravenously. If the tachycardia does not subside or if the systolic blood pressure does not rise above 160 mm Hg, another 1 mg may be given. The drug may also be given as a rapid intravenous infusion containing 5 mg in 100 ml of 5% glucose in water. The blood pressure is monitored during the administration aiming to raise the level to about 160–180 mm. Phenylephrine hydrochloride has been found quite effective in many cases. However, it should not be used in older individuals, patients with organic heart disease, hypertension, marked sinus bradycardia, or partial AV block. Occasionally profound sinus bradycardia, even asystole, as well as short runs of tachycardia, have been observed following its use.

DIGITALIS

If the previously described simple therapeutic approaches are ineffective, digitalis is considered by most the drug of choice. This is usually given parentally in the form of a rapidly acting glycoside. Digoxin (Lanoxin) 0.5–0.75 mg is usually given as the first dose intravenously, and is followed by 0.25 mg every 3–4 hours. The total amount required is usually 0.75 to 1.25 mg. An oral preparation of digoxin may also be employed with an initial dose of 0.5–1.0 mg, and is followed by 0.25–0.5 mg at 4–6 hour intervals, if needed. The average total dose for digitalization with this oral glycoside is 1.0–1.5 mg. Deslanaside (Cedilanid-D) intravenously may also be used. The initial dose is usually 0.8 mg and is followed by additional doses of 0.4 mg every 3–4 hours until the patient is digitalized. In the majority of instances the total amount of deslanaside required does not exceed 1.6 mg. In many patients the conversion can be accomplished before an average digitalizing dose has been administered. Digitalis is especially favored when there is an evidence of underlying heart disease and continuing digitalis therapy is expected. The mechanism involved in the conversion of paroxysmal atrial tachycardia by digitalis is to increase vagal tone or sensitize the carotid sinus reflex, and to prolong the conduction in the AV node. Therefore, in some patients the conversion may be accomplished by applying carotid sinus pressure after the patient is digitalized when either one of the procedures alone is unsuccessful.

QUINIDINE

Quinidine may be employed alone or after the patient is digitalized. It terminates an attack by increasing the refractory period of the atrial muscle and by depressing the ectopic pacemaker. The drug may be given every 6 hours at the dosage of 0.3–0.4 g. Special effort should be made to detect the toxic manifestations of quinidine. Although the most common reason for the discontinuance of the drug is the development of gastrointestinal symptoms such as nausea, vomiting, and diarrhea, its most serious complications are those related to the cardiovascular systems (25, 27) Depression of the sinus node, impairment of intraatrial, atrioventricular and intraventricular conduction as well as ventricular premature contractions, ventricular tachycardia, and fibrillation may occur. Electrocardiograms should be obtained before the therapy is begun and repeated frequently later. An increase of 0.02 sec or more in the duration of the QRS complex is an indication for reducing the dosage or stopping the drug. Quinidine blood levels should be obtained and a concentration ranging between 4–6 mg/liter is desired. A level above 8 mg/liter is considered dangerous. Because of the possibility of serious complications many clinicians have been reluctant to use more than an average dose of quinidine for the conversion of cardiac arrhythmias. Usually, if the measures described previously have failed, we try DC electric shock before using quinidine.

PROCAINE AMIDE, PROPRANOLOL AND DIPHENYLHYDANTOIN

Procaine amide (Pronestyl) has also been used in the treatment of supraventricular tachycardia with reasonable success. The drug may be given intramuscularly in a dose of 500 mg and repeated in 2 hours, if necessary. It may also be administered intravenously with a rate not faster than 100 mg/min. The total amount should not exceed 1000 mg. Its oral dose is from 250–750 mg every 3–4 hours. This route of administration is less dependable for the termination of acute attacks. The toxic effects of procaine amide include hypotension, widening of the QRS complex, ventricular tachycardia or fibrillation. Electrocardiographic and blood pressure monitoring are therefore required.

Propranolol (Inderal), a β-adrenergic blocking agent, has been used in recent years in the treatment of various forms of tachyarrhythmias, especially those resistant to the more conventional drugs. Although its antiarrhythmic property depends mostly on the blocking of β-adrenergic receptors, a quinidinelike action also is believed to exist. It increases the refractory period at the SA and AV junctions and depresses the automaticity of the sinoatrial and ectopic myocardial pacemakers (26). It is found particularly useful in the treatment and prevention of paroxysmal supraventricular tachycardia associated with the W–P–W syndrome and in patients whose episodes are provoked by exertion or emotion (29). The drug may be given orally or intravenously. For oral administration the usual amount is 40–160 mg/day in four divided doses. The intravenous dose recommended for the treatment of arrhythmias is 1–3 mg. A second dose may be repeated after 2 minutes, if needed. It is usually not advisable to exceed a total amount of 0.1 mg/kg of body weight at any one time. Additional medication should not be given in less than 4 hours. When the intravenous method is used, it should be given under electrocardiographic monitoring and the rate of administration should not exceed 1 mg each 3 min. The drug is contraindicated in patients with bradycardia, congestive heart failure, hypotension, asthma, diabetic patients taking insulin, and patients on adrenergic-augmenting psychotropic drugs (including monoamine oxidase MAO inhibitors). We would usually try DC electric shock therapy before using intravenous propranolol because of the danger of cardiac arrest with the latter.

Diphenylhydantoin (Dilantin) has been used in the treatment of paroxysmal atrial tachycardia with moderate success by some observers (1). However, others were not able to obtain comparable encouraging results in the treatment of atrial arrhythmias other than those induced by digitalis. The drug may be given intravenously at the dosage of 250 mg or orally 100 mg 3 times per day. With intravenous administration, its potential toxic effects are similar to those due to procaine amide and the same precautions should be taken.

DIRECT CURRENT COUNTERSHOCK AND RAPID ATRIAL STIMULATION

If the tachycardia is refractory to the various maneuvers and drug therapy, conversion may be obtained by using synchronized direct current countershock. This method is especially indicated when the patient is in congestive heart failure or shock, and prompt termination of the arrhythmia is needed. When properly prepared the procedure is relatively safe and is preferred over large doses of antiarrhythmic drugs when serious toxic effects are feared. Its rate of success in supraventricular tachycardia is about 72% (16). The procedure should not be applied to patients in whom the arrhythmia is likely the result of digitalis toxicity, since serious ventricular arrhythmias may occur.

Recently, rapid atrial stimulation has been employed for the conversion of atrial and AV junctional tachycardia, as well as atrial flutter (15). A bipolar electrode catheter is introduced transvenously into the right atrium. The position of the catheter is guided by fluoroscopy or intracavitary electrogram. The atria are paced by a Medtronic pulse generator at a rate slightly greater than the patient's atrial rate. The mechanisms thought to be responsible for the termination of the tachycardia are: overdrive and suppression of an ectopic supraventricular pacemaker; alteration in the type of supraventricular arrhythmia and the resulting new arrhythmia is not self-perpetuating; the interruption of a fixed circus movement by atrial paced beats. The procedure has the advantages of being applicable to patients who were receiving digitalis. Anesthesia is not necessary, as in the case of DC countershock. In cases of recurrent tachycardia at short intervals, the right atrial electrode catheter can be left in place and rapid atrial stimulation can be applied repeatedly with no discomfort to the patient.

PREVENTION OF RECURRENT ATTACKS

In patients whose repeated attacks of paroxysmal tachycardia appear to be related to emotional stress or other factors listed previously, avoidance of such precipitating causes should be stressed. Mild sedatives may be helpful in certain instances. The most reliable drug is digitalis. A maintenance dose of digoxin 0.125 to 0.5 mg, usually 0.125 mg–0.375 mg/day may be given after the patient is fully digitalized. Quinidine sulfate 0.2–0.4 g or propranolol 10–40 mg every 6 hours may also be used. Procaine amide is usually avoided because of the high incidence of a lupuslike syndrome associated with its long-term use (6). Various combinations of the above-mentioned drugs may be used in resistant cases.

PAROXYSMAL ATRIAL AND NODAL TACHYCARDIA IN CHILDREN

Although the total incidence of paroxysmal tachycardia in children is low, the supraventricular variety is the most common type. The majority of patients are infants under 4 months of age. They are usually male and without organic heart disease. In these infants it often presents as a cardiac emergency and is associated with pallor or cyanosis, vomiting, symptoms and signs of congestive heart failure such as rapid respiration, enlargement of the heart and liver, and pulmonary congestion. Death may result if treatment is not given promptly. In older infants and children the tachycardia occurs in males and females in about equal frequency, and it may or may not be associated with organic heart disease. In the series reported by Nadas (20) slightly over 10% of the patients had the Wolff–Parkinson–White syndrome. Twenty percent had congenital heart disease. Another 20% of the patients had infections, injuries, heart tumors, or were under the influence of drugs. No etiology could be found in the other 50%.

The characteristics of the arrhythmia are similar to those seen in adult subjects, except the heart rate is generally faster and varies between 160–330 beats/min. This is especially true in young infants.

TREATMENT

To terminate the attack vagal stimulation by carotid sinus pressure should be tried first. In young infants this method is frequently unsuccessful. If drug therapy is needed, digitalis preparation is the drug of choice. Digoxin (Lanoxin) may be given orally or parenterally depending on the urgency of the case. For oral administration the total digitalizing dose is 0.03–0.04 mg/pound of body weight for children under 2 years of age, and 0.02–0.03 mg/pound for those over 2. One-half of the total dose may be given initially and the remainder is given in 2 divided doses at 4– or 8–hour intervals. If digoxin is to be used intramuscularly or intravenously, the total dosage should be one-half to two-thirds of the amount calculated for oral administration. If the tachycardia is successfully terminated, daily maintenance digoxin in the amount of one-fourth of the digitalizing dosage should be given for 3–6 months. Recurrence is usually infrequent beyond one year after the initial episode. In the older infant and child the tachycardia may recur for several years, especially in patients with the Wolff–Parkinson–White syndrome. If the tachycardia cannot be terminated with the calculated digitalizing dose of digoxin, additional digoxin about one-sixth of the calculated amount may be administered every 4 hours until either the desired effect is obtained or evidence of digitalis toxicity appears. Carotid sinus stimulation may be applied after full digitalization and may be effective in certain instances.

If digoxin alone fails, quinidine sulfate, 3 mg/pound of body weight, may be given every 3–5 hours orally. Quinidine gluconate may be administered intramuscularly in a similar dosage.

Often in resistant cases propranolol (Inderal) has been found effective in the conversion of paroxysmal supraventricular tachycardia and the maintenance of a normal sinus rhythm, especially in patients with the Wolff–Parkinson–White syndrome. If the usual pharmacologic agents are not effective, or the patient is desperately ill requiring prompt conversion, synchronized DC countershock is indicated. In some infants a very small energy level is required for the successful conversion of arrhythmias (24).

PAROXYSMAL SUPRAVENTRICULAR TACHYCARDIA IN PATIENTS WITH THE WOLFF–PARKINSON–WHITE SYNDROME

The frequent association of paroxysmal supraventricular tachycardia and W–P–W syndrome is well known. In its classical form the preexcitation syndrome is characterized by the electrocardiographic findings of short PR interval, wide QRS complex with an initial slowing of the QRS complex, the delta wave. The syndrome has been attributed to the presence of abnormal muscular bridges between the atrium and ventricle (bundles of Kent) causing premature activation of an area of the ventricle. Detailed pathologic examinations have verified the presence of such muscular bridges in the majority of patients examined who have had the W–P–W syndrome. Electrophysiologic studies by epicardial mapping at the time of surgery has verified further the nature of the excitation anomaly (2,3,9)

The reported incidence of supraventricular arrhythmias in patients with the W–P–W syndrome varies from 13–80%. Paroxysmal atrial tachycardia is by far the most common type, with atrial fibrillation and atrial flutter being less frequent. Ventricular tachyarrhythmia is rare. The frequent association of recurrent paroxysmal supraventricular tachycardia has been explained on the basis of a circus movement of the excitatory wave. It has been postulated that during the paroxysm the atrial impulse is usually conducted through the AV node and bundle of His to the ventricles, and then returns to the atrium by a retrograde conduction via the bundle of Kent. This hypothesis has been confirmed by recent electrophysiologic observations during epicardial exploration at surgery. In these patients the electrocardiogram during tachycardia showed normal QRS complexes. Not infrequently, especially in patients with atrial flutter or fibrillation, the antegrade conduction is by way of the bundle of Kent, the QRS complexes are abnormally wide and the tracing mimics ventricular tachycardia.

Several variants of the W–P–W syndrome have been recognized and they are also associated with increased incidence of tachycardias (7). Lown, Ganong, and Levine described the syndrome of short PR interval with normal QRS complex (17). Recent observation suggests that this phenomenon may be explained by the existence of a bypass tract described by James. Some of the specialized conduction pathways connecting the SA and AV nodes may bypass the upper and central portions of the AV node and enter the lower third, or may even connect directly with the common bundle of His. Conduction over such a bypass tract would result in a short PR interval since the normal conduction delay at the upper part of the AV node would be avoided. Since the ensuing ventricular excitation proceeds as usual, the QRS is normal in configuration. Another variant of the preexcitation syndrome is represented by the presence of a delta wave with prolongation of the QRS duration, but the PR interval is normal. This anomaly has been attributed to the existence of Mahaim fibers connecting the bundle of His with the interventricular septum allowing premature activation and the production of delta waves. The conduction of the atrial impulse through the AV node is as usual and therefore the PR interval remains normal.

The treatment of paroxysmal supraventricular tachycardia associated with the W–P–W syndrome is similar to those described for the tachycardia in general. Many of the refractory tachycardias are encountered in this type of patient. Under the circumstance propranolol is often successful in the termination of the arrhythmia and prevention of recurrences when other drugs have failed. In patients whose recurrent episodes could not be controlled by all available medical means, surgical interruption of the bundle of Kent has been performed and has been successful in preventing recurrence in the majority of cases (9). In one instance the AV bundle was severed and the ventricles were paced electronically (4).

NONPAROXYSMAL AV JUNCTIONAL TACHYCARDIA

Although nonparoxysmal AV nodal tachycardia (22) is also the result of an abnormal enhancement of impulse formation at the AV junction, the arrhythmia differs from the paroxysmal variety in many aspects. The rate of the junctional discharge is only moderately increased, being about 70–130/min instead of 150–220/min. The ectopic rhythm lacks the sudden onset and termination which is characteristic of the paroxysmal type. While paroxysmal junctional tachycardia is seen mainly in patients without demonstrable heart disease, the reverse is true in the nonparoxysmal form. The latter arrhythmia is most commonly the result of digitalis intoxication, acute myocardial infarction, intracardiac surgery, myocarditis (for example, rheumatic). In rare instances the etiology of the arrhythmia cannot be found.

Depending on the state of antegrade and retrograde conduction at the AV junction and the atrial and ventricular rates, various manifestations of rhythm disturbances may be observed. If the enhanced automaticity of the AV junctional pacemaker leads to retrograde activation of the atria, a constant relationship will exist between the P wave and the QRS complex (Fig. 5–3A). If there

Fig. 5–3. **A. Nonparoxysmal junctional tachycardia with retrograde capture of atria due to digitalis intoxication. B. Interference dissociation. Tracing was recorded from same patient 1 day later. It shows the dissociation of atrial and ventricular activities with occasional ventricular captures.**

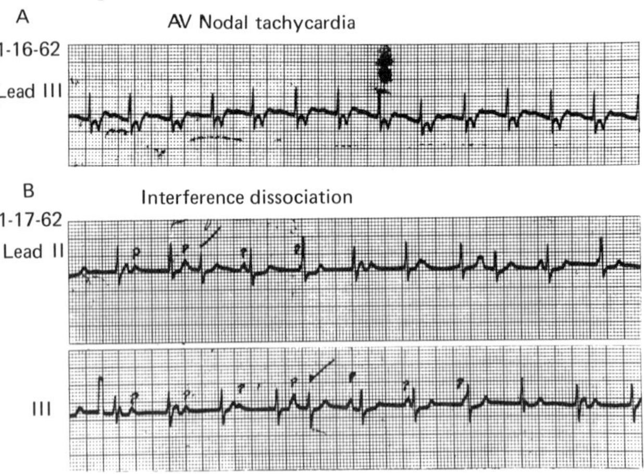

is an impairment of the retrograde conduction, the atria will remain under the control of the sinus impulse. The independent atrial and ventricular activities result in AV dissociation. The ventricular rate is generally faster than the atrial rate except when nonparoxysmal junctional tachycardia develops in the presence of atrial tachycardia, atrial fibrillation or flutter. If the atrial impulse arrives at the AV junction outside of its refractory phase and there is no antegrade AV block, it may capture the ventricles and "premature" conducted beat or beats are seen. The rhythm is then called interference dissociation or AV dissociation with interference (Fig. 5–3B). In some instances the rate of the dissociated pacemakers is very similar and the P waves and the QRS complexes are closely grouped. Because of the slight variation of the sinus rate, the P wave may periodically appear before, be buried in, and then reappear after the QRS, a phenomenon called isorhythmic AV dissociation with accrochage.

The treatment of nonparoxysmal AV junctional tachycardia depends on the etiology of the arrhythmia. In patients receiving digitalis the drug should be discontinued. Electrolyte imbalance such as hypokalemia, should be corrected. In the absence of impaired renal function or hyperkalemia, administration of potassium may be beneficial even though its serum level is within normal range. Potassium chloride may be given orally 40–80 mEq/day, or by intravenous drip with 40 mEq given over a 2 hour period initially. In most patients no additional drug therapy is needed. However, if the ventricular rate is very rapid and evidence of congestive heart failure is present, diphenylhydantoin (Dilantin), procaine amide, or quinidine sulfate may be tried. β-adrenergic blocking agents, such as propranolol, may also be useful but are contraindicated in the presence of congestive heart failure. Direct current countershock is contraindicated in patients with digitalis intoxication, as serious or even fatal ventricular arrhythmias may develop.

In nonparoxysmal junctional tachycardia occurring in patients with acute myocardial infarction, myocarditis, or in association with intracardiac surgery, the complication is often transient and benign and requires no specific treatment. However, if the ventricular rate is rapid or congestive heart failure appears and the patient has not received digitalis, digitalization is indicated. Other antiarrhythmic drugs described previously may be employed if digitalis alone is ineffective. In emergency situations DC countershock may be used.

PAROXYSMAL ATRIAL TACHYCARDIA WITH BLOCK

This subject is discussed in the chapter of digitalis-induced arrhythmias. In the majority of cases paroxysmal atrial tachycardia with block (PAT with block) is caused by digitalis, especially if hypokalemia is present. The treatment is to discontinue the drug and correct the electrolyte imbalance. However, PAT with block is also seen in patients with organic heart disease who do not receive digitalis. In these patients the arrhythmia may be treated with digitalis (19). Quinidine or pronestyl may also be used. Direct current countershock has been successful in the conversion of the rhythm (18). Since the ventricular rate in

PAT with block is usually not very fast, emergency measures are seldom necessary.

CHAOTIC ATRIAL TACHYCARDIA

Choatic atrial tachycardia is also called multifocal atrial tachycardia. It has been recognized as a distinctive electrocardiographic and clinical entity only in recent years (14, 21, 28). It is characterized by an atrial rate greater than 100/min with discrete P waves of varying morphology from at least three different focuses. The PP, RR, and PR intervals are variable (Fig. 5–4). The arrhythmia is usually transient, lasting not more than a few days, but recurrences are common. It is often preceded by sinus rhythm with unifocal or multifocal premature atrial contractions. In distinction to the latter it does not have a single persistent dominant atrial pacemaker. The rhythm frequently progresses to atrial fibrillation or flutter; it may superficially resemble the former.

Chaotic atrial tachycardia is mainly seen in elderly and very ill patients. There is a high incidence of chronic obstructive lung disease in patients with this arrhythmia, although its association with coronary and other heart diseases has also been demonstrated.

Treatment of the arrhythmia should be directed toward the underlying clinical derangements. It is important to improve the ventilation and oxygenation, and to correct the electrolyte and metabolic disturbance in the restoration of sinus rhythm. Digitalis therapy usually has no effect on the course of the rhythm. Although the drug should be used if it is otherwise indicated, attempts

Fig. 5–4. **Chaotic atrial tachycardia in a 61-year-old man with chronic obstructive lung disease.**

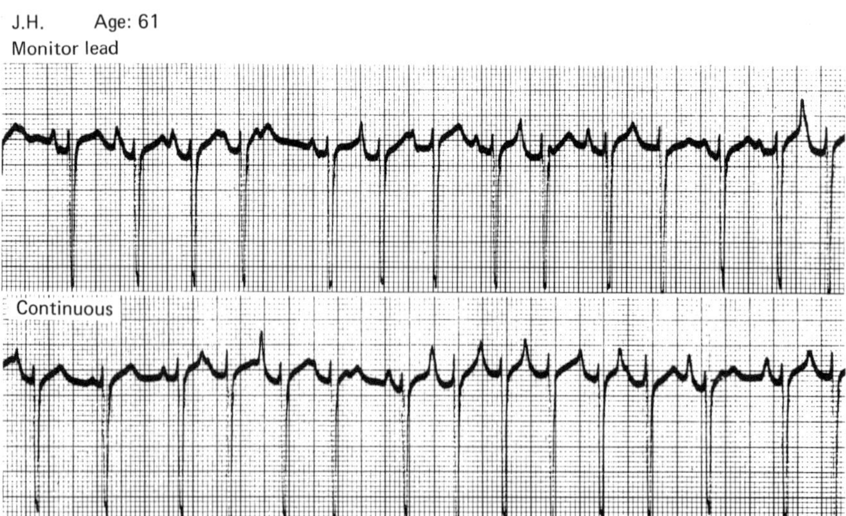

to control the ventricular rate by increasing the dosage should be discouraged. There is usually little response and serious digitalis-induced arrhythmias may occur. The use of other antiarrhythmic agents has not been shown to be beneficial.

REFERENCES

1. Bernstein H, Gold H, Lang T, Pappelbaum S, Bazika V, Corday E: Sodium diphenylhydantoin in the treatment of recurrent cardiac arrhythmias. JAMA 191:695, 1965
2. Burchell HB, Frye RL, Anderson MW, McGoon DC: Atrioventricular and ventriculoatrial excitation in Wolff-Parkinson-White syndrome (Type B). Circulation 36:663, 1967
3. Cobb FR, Blumenschein SD, Sealy WC, Boineau JP, Wagner GS, Wallace AG: Successful surgical interruption of the bundle of Kent in a patient with Wolff-Parkinson-White syndrome. Circulation 38:1018, 1968
4. Dreifus LS, Nichols H, Morse D, Watanabe Y, Treux R: Control of recurrent tachycardia of Wolff-Parkinson-White syndrome by surgical ligature of the A–V bundle. Circulation 38:1030, 1968
5. Easley RM Jr, Goldstein S: Differentiation of ventricular tachycardia from junctional tachycardia with aberrant conduction. The use of competitive atrial pacing. Circulation 37:1015, 1968
6. Fakhro AM, Ritchie RF, Lown B: Lupus-like syndrome induced by procainamide. Am J Cardiol 20:367, 1967
7. Ferrer MI: New concepts relating to the preexcitation syndrome. JAMA 201:162, 1967
8. Gallagher JJ, Damato AN, Lau SH: Electrophysiologic studies during accelerated idioventricular rhythms. Circulation 44:671, 1971
9. Gallagher JJ, Gilbert M, Svenson RH, Sealy WC, Kasell J, Wallace AG: Wolff-Parkinson-White syndrome: the problem, evaluation, and surgical correction. Circulation 51:767, 1975
10. Goldreyer BN: Intracardiac electrocardiography in the analysis and understanding of cardiac arrhythmias. Ann Intern Med 77:117, 1972
11. Grossman JI, Cooper JA, Frieden J: Hemodynamic and antiarrhythmic effects of edrophonium chloride (tensilon). Circulation 40 (Supp. III):97, 1969
12. Hoffman BF, Cranefield PF: Physiological basis of cardiac arrhythmias. Am J Med 37:670, 1964
13. Holter NJ: New methods for heart studies. Science 134:1214, 1961
14. Lipson MJ, Naimi S: Multifocal atrial tachycardia (Chaotic atrial tachycardia). Clinical associations and significance. Circulation 42:397, 1970
15. Lister JW, Cohen LS, Bernstein WH, Samet P: Treatment of supraventricular tachycardias by rapid atrial stimulation. Circulation 38:1044, 1968
16. Lown B: Electrical reversion of cardiac arrhythmias. Br Heart J 29:469, 1967
17. Lown B, Ganong WF, Levine SA: Syndrome of short P–R interval, normal QRS complex and paroxysmal rapid heart action. Circulation 5:693, 1952
18. Mark H, Sham R: Non digitalis induced paroxysmal atrial tachycardia with block. I. Management with cardioversion. J Electrocardiol 2:171, 1969
19. Morgan WL, Breneman GM: Atrial tachycardia with block treated with digitalis. Circulation 25:787, 1962
20. Nadas AS, Daeschner CW, Roth A, Blumenthal SL: Paroxysmal tachycardia in infants and children. Pediatrics 9:167, 1952
21. Phillips J, Spano J, Burch G: Chaotic atrial mechanism. Am Heart J 78:171, 1969
22. Pick A, Dominguez P: Nonparoxysmal A–V nodal tachycardia. Circulation 16:1022, 1957
23. Pick A, Lagendorf R: Recent advances in the differential diagnosis of A–V junctional arrhythmia. Am Heart J 76:553, 1968
24. Pryor R, Blount SG Jr: Refractory supraventricular tachycardia in infancy. Am J Dis Child 107:428, 1964

25. Rokseth R, Storstein O: Quinidine therapy of chronic auricular fibrillation. Arch Intern Med 111:184, 1963
26. Schamroth L: Immediate effects of intravenous propranolol on various cardiac arrhythmias. Am J Cardiol 18:438, 1966
27. Selzer A, Wray HW: Quinidine syncope. Paroxysmal ventricular fibrillation occurring during treatment of chronic atrial arrhythmias. Circulation 30:17, 1964
28. Shine KI, Kastor JA, Yurchak PM: Multifocal atrial tachycardia. Clinical and electrocardiographic features in 32 patients. N Engl J Med 279:344, 1968
29. Stock JPP: Beta adrenergic blocking drugs in the clinical management of cardiac arrhythmias. Am J Cardiol 18:444, 1966
30. Wood P: Polyuria in paroxysmal tachycardia. Br Heart J 25:273, 1963

6 | Atrial Fibrillation

NOBLE O. FOWLER

Except for extrasystoles, atrial fibrillation is the commonest of the disorders of the heart beat. Sir Thomas Lewis believed that atrial fibrillation was produced by a circus movement of the atrial depolarization wave (12). Scherf believed, however, that atrial fibrillation orginated from a single ectopic atrial focus or multiple focuses, like atrial flutter (16). Prinzmetal, using 2000 frame/sec cinematography, found atrial fibrillation in the dog to consist of two types of waves: large waves (L waves) at a rate of approximately 400–600/min, and a sea of small wavelets (M waves) (15). There was no evidence of a circus movement in Prinzmetal's studies. In the standard twelve lead electrocardiogram of a patient with atrial fibrillation one can often discern fibrillary waves, especially in Lead V_1. These waves are usually of irregular rhythm and varying form. Their rate is ordinarily somewhat in excess of 300/min.

ETIOLOGY

Most but not all patients with atrial fibrillation have additional clinical evidence of heart disease. Atrial fibrillation is most common in diseases which enlarge the left atrium, and is relatively uncommon in isolated aortic valve disease. Atrial fibrillation may be of either the paroxysmal or established (chronic) variety. Atrial fibrillation is usually considered established when it is of more than 6 weeks duration, since it is then relatively uncommon for spontaneous reversion to sinus rhythm to occur. Rheumatic mitral stenosis or insufficiency are commonly complicated by atrial fibrillation. When fibrillation occurs in this setting the valvular disease is usually of some years standing, and the left atrium is considerably enlarged. In our patients with tight mitral stenosis approximately one-third had established atrial fibrillation. Atrial fibrillation is said to be an uncommon complication of the left atrial enlargement of left atrial myxoma, but it may occur. In our series of patients with idiopathic nonobstructive cardiomyopathy, atrial fibrillation occurred in approximately one-third at some time before death. Atrial fibrillation may occur in idiopathic hypertrophic subaortic stenosis, but less often than in nonobstructive cardiomyopathy. Paroxysmal atrial fibrillation is common in cor pulmonale caused by chronic obstructive lung disease, but established atrial fibrillation is rare. We found established fibrillation had existed in only one of 70 patients with chronic cor pulmonale who came to autopsy at the Cincinnati General Hospital. Atrial fibrillation is uncommon in congenital heart disease except in older patients with atrial septal defect. Atrial fibrillation is found in approximately 10–15% of adults over 45 years of age with persistent ostium secundum atrial septal defect (2). Atrial fibrillation is a not uncommon complication of acute cardiac infarction; as many as 10% of such patients either have or develop this arrhythmia (3). Patients with enlarged hearts caused by chronic hypertension or coronary artery disease commonly develop atrial fibrillation. Atrial fibrillation is common in chronic constrictive pericarditis. As many as 25% of patients with chronic constrictive pericarditis have atrial fibrillation. Atrial fibrillation may occur in patients with acute myocarditis, including rheumatic myocarditis. In thyrotoxicosis, Williams found atrial fibrillation in 10% of 225 hyperthyroid patients (18). Atrial fibrillation is often of the paroxysmal variety in thyrotoxic patients. Atrial fibrillation is said to exist in the majority of patients with thyrotoxicosis who have congestive heart failure. Atrial fibrillation is not uncommon in patients with the Wolff–Parkinson–White syndrome. Atrial fibrillation also occurs in the absence of clinical evidence of heart disease. Each year the writer observes a few patients in whom paroxysmal fibrillation is the only evidence of heart disease. In many such instances there is a background of infection, especially pneumonia, or fatigue, smoking, emotional tension, or an acute alcoholic debauch.

DIAGNOSIS

The presence of atrial fibrillation is usually suspected from the rapid and irregular pulse and irregular irregularity of the heart sounds on auscultation of the precordium. In untreated atrial fibrillation, the ventricular rate is usually between 100 and 200 beats/min; however, when there is disease of the atrioventricular conducting system the ventricular rate may be as slow as 50–80 beats/min. At times it is difficult or impossible to distinguish atrial fibrillation from other irregular cardiac rhythms by means of physical examination alone.

As a rule the recognition of atrial fibrillation from the standard electrocardiogram presents few problems but there are exceptions to this statement. The electrocardiogram of atrial fibrillation is characterized by three principal features: the absence of normal P waves; the irregular irregularity of the QRS complexes, and the presence of fibrillary waves (Fig. 6–1). When fibrillary waves are clearly demonstrable the diagnosis of atrial fibrillation can be regarded as proved. When there are no discernible P waves, and the QRS complexes are irregular, but fibrillary waves are not identified, the diagnosis of atrial fibrillation is in some question.

ERRORS IN ELECTROCARDIOGRAPHIC DIAGNOSIS

The following errors may occur with regard to the electrocardiographic diagnosis of atrial fibrillation:

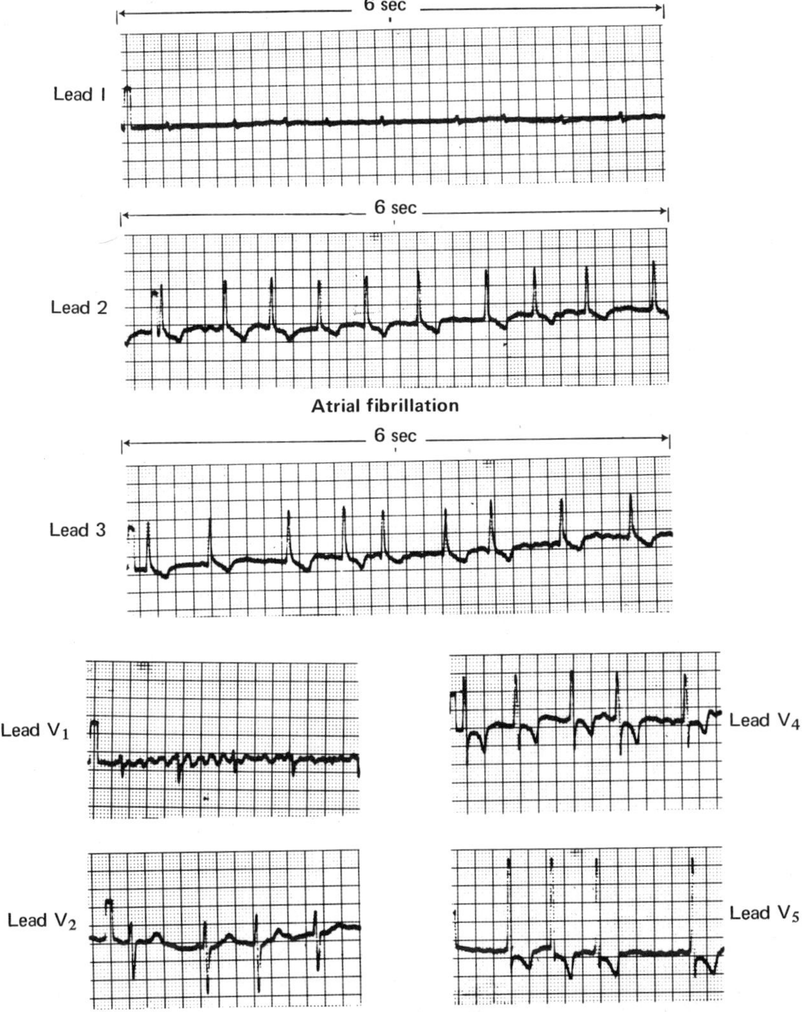

Fig. 6–1. **Fibrillary waves in atrial fibrillation. Fibrillary waves are best seen in Leads II, III, V$_1$, and V$_5$. [From Fowler (5).]**

1. Paroxysmal atrial tachycardia with varying AV block may be mislabeled as atrial fibrillation, especially when the P waves are very small or invisible. Careful study will reveal that the arrhythmia is not totally irregular. A right atrial lead may be needed to demonstrate the P waves.

2. Chaotic atrial activity with the atrial mechanism being that of multifocal atrial premature contractions or multifocal atrial tachycardia, with only occasional sinus activated P waves, resembles atrial fibrillation. Careful study will show only one P wave before each QRS complex, although the form of the P wave may vary from beat to beat (Fig. 6–2).

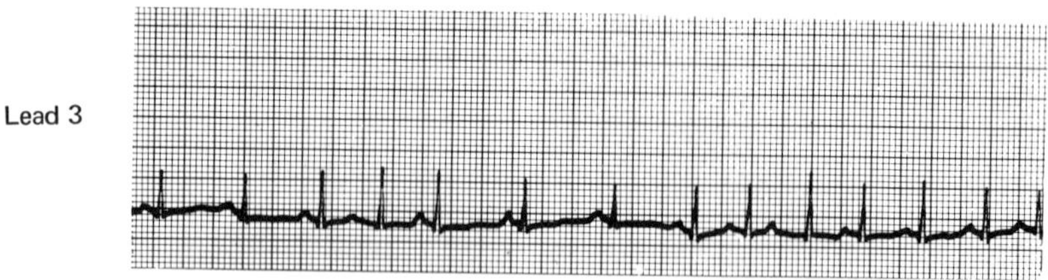

Fig. 6–2.   Chaotic atrial activity. Lead III. There are numerous premature atrial contractions. Clinically, the irregularity simulates atrial fibrillation.

Fig. 6–3.   Atrial fibrillation with regular atrial activity simulating atrial flutter in Lead V₁. Lead III shows that rhythm is atrial fibrillation rather than atrial flutter. [From Fowler (6).]

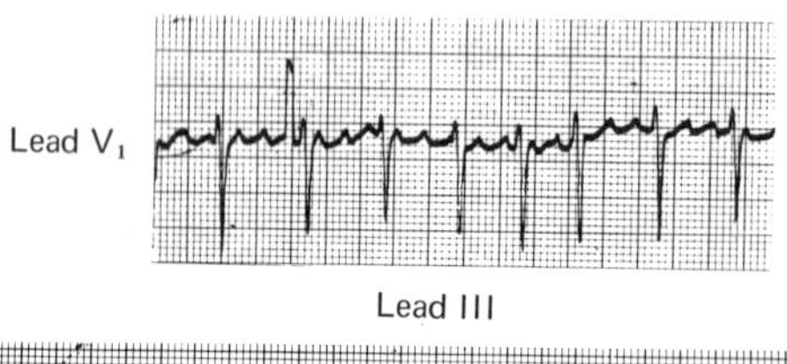

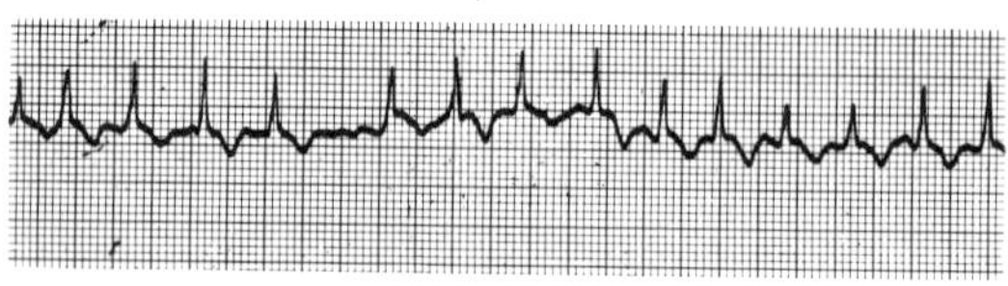

Fig. 6–4

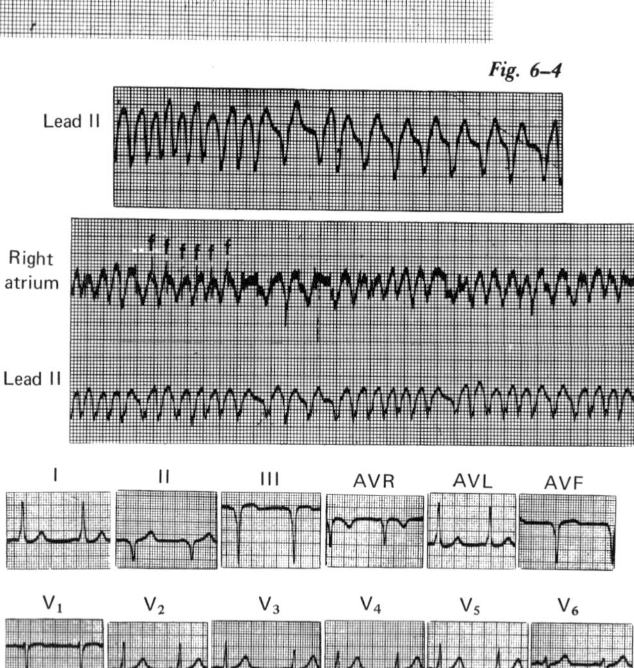

3. Atrial fibrillation may be mislabeled as atrial flutter. In a small percentage of patients with atrial fibrillation there are regular atrial depolarization waves at a rate of approximately 300/min in Lead V_1, but in no other leads. These waves simulate the appearance of atrial flutter, but usually in Lead V_1 only (Fig. 6–3). In standard leads atrial flutter is clearly not present.

4. Ventricular tachycardia may erroneously be thought to be present in patients with atrial fibrillation and broad QRS complexes, related either to aberrant intraventricular conduction, preexisting bundle branch block, or the Wolff–Parkinson–White syndrome. With Wolff–Parkinson–White syndrome the ventricular rate is often in excess of 200/min; thus aberrant intraventricular conduction is common (Fig. 6–4). The QRS pattern in Fig. 6–4 is characteristic of atrial fibrillation in which the abnormal pathway of the Wolff–Parkinson–White syndrome is activated before the normal pathway. As a rule the ventricular complexes are not irregular in ventricular tachycardia, unless there are fusion beats or captured beats. When there is serious doubt right atrial leads are useful to establish the atrial n.echanism (Fig. 6–4).

5. Patients with atrial fibrillation may have complete AV block, with a junctional or ventricular pacemaker activating the ventricles. Usually the ventricular rate is 40–100/min: the QRS complexes of the electrocardiogram are of supraventricular form and the ventricular rhythm is regular. Digitalis intoxication is often responsible for the complete AV block. When the fibrillary waves are small, or invisible, it may be difficult to know whether there is atrial fibrillation or atrial arrest. Right atrial leads will usually settle the issue.

CIRCULATORY EFFECTS OF ATRIAL FIBRILLATION

Atrial fibrillation has a number of undesirable effects upon the circulation. It causes a loss of the atrial aid to ventricular filling. It tends to accelerate the ventricular rate, and the irregularity of ventricular rhythm results in an inadequate time for ventricular diastolic filling during some cardiac cycles. The result is a tendency for a decreased circulatory reserve. Persons with relatively normal hearts tend to maintain a normal cardiac output at rest, but have a decreased ability to increase the cardiac output with severe exercise (14). Patients who have slight or moderate heart disease may or may not have a

◀ *Fig. 6–4.A.   Top,* **Atrial fibrillation in a patient with Wolff–Parkinson–White syndrome. Standard Lead II (upper strip) reveals broad QRS complexes and irregular irregularity of ventricular rhythm. Atrial activity is not visualized. In right atrial lead (middle strip) are visualized fibrillary waves (labeled F), giving evidence that rhythm is atrial fibrillation. It may be seen from simultaneously recorded Lead II (bottom strip) that there are periods of 1:1 conduction in which every large fibrillary wave is followed by a QRS complex. Hence, for very brief periods the ventricular rate is 300 beats/min or slightly faster.**

◀ *Fig. 6–4B.   Bottom,* **Standard 12 Lead electrocardiogram of same patient during normal sinus rhythm. There is a short PR interval with a delta wave in Lead I characteristic of the Wolff–Parkinson–White syndrome. Negative delta waves are present in Leads II, III, and AVF. It can be seen how an incorrect diagnosis of previous inferior infarction may be made in some patients with Wolff–Parkinson–White syndrome. [From Fowler (6).]**

normal cardiac output at rest with atrial fibrillation, but this is likely to be maintained at the expense of an increased cardiac filling pressure (14). The exercise response of the cardiac output is impaired. With more severe heart disease the cardiac output falls at rest despite an increased atrial pressure, and congestive failure may occur. A striking reduction in resting cardiac output with an elevation of left atrial pressure, perhaps leading to pulmonary edema, is a special danger in the patient with severe mitral stenosis. The rapid ventricular rate shortens diastole more than systole, and thus reduces the time available for blood to flow across the narrowed mitral orifice.

Atrial fibrillation has other undesirable effects. In many patients the irregularity causes annoying palpitation. If the ventricular rate is extremely rapid, syncope or angina pectoris may occur. Atrial fibrillation increases the risk of atrial mural thrombi and of systemic or pulmonary embolism. In patients with mitral stenosis, systemic arterial embolism to the brain, splanchnic area, kidney, or extremities seldom occurs unless atrial fibrillation is present.

TREATMENT

The treatment of atrial fibrillation may be discussed under the following headings:

1. Treatment of the underlying heart disease (if any), or the precipitating cause.
2. Control of the ventricular rate.
3. Termination of the arrhythmia.
4. Prevention of recurrences.
5. Prevention of thromboembolism.

In planning the treatment of atrial fibrillation it is necessary to consider the underlying disease. If thyrotoxicosis is present it will be necessary to employ thyroidectomy or radioactive iodine, but satisfactory decrease of the ventricular rate can usually be achieved with digitalis. Somewhat greater than customary amounts may be required. When there is rheumatic mitral disease of sufficient severity to require cardiac surgery, often no attempt is made to terminate the arrhythmia until 4–6 weeks postoperatively. If the patient has no organic heart disease, attention may need to be directed toward such precipitating factors as infection, excessive use of tobacco, emotional tension, or fatigue.

CONTROL OF VENTRICULAR RATE

The resting cardiac output is less likely to be greatly decreased by atrial fibrillation when the resting ventricular rate is 70–80/min, rather than in the usual range of 100–200/min in the untreated case. In general the first therapeutic goal is to decrease the ventricular rate when a patient is first seen with atrial fibrillation and a rapid ventricular rate, and especially when the atrial fibrillation is of recent onset or of unknown duration. Digitalis preparations are used for this purpose. Digitalis slows the ventricular rate in atrial fibrillation by increasing AV block both by vagal stimulation and by extravagal action (7). Often when the atrial fibrillation is of recent onset, digitalization is followed by a return to sinus rhythm, and a consideration of cardioversion by DC shock becomes unnecessary. The return of sinus rhythm following digitalization may be the result of improved hemodynamics or may be coincidental, since the pharmacologic action of digitalis upon the fibrillating atria does not tend to restore sinus rhythm. Further, many patients will need digitalization in any event, because of associated cardiac enlargement and decompensation. Finally, digitalization will permit time for complete diagnostic evaluation to determine whether or not an attempt to terminate the arrhythmia is desirable.

DIGITALIS

When the patient with atrial fibrillation and a ventricular rate of 100–200/min is in no distress and is without cardiac decompensation, digitalization should be undertaken with an oral preparation. Optimally the patient is hospitalized for better observation and for complete diagnostic evaluation. In the patient who has not received digitalis, an initial dose of 1 mg digoxin is given orally; this is followed at 8-hour intervals by 2 or 3 doses of 0.25 to 0.5 mg digoxin, with the therapeutic goal a resting ventricular rate of 70–80/min if there is no evidence of toxicity. If the ventricular rate is still above 80/min and an electrocardiogram shows that new premature ventricular contractions or other clinical or electrocardiographic signs of digitalis toxicity have not appeared, the digoxin dosage is reduced to 0.25 mg every 8 hours until the desired ventricular rate is attained. Then the digoxin dosage is reduced to a maintenance level, usually 0.25 mg once or twice/day, selected at the amount sufficient to control the ventricular rate. In some patients difficulty is encountered in controlling the ventricular rate with digitalis alone. One study reported that this was true in the majority of patients with atrial fibrillation and an acute illness, such as infection, hypoxia, or recent thoracotomy (8). Four of 14 patients with chronic atrial fibrillation and without an acute illness had uncontrolled ventricular rates (> 95/min) even with serum dixogin levels in the usual therapeutic range (0.8–2 ng/ml). In 4 of 16 patients with chronic atrial fibrillation and an acute illness, even serum digoxin levels usually considered toxic (2–5 ng/ml) failed to control the ventricular rate. In 30 patients with acute atrial fibrillation, most having a concomitant serious disorder such as recent cardiac infarction, congestive heart failure, recent operation, or infection, only 12 had satisfactory control of ventricular rate with therapeutic serum levels of digoxin. Thus in many patients with atrial fibrillation, especially with an acute illness, in addition to the use of often larger than usual doses of digoxin, one must consider the treatment of the associated condition, the addition of propranolol, or an attempt to revert the arrhythmia to sinus rhythm, probably with cardioversion. Control of ventricular rate is often a problem in thyrotoxicosis, when unusually large doses may be needed. In some instances the addition of propranolol (Inderal), 10–40 mg three or four times/day, will permit satisfactory control of the ventricular rate. One should be extremely cautious in the use of propranolol in patients with enlarged hearts, since congestive heart failure may be a complication of propranolol therapy in such patients. When the onset of atrial fibrillation with a rapid ventricular rate has precipitated pulmonary edema in the undigitalized patient, an intravenous digitalis preparation is used. One may give ouabain, 0.3 mg intravenously, followed by 0.1 mg at hourly intervals until a satisfactory response is obtained. The total dosage of ouabain should not exceed 0.7–0.8 mg within 24 hours. This method is effective in approximately 80–92% of patients (2). Alternatively one may give digoxin, 0.75 mg intravenously, with supplemental doses of 0.25 mg after 2 and 4 hours, if needed. Or one may use lanatoside C, 0.8 mg intravenously with supplemental doses of 0.4 mg after 2 and 4 hours, if needed.

When the ventricular rate does not decrease adequately after the initial dose of digitalis glycoside and a rapid effect is desired, an increase in AV block with decrease in ventricular rate can usually be achieved by the intravenous administration of 0.5–1 mg of propranolol. This dosage may be repeated at 3 minute intervals for a maximum of 5 doses. Alternatively, one may infuse 0.1 mg/kg body weight over a period of 10–30 minutes (9). Larger doses should not be used because of the negative inotropic effects of this drug and the danger of pulmonary edema. This regimen should probably not be used if there is cardiac enlargement, heart failure, or recent myocardial infarction.

Digitalis should generally not be used in two groups of patients with atrial fibrillation. One group is that in which the ventricular rate is already somewhat slow (50–80/min) without digitalis. The other is that in which there is an aberrant QRS, usually with a very rapid rate in excess of 200/min in a patient with atrial fibrillation and the Wolff–Parkinson–White syndrome (Fig. 6–4). In such patients digitalis tends to block conduction over the normal AV pathway; rapid conduction over the aberrant pathway may favor the development of fatal ventricular fibrillation (4).

TERMINATION OF ARRHYTHMIA

When it is considered desirable to attempt to restore the sinus mechanism in a patient with atrial fibrillation, direct current electric shock is the method of choice. As an alternative quinidine may be used in the manner employed for the treatment of atrial flutter as described in that section. Since quinidine is more hazardous and generally less effective than electric shock, its routine use cannot be recommended. The use of quinidine for the termination of atrial fibrillation probably has a mortality rate of 1–2%. The risk of electric shock is much lower, especially if its use is avoided in patients with digitalis toxicity. The risk of systemic embolism is about the same, averaging 1.5% with either method (13).

Since atrial fibrillation tends to reduce cardiac output and to increase the risk of systemic embolism, it might be thought that DC electric shock should be employed in all patients. There are certain categories of patients, however, in whom the procedure should be delayed or not used at all, and others in whom its benefit is doubtful (13). These are listed as follows:

1. The patient who cannot tolerate quinidine, which will be needed to help in preventing the return of the arrhythmia if the conversion attempt is successful.
2. The patient who is over 70 years of age.
3. The patient who has had atrial fibrillation for 3 years or more. In such patients, the rhythm is difficult to revert, and is unlikely to remain reverted (10).
4. The patient with considerable cardiac enlargement, especially if the left atrium is very large.
5. The patient who has atrial fibrillation with complete, or nearly complete, AV block, or who has a ventricular rate below 70–80/min in the absence of digitalis.
6. The patient who is to undergo mitral valve surgery. In such patients atrial fibrillation is likely to recur during the operation or shortly thereafter. It is better to attempt cardioversion 4–6 weeks after the operation.
7. The patient who has been unable to maintain a sinus rhythm with adequate quinidine therapy despite repeated reversions of atrial fibrillation to sinus rhythm.
8. The patient who had an unstable sinus mechanism prior to the onset of atrial fibrillation.
9. The patient with repetitive paroxysmal atrial tachycardia or atrial flutter refractory to drug treatment predating the atrial fibrillation.

METHOD OF CARDIOVERSION FOR PATIENTS WITH ATRIAL FIBRILLATION

The patient is hospitalized. If he is receiving digitalis, digitalis is omitted for 1 or 2 days to lessen the likelihood of a digitalis-related postcardioversion arrhythmia (11). Quinidine, 0.3 g every 6 hours, is given the day prior to the cardioversion attempt and is continued if sinus rhythm is restored. In perhaps 10% of patients this maintenance dosage of quinidine restores sinus rhythm and the DC shock is unnecessary. The patient may be anesthetized with intravenous sodium pentothal, unless already unconscious. At present we more often use Valium, 5–10 mg intravenously. The paddles of the shock apparatus are placed on the chest in front of the heart and behind it. The initial shock is 100 w-sec. If this fails, the amount is increased by 100 w-sec until the full current of 400 w-sec is reached. Anticoagulants are used for 2 weeks prior to the cardioversion attempt but only in patients with rheumatic mitral disease, or in those with a history of systemic arterial embolism.

PREVENTION OF RECURRENCE

If sinus rhythm is restored, maintenance quinidine, 0.3 g–0.4 g every 6 hours is continued indefinitely unless the signs of quinidine toxicity described earlier in this book appear. The blood quinidine level should be 3–6 mg/liter just before a dose of quinidine. Procaine amide, 0.25–0.5 g every 6 hours orally, may be used as an alternative to quinidine, but is considered less effective. Studies following successful cardioversion show that atrial fibrillation has returned in approximately two-thirds of the patients after one year has elapsed (13). A recent report suggests that quinidine therapy does decrease the relapse rate of atrial fibrillation (17).

PREVENTION OF EMBOLISM

In one study approximately 13.5% of patients with arteriosclerotic heart disease and atrial fibrillation developed embolism (1). In those with rheumatic heart disease, 42% of those with atrial fibrillation developed arterial embolism. The prevalence of systemic embolism can be decreased by the use of oral anticoagulants. Hence, if cardioversion is not to be used or is unsuccessful in the patient with atrial fibrillation, long-term oral anticoagulants should be employed unless there is a contraindication to their use. In patients with mitral stenosis, some consider that the onset of atrial fibrillation indicates that anticoagulants should be started as an emergency measure. The goal is to prevent disabling or fatal cerebral or aortoiliac embolism.

ATRIAL FIBRILLATION WITH INTERMITTENT OR PERSISTENT BRADYCARDIA

Some patients have paroxysmal atrial fibrillation; at other times they may have sinoatrial bradycardia. This is one manifestation of the sick sinus syndrome (10). Other patients with atrial fibrillation may have a high degree of AV block, with ventricular rates as slow as 40–80/min without drug treatment. As a rule such patients should not be treated with digitalis, quinidine, or DC shock. When these patients have symptoms which reflect a decreased cardiac output, *e.g.*, syncope, dizziness, renal failure, or congestive heart failure, a right ventricular pervenous demand electronic pacing unit should be inserted. Then digitalis or quinidine may be used to treat atrial fibrillation in such patients.

REFERENCES

1. Beer DT, Ghitman B: Embolization from the atria in arteriosclerotic heart disease. JAMA 127:83, 1961
2. Campbell M, Neill C, Suzman S: Prognosis of atrial septal defect. Br Med J 1:1375, 1957
3. DeSanctis RW, Block P, Hutter AM Jr: Tachyarrhythmias in myocardial infarction. Circulation 45:681, 1972
4. Dreifus LS, Haiat R, Watanabe J et al.: Ventricular fibrillation. A possible mechanism of sudden death in patients with Wolff–Parkinson–White syndrome. Circulation 43:520, 1971
5. Fowler NO: Physical Diagnosis of Heart Disease. New York, Macmillan, 1962
6. Fowler NO: Cardiac Diagnosis and Treatment. Hagerstown, Harper & Row, 1976
7. Gold H, Kwit NT, Otto H et al.: On the vagal and extravagal factors in cardiac slowing by digitalis in patients with atrial fibrillation. J Clin Invest 18:429, 1939

8. Goldman S, Probst P, Selzer A: Inefficacy of "therapeutic" serum levels of digoxin in controlling the ventricular rate in atrial fibrillation. Am J Cardiol 35:651, 1975

9. Harrison DC, Griffin JR, Fiene TJ: Effects of beta-adrenergic blockade with propranolol in patients with atrial arrhythmias. N Engl J Med 273:410, 1965

10. Kaplan BM, Langendorf R, Lev M et al.: Tachycardia-bradycardia syndrome (so-called "sick sinus syndrome"). Am J Cardiol 31:497, 1973

11. Kleiger R, Lown B: Cardioversion and digitalis. II. Clinical studies. Circulation 33:878, 1966

12. Lewis T: The Mechanism and Graphic Registration of the Heart Beat. London, Shaw & Sons, 1925, p 340

13. Meltzer LE, Kitchell JR: Cardiac Pacing and Cardioversion. Philadelphia, Charles Press, 1967

14. Mitchell JH, Shapiro W: Atrial function and the hemodynamic consequences of atrial fibrillation in man. Am J Cardiol 23:556, 1969

15. Prinzmetal M, Corday E, Britt IC et al.: Mechanism of the auricular arrhythmias. Circulation 1:241, 1950

16. Scherf D, Boyd LJ: Cardiovascular Diseases, 3rd ed. New York, Grune & Stratton, 1958, p 646

17. Sodermark T, Jonsson B, Olsson A et al.: Effect of quinidine in maintaining sinus rhythm after conversion of atrial fibrillation or flutter. Br Heart J 37:486, 1975

18. Williams RH: Textbook of Endocrinology, 5th ed. Philadelphia, WB Saunders, 1974, p 158

7 | Atrial Flutter

NOBLE O. FOWLER

Atrial flutter is a disorder of the heartbeat in which the atria beat regularly at a rapid rate that is usually near 300/min, but may range from below 200/min to as much as 400/min. There is usually 2:1 AV block or a greater degree of AV block, so that the ventricular rate is most commonly 150/min or less.

ETIOLOGY

Atrial flutter is usually associated with underlying organic heart disease. In occasional patients, the underlying disease is not demonstrable or is obscure. We found no evidence of organic heart disease in 4 of 31 consecutive patients with atrial flutter (7). Atrial flutter occurs in approximately 5% of patients with acute cardiac infarction (6) or may occur with chronic coronary artery disease. Hypertensive patients and those with rheumatic mitral disease may develop atrial flutter. Atrial flutter may occur in patients with obstructive and nonobstructive cardiomyopathy. We have observed several instances of atrial flutter complicating acute pericarditis. Paroxysmal atrial flutter may complicate pneumonia or pulmonary embolism. Patients with chronic obstructive pulmonary disease and cor pulmonale not uncommonly develop atrial flutter during periods of respiratory decompensation, but the arrhythmia is seldom persistent. Atrial flutter may occur in the older adult with ostium secundum atrial septal defect (3); it may develop as a complication of cardiac surgery. A small percentage of patients with thyrotoxicosis develop atrial flutter. Digitalis intoxication may produce atrial flutter (4), but this is a relatively uncommon event. Atrial flutter may occur in patients with the Wolff–Parkinson–White syndrome.

DIAGNOSIS

Atrial flutter is a relatively common arrhythmia, but is often overlooked. Since the atrial rate is usually near 300/min and almost 70% of patients have 2:1 AV conduction initially, the characteristic patient develops a sudden regular paroxysmal tachycardia with a ventricular rate of approximately 150/min. Hence, atrial flutter must be considered as a strong possibility whenever there is a paroxysmal arrhythmia with a regular ventricular rhythm and a ventricular rate near 150/min. The difficulty in diagnosis of atrial flutter lies in the fact that 2:1 AV conduction is the most common mechanism. When there is a higher degree of AV block the diagnosis is usually made easily from the characteristic saw-tooth pattern of the flutter waves in Leads II and III (Fig. 7–1). In Lead I the flutter waves are small and usually not of saw-tooth configuration. In Lead V_1 flutter waves are usually easily seen, and at times can be recognized there when not apparent in Leads II and III. In Lead V_1 the flutter waves are usually not of saw-tooth pattern, but appear as small positive waves.

When atrial flutter is suspected and there is 2:1 AV block, the flutter waves may be obscured by the QRS complexes of the electrocardiogram; and one cannot then be certain of the diagnosis (Fig. 7–2). There are several ways of confirming the impression of atrial flutter under these circumstances. In some patients inspection of the neck veins will reveal the rapid atrial flutter activity, with regular pulsations occurring approximately 300/min. Carotid sinus pressure may be quite valuable in the recognition of atrial flutter. Carotid sinus pressure may temporarily increase the AV block, thus enabling the flutter waves to be recognized in the electrocardiogram (Fig. 7–2). When the QRS complexes are broad because of previous bundle branch block or aberrant intraventricular conduction, atrial flutter with 2:1 AV block may simulate ventricular tachycardia. Carotid sinus pressure is often helpful in unmasking the flutter waves (Fig. 7–3). Carotid sinus pressure, when effective, temporarily increases AV block of atrial flutter and slows the ventricular rate. Upon release of the carotid sinus pressure, the original pattern of AV conduction is resumed and the ventricular rate returns to its previous level. This characteristic response of atrial flutter to carotid sinus pressure often permits the bedside recognition of this arrhythmia. Other means of vagal stimulation may be effective in increasing the AV block in patients with atrial flutter. These include the Valsalva maneuver, the intravenous administration of 0.5 mg neostigmine (Prostigmin), and the use of digitalis. Carotid sinus pressure, when previously ineffective, may become effective following the administration of digitalis. Carotid sinus pressure does not convert atrial flutter to another mechanism.

FEATURES OF ATRIAL FLUTTER

Atrial flutter is recognized from three features: 1) the atrial rate, which is usually near 300/min, 2) the regularity of the atrial mechanism, and 3) the characteristic saw-tooth pattern of the flutter waves in Leads II and III. Only the last is diagnostic; the atrial rate may be below 200/min and overlap the range of atrial rates found in paroxysmal atrial tachycardia. When the atrial rate is between 200–250/min either paroxysmal atrial tachycardia or atrial flutter may be present. Vassaux and Lown stated that the atrial rate is seldom below 200/min with atrial flutter, and not often above 220/min with paroxysmal atrial tachycardia with AV block (16). Two to one AV block may be present with either disorder; when there is AV block with paroxysmal atrial tachycardia, the arrhythmia typically responds to carotid sinus pressure with temporary increased AV block and ventricular slowing, much like atrial flutter, and unlike the usual response of paroxysmal atrial tachycardia without AV block. When there is paroxysmal atrial tachycardia without AV block, carotid sinus pressure

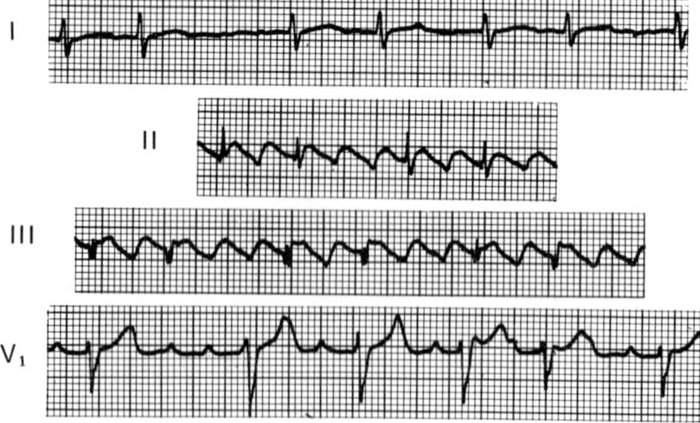

Fig. 7–1.   **Atrial flutter with varying AV block, showing characteristic saw-tooth pattern of the flutter waves in Leads II and III. Flutter activity is poorly seen in Lead I. In Leads II and III there is constant activity of the base line with no isoelectric interval. In Lead V₁, however, the flutter waves are small positive spikes appearing somewhat like normal P waves and there is an isoelectric interval between the flutter waves. This is rather characteristic of atrial flutter. There is an atrial rate of 250/min with varying atrioventricular conduction so that the ventricular rhythm is irregular. [From Fowler (8).]**

Fig. 7–2.   **Atrial flutter with 2:1 AV block is shown in the upper electrocardiogram. Flutter waves are not discernible. The lower electrocardiogram shows increased AV block during carotid sinus pressure; the saw-tooth flutter waves are now clearly demonstrated.**

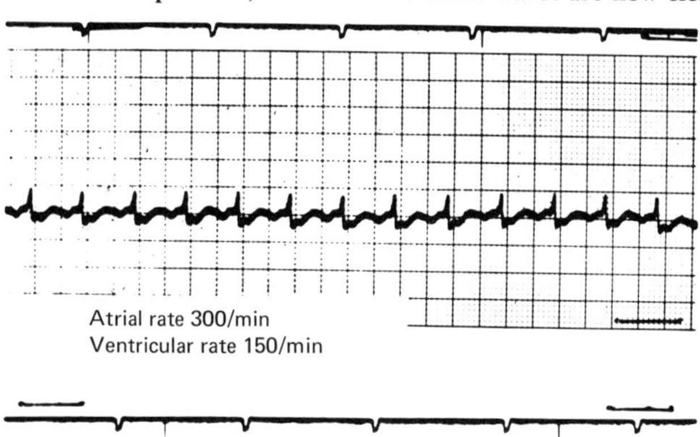

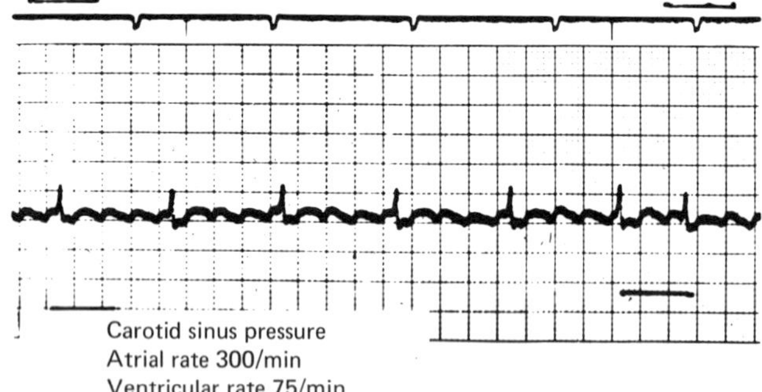

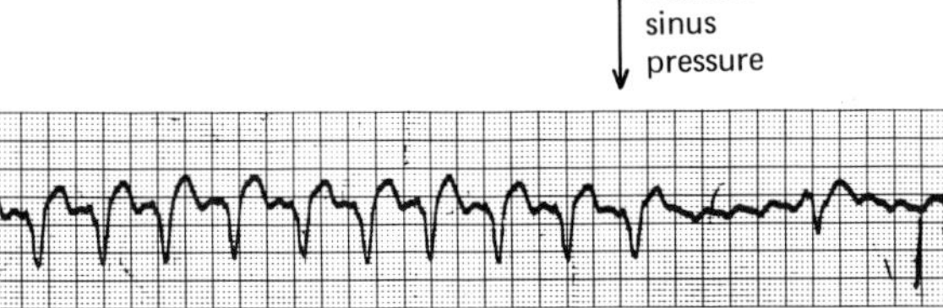

Fig. 7–3.   **Carotid sinus pressure unmasking atrial flutter in a patient with atrial flutter and 2:1 atrioventricular block. In the absence of carotid sinus pressure, atrial activity cannot be visualized with certainty. Ventricular rate is 120 beats/min with regular rhythm. Broad QRS complexes are caused by bundle branch block. With carotid sinus pressure the atrioventricular block is increased, and the characteristic saw-tooth pattern of the flutter waves is visualized. Atrial rate is 240 beats/min. [From Fowler (8).]**

ordinarily produces no response, or terminates the arrhythmia. When the atrial rate is 200–250/min and there is AV block, the distinction between atrial flutter and paroxysmal atrial tachycardia with AV block depends upon the configuration of the atrial activity. When there is a saw-tooth configuration of the atrial activity in Leads II and III, the diagnosis of atrial flutter can be made. In some instances the distinction remains in doubt even when the atrial waves have been identified. In this setting the management of the arrhythmia depends upon the circumstances. In patients with paroxysmal atrial tachycardia with AV block, digitalis intoxication is responsible in perhaps 50% of instances. Digitalis intoxication is rarely responsible for atrial flutter. When the distinction between atrial flutter and paroxysmal atrial tachycardia is in doubt, if digitalis overdosage seems possible then digitalis should be discontinued. On the other hand, if the patient has not received digitalis, the arrhythmia should be managed as if it were atrial flutter; digitalis may be useful.

STEPS IN DIAGNOSIS

The diagnosis of atrial flutter depends upon the following steps:

1. Recognition of the characteristic saw-tooth pattern of the flutter waves in Leads II and III, which is readily done if there is more than 2:1 AV block.
2. A high index of suspicion of atrial flutter when the ventricular rate is regular and near 150/min and the atrial mechanism is not identified.
3. Use of carotid sinus pressure to increase AV block and then to reveal the flutter waves.
4. When there is no response to carotid sinus pressure.
   a. Use a right atrial lead to amplify the flutter waves (Fig. 7–4).
   b. Use digitalis and if the AV block is not increased, repeat carotid sinus pressure to increase the AV block.

In some patients with atrial fibrillation there is regular atrial activity at a rate of approximately 300/min visible in Lead V_1 of the electrocardiogram. Hence, Lead V_1 resembles the pattern of atrial flutter (Fig. 7–5). In the limb leads there are small and uneven fibrillary waves rather than saw-tooth flutter waves, and there should be no confusion with atrial flutter.

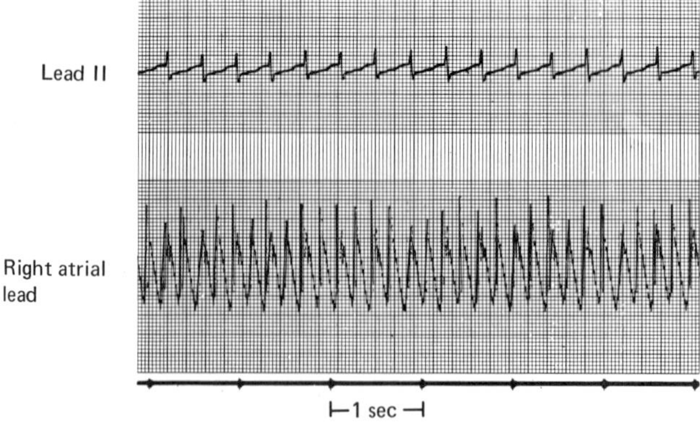

Fig. 7–4.   **Atrial flutter with 2:1 atrioventricular block in a patient with cor pulmonale. Ventricular rate is 155 beats/min with regular rhythm. Atrial flutter activity was not visible in standard electrocardiogram (see Lead II). Right atrial lead shows regular atrial activity at a rate of 310 beats/min consistent with atrial flutter. [From Fowler (8).]**

Fig. 7–5.   **Atrial fibrillation simulating atrial flutter in lead V_1. Note irregular irregularity of the ventricular response. The fibrillary waves appear as small waves at a rate slightly in excess of 300/min in Lead V_1, thus superficially resembling the pattern often seen with atrial flutter. In Lead III the characteristic saw-tooth pattern of atrial flutter is not seen. Compare Figure 7-1. [From Fowler (8).]**

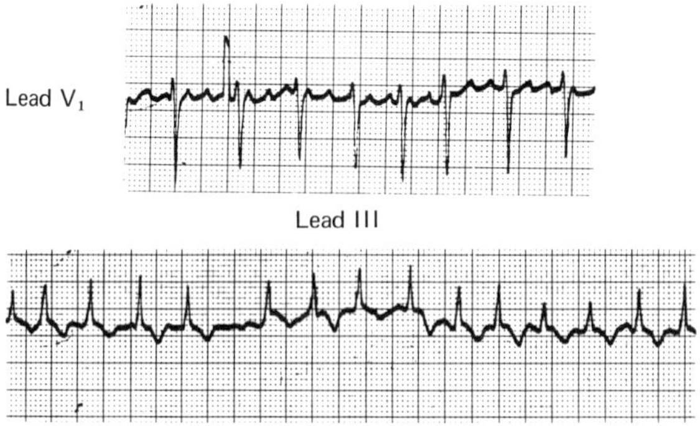

OTHER VARIETIES OF AV CONDUCTION IN ATRIAL FLUTTER

Although approximately 70% of patients with atrial flutter originally have 2:1 AV conduction, many other patterns are possible. Rarely, there is conduction of all atrial impulses to the ventricles, and there is a rapid regular ventricular rhythm at a rate of 240–300/min; this is more likely when the atrial rate is below 300/min, since the junctional tissue will not usually conduct rapidly enough to permit a ventricular rate much above 270/min. Quinidine therapy, through its vagolytic effects upon the junctional tissue, may lessen AV block during flutter, and result in 1:1 AV conduction. It may also decrease the atrial rate to facilitate 1:1 AV conduction. Patients with atrial flutter may have 4:1 AV block, with a regular ventricular rhythm at a rate of approximately 75/min. Three to one AV block is said to be uncommon in atrial flutter. There may be varying AV block, with a very irregular ventricular rhythm, so that the irregular ventricular rhythm resembles that of atrial fibrillation (Fig. 7–1). There may be complete AV block during atrial flutter; in this event the ventricular rhythm is regular and the ventricular rate depends upon the site of the ventricular pacemaker. It is usually 50–70/min if there is an AV junctional pacemaker; it is near 40/min when there is a ventricular pacemaker.

TREATMENT

The treatment of atrial flutter may be considered under the following divisions.

1. Treatment of the underlying cause
2. Termination of the atrial arrhythmia
3. Increasing the degree of AV block
4. Prevention of recurrences

TREATMENT OF UNDERLYING CAUSE

When atrial flutter is associated with thyrotoxicosis, rheumatic mitral disease, atrial septal defect or (rarely) digitalis intoxication, the underlying disease should be corrected, if possible. One should improve ventilation in patients with chronic obstructive lung disease and cor pulmonale. There is, unfortunately, little evidence that surgical correction of an atrial septal defect will prevent attacks of atrial arrhythmia, including atrial flutter. On the contrary, we have patients in whom refractory atrial flutter appeared for the first time following surgical correction of the atrial septal defect.

TERMINATION OF ATRIAL ARRHYTHMIA

In general it is desirable to convert atrial flutter to sinus rhythm, or failing that, to atrial fibrillation. Although some benefit can be achieved by increasing the AV block with digitalis and thus slowing the ventricles, it is difficult to prevent excessive ventricular rates with exercise and/or at other times. Hence, the goal of therapy is to terminate the arrhythmia and to prevent recurrences, if possible.

There are four methods of converting atrial flutter which have met with sufficient success to warrant discussion. Electric countershock and digitalization are each quite effective and may be considered primary methods. Electric pacing of the right atrium and quinidine may be used as secondary methods. Because of its risk and the fact that it is less successful than electric DC shock, quinidine enjoys little popularity today as a method of terminating atrial flutter, but is useful to prevent recurrences.

DC ELECTRIC SHOCK

Electric DC shock is successful in terminating atrial flutter in better than 95% of instances (12). In one series of 60 patients, atrial flutter was converted by countershock to sinus rhythm in 58, without serious complications (2). One may begin with a DC shock of 25 w-sec., with the two paddles of the shock apparatus in place. One is over the precordium and the other directly opposite the precordium on the posterior chest. The patient is anesthetized with intravenous pentothal, or with diazepam (Valium), 10 mg intravenously. It is safest to give diazepam in divided doses of 2.5 mg each. One should observe the effect of one 2.5 mg dose for 5 minutes before giving the next dose. Respiratory arrest may occur; when diazepam is used one must be prepared for tracheal intubation and artificial respiration. If initially unsuccessful, the DC shock may be increased stepwise to a maximum of 400 w-sec. If the patient has already received full doses of digitalis it is desirable to omit the drug for 1 or 2 days before electric shock, if possible, in order to obviate the risk of digitalis-related arrhythmias with electric shock (9). Alternatively, in the digitalized patient one may elect to use shock therapy without delay. When this is done the initial DC shock should not exceed 5 w-sec at a time, up to 25 w-sec. Then if there is still no effect, one may try 50, 75 and 100 w-sec. When this is done, the electrocardiogram should be observed carefully after each shock for evidence of digitalis intoxication; ventricular premature beats or short runs of ventricular tachycardia may appear. If this occurs one should not proceed immediately with further DC shocks; however, one may give a bolus of 25–50 mg lidocaine intravenously and then repeat the DC shock. If the ventricular premature beats are suppressed it may then be safer to use higher electric energies. One is reluctant to advise this if there are alternative forms of therapy. In the digitalized patient some prefer to limit the maximum shock to 100 w-sec. We have employed 400 w-sec DC shock successfully and without complications in the treatment of atrial flutter in a patient who was receiving large amounts of digitalis. Once the arrhythmia is terminated it is often desirable to digitalize the patient. The use of digitalis has several goals. The patient may need digitalis because of congestive failure or cardiac enlargement. Digitalis may possibly aid in preventing recurrences of the arrhythmia. If the atrial flutter does recur digitalization may produce sufficient AV block to prevent excessively rapid ventricular rates.

DIGITALIS

Digitalis may be used as an alternative to electric shock in the treatment of atrial flutter. In paroxysmal flutter of less than a few weeks duration, we found digitalization to be followed by reversion to sinus rhythm in 28 of 31 patients (7). It is not unlikely that the arrhythmia might terminate spontaneously in some of these patients with paroxysmal atrial flutter. However digitalis tends to increase the AV block and decrease the ventricular rate, thereby improving cardiac performance, which is not only desirable in itself but may also create a more favorable climate for reversion. In the undigitalized patient we used digoxin, 1 mg orally, followed by 0.5 mg every 8 hours for 5 days or until there was increased AV block.* Contrary to what is often stated, it is not necessary to discontinue digoxin in order for reversion to a sinus mechanism to occur. The dosage was then reduced to 0.25 mg every 6 hours until reversion occurred. When atrial fibrillation or sinus rhythm occurred, the digoxin was reduced to 0.25 mg twice daily. If reversion to sinus rhythm did not occur after 8–10 days, then quinidine was employed (this study was made prior to the availability of electric shock, which would be preferred to quinidine). If the patient had already been receiving digitalis the initial dose of digoxin was 0.5 mg and the therapy was then the same as described for the undigitalized patient. It is essential that the patient be examined for evidence of change in rhythm or of digitalis toxicity before each dose of digoxin. This regimen was employed in 31 patients; only one developed mild digitalis intoxication, and in this patient the physician failed to observe that the atrial flutter had already been converted to a sinus mechanism when additional digoxin was given. In the undigitalized patient with atrial flutter, who initially has 2:1 AV block, relatively large amounts of digoxin may be needed to convert the arrhythmia or to achieve a satisfactory degree of AV block. Many of these patients seem to be able to tolerate more digitalis than the average cardiac patient. Certain patients are poor candidates for treatment of atrial flutter by this method, which employs rather large doses of digitalis. Among them are patients with renal failure, patients with ventricular rates below 80–90/min in the absence of digitalis, elderly patients. Serious digitalis intoxication may result when this method is used in such patients.

When it is desirable to increase the degree of AV block quickly, one may give propranolol, 0.5 mg every 15 min, intravenously, the total dose not to exceed 2 mg. Practolol, a cardioselective β-adrenergic blocking agent, may be useful in slowing the ventricular rate in patients with atrial flutter (14). It is not approved for use in the United States.

ELECTRONIC PACING

Atrial flutter may be terminated by electronic pacing of the right atrium, employing a pervenous bipolar pacing catheter and a Medtronics or Electrodyne battery-powered pacing unit (13). Pacing the right atrium at a rate slower than the atrial rate may convert the arrhythmia to atrial fibrillation when the pacing impulse falls within the critical period to interrupt a reentry mechanism (10), (Fig 7–6). The atrial fibrillation may then spontaneously convert to sinus rhythm when the pacing is stopped. Alternatively, the atrium may be paced at a more rapid rate of 200–375/min or more in order to terminate the arrhythmia (11,17). In patients unable to tolerate anesthesia, withdrawal from digitalis, or large doses of antiarrhythmic drugs, right atrial stimulation may

---

*At present we would employ only one-half this dosage.

be the preferred initial treatment (17). Electronic pacing may be the treatment of choice in patients with atrial flutter who are elderly, who have severe chronic obstructive airway disease, or who have digitalis intoxication. This method may be successful in as many as 70% of patients (5).

QUINIDINE

Quinidine is not popular today as an agent to terminate atrial flutter. It is less effective than electric DC shock, and is also more hazardous. Quinidine should not be employed without first digitalizing the patient; otherwise AV conduction may be improved and the ventricular rate may become excessively rapid. Quinidine may be given in doses that begin at 0.2 g four times daily orally; the

Fig. 7–6.   **Upper two electrocardiograms demonstrate simultaneous recordings of Lead II and a right atrial lead of a patient with atrial flutter and 2:1 AV block. Flutter waves occur at approximately 300/min, and appear as sharp negative spikes in the intraatrial lead. Third strip (1:21 PM) shows electrocardiographic Lead II during atrial pacing at a rate of 120/min; at arrow, the atrial flutter is converted to atrial fibrillation. Fourth and fifth strips (1:22 PM) are of Lead II and the right atrial lead and demonstrate atrial fibrillation. Atrial pacing has been discontinued. Lower two electrocardiographic strips are made 8 minutes later and show conversion to sinus rhythm. Large principally negative complexes in the intraatrial lead are the P waves. (By courtesy of Gene Conway, M.D.)**

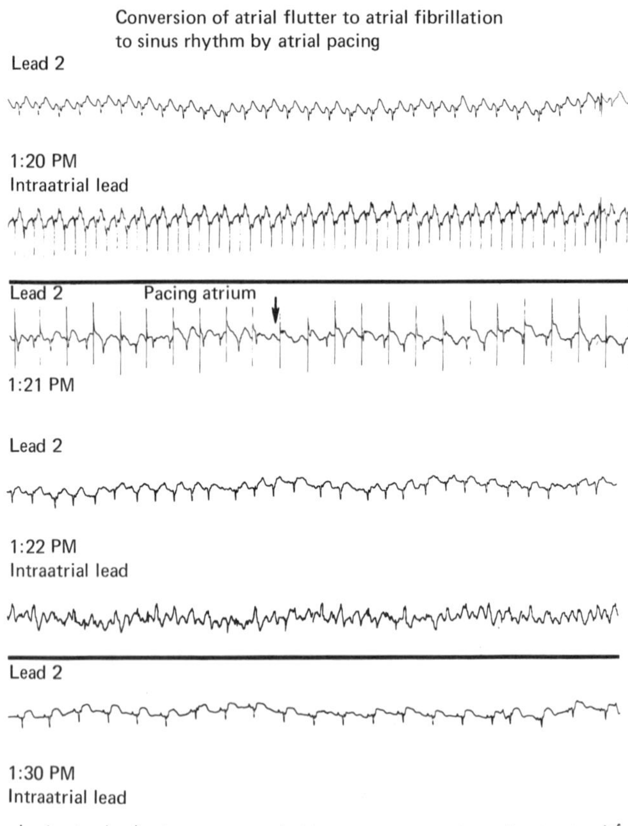

four times daily dose may be increased successively to 0.3 g, 0.4 g, 0.5 g, and 0.6 g, if there is no success with the smaller doses. As much as 0.8–1 g four times daily has been given. The risk is increased at these doses, however, and is probably not warranted today in view of the availability of DC countershock. Further, the use of quinidine in a patient who is receiving digitalis may increase the risk of quinidine syncope over that when quinidine is used alone (15). We prefer to measure blood levels of quinidine daily, and the quinidine blood level should probably not be allowed to exceed 6–8 mg/liter. The usual effective therapeutic range is 3–6 mg/liter (1). The maximum blood level of quinidine may not be attained until after 3 days of medication on a fixed daily regimen; hence one may prefer not to increase the dosage until there has been no success at that level for 3 days.

PREVENTING RECURRENCE OF ATRIAL FLUTTER

Although DC electric shock will terminate more than 95% of instances of atrial flutter, in many patients the arrhythmia recurs. Recurrence is especially likely when there is chronic atrial flutter of greater than 6 weeks duration, and when there is an underlying cause, such as thyrotoxicosis, rheumatic mitral disease, or atrial septal defect, or cardiomyopathy. If the patient is not already digitalized, he should be digitalized following conversion of the arrhythmia to a sinus mechanism. In the previously undigitalized adult patient, we usually employ oral digoxin, 1 mg initially, followed by 2 or 3 successive oral doses of 0.25 mg each at 8 hourly intervals. The maintenance dosage is usually 0.25 mg/day, orally, or 0.25 mg in the morning and 0.125 mg at night; some patients require as much as 0.25 mg digoxin 3 times daily, others as little as 0.05 mg/day. If the arrhythmia recurs despite digitalization, quinidine orally, 0.3–0.4 g four times daily may be added. We estimate the quinidine blood level and prefer to keep it at 3–6 mg/liter. Patients receiving quinidine should be observed for evidence of toxic reactions. These include: tinnitus, deafness, purpura, diarrhea, anorexia, nausea, fever, AV block; intraventricular conduction disturbances; premature ventricular contractions; ventricular tachycardia, and syncope owing to ventricular fibrillation (15). If sinus rhythm cannot be maintained despite digitalis and quinidine, one may attempt to convert the atrial flutter to atrial fibrillation by pacing the right atrium electronically at a rate of 120–140/min in the hope of producing permanent atrial fibrillation. With atrial fibrillation the ventricular rate can usually be more readily controlled with digitalis than with atrial flutter. In a small percentage of patients one must be resigned to persistent atrial flutter, and the ventricular rate is controlled by producing the optimal degree of atrioventricular block with digitalis.

REFERENCES

1. Atkinson AJ: Clinical use of blood levels of cardiac drugs. Mod Concepts Cardiovasc Dis 42:1, 1973

2. Castellanos A Jr, Lemberg L, Gosselin A et al.: Evaluation of countershock treatment of atrial flutter. Arch Intern Med 115:42, 1965

3. Craig RJ, Selzer A: Natural history and prognosis of atrial septal defect. Circulation 37:805, 1968

4. Delman AJ, Stein E: Atrial flutter secondary to digitalis toxicity. Circulation 29:593, 1964

5. DeSanctis RW: Diagnostic and therapeutic uses of atrial pacing. Circulation 43:748, 1971

6. DeSanctis RW, Block P, Hutter AM Jr: Tachyarrhythmias in myocardial infarction. Circulation 45:681, 1972

7. Fowler NO, Gueron M: Conversion of atrial flutter with digoxin alone. Circulation 27:716, 1962

8. Fowler NO: Cardiac Diagnosis and Treatment. Hagerstown, Harper & Row, 1976

9. Gilbert R, Cuddy RP: Digitalis intoxication following conversion to sinus rhythm. Circulation 32:58, 1965

10. Hunt NC, Cobb FR, Waxman MB et al.: Conversion of supraventricular tachycardias with atrial stimulation: evidence of re-entry mechanisms. Circulation 38:1060, 1968

11. Lister JW, Cohen LS, Bernstein WH et al.: Treatment of supraventricular tachycardias by rapid atrial stimulation. Circulation 38:1044, 1968

12. Lown B: Cardioversion of arrhythmias (II). Mod Concepts Cardiovasc Dis 33:869, 1964

13. Pittman DE, Makar JS, Kooros KS et al.: Rapid atrial stimulation: successful method of conversion of atrial flutter and atrial tachycardia. Am J Cardiol 32:700, 1973

14. Pribble AH, Conn RD: The use of practolol in supraventricular arrhythmias associated with acute illness. Am J Cardiol 35:645, 1975

15. Selzer A, Wray HW: Quinidine syncope. Paroxysmal ventricular fibrillation occurring during treatment of chronic atrial arrhythmias. Circulation 30:17, 1964

16. Vassaux C, Lown B: Cardioversion of supraventricular tachycardia. Circulation 39:791, 1969

17. Zeft HJ, Cobb FR, Waxman MB, et al: Right atrial stimulation in the treatment of atrial flutter. Ann Intern Med 70:447, 1969

NOBLE O. FOWLER

Ventricular tachycardia is usually a serious disorder of the heart-beat. Ventricular tachycardia may presage ventricular fibrillation, or in itself produce an ineffective cardiac pumping mechanism. Shock or pulmonary edema are more likely than with supraventricular tachycardia. This is true because ventricular tachycardia most commonly occurs in the presence of organic heart disease. In addition the atrial aid to ventricular filling is lost, and the course of ventricular depolarization is abnormal. Schlant and associates emphasized the importance of an orderly sequence of ventricular depolarization in the development of the optimal force of ventricular systole (26). The optimum treatment of ventricular tachycardia requires attention to several factors. These include:

1. Measures to exclude supraventricular tachycardia with abnormal intraventricular conduction, if time permits (15)
2. The etiology of the arrhythmia
3. The ventricular rate
4. Attendant complications, such as shock, pulmonary edema, or ventricular fibrillation
5. The presence or absence of previous attacks
6. Previous measures employed in therapy
7. The possible role of drugs, such as digitalis or quinidine in the production of the arrhythmia
8. The existence of mechanical factors, electric currents, electrolyte imbalance, or emotional factors which may have precipitated the arrhythmia

Ventricular tachycardia is associated with organic heart disease in 90–95% of instances (19). The writer has observed several instances of ventricular tachycardia in otherwise apparently healthy young adults in the third decade of life. At times there were repeated bouts of ventricular fibrillation and syncope associated with the arrhythmia. Six patients with idiopathic ventricular tachycardia were recently reported (4).

The most common underlying disease is coronary artery disease, which was the cause in 72% of one series (19). Ventricular tachycardia occurs in approximately 10% of patients with acute cardiac infarction (5); at times the arrhythmia lasts only a few seconds or minutes and subsides without producing clinical symptoms. Often the underlying heart disease is chronic coronary disease, with or without angina pectoris or previous infarction. Perhaps the second commonest cause of ventricular tachycardia is digitalis intoxication; this was observed in 22% of one series of 83 patients with ventricular tachycardia (19). Ventricular tachycardia was associated with rheumatic heart disease in 11% of this series. In this writer's experience, myocardiopathy rather than rheumatic disease is more commonly the underlying disease. Ventricular tachycardia and fibrillation may lead to sudden death in the mitral valve prolapse-click syndrome (12a). Selzer has documented that quinidine may produce ventricular tachycardia or fibrillation, even in doses that are ordinarily nontoxic (27). Ventricular tachycardia may result from mechanical stimuli; handling the heart during surgery and cardiac needling, catheterization, or coronary arteriography are examples. Ventricular tachycardia has been reported as a complication of fright (1). Other examples of sympathetic influences which may produce ventricular tachycardia are overdosage of isoproterenol (Isuprel) or epinephrine, and the occasional occurrence of ventricular fibrillation in patients with pheochromocytoma (21). Hereditary prolongation of the QT interval with or without (Romano–Ward syndrome) deafness may be associated with syncope due to ventricular ectopic activity (23a). Ventricular tachyarrhythmias may occur with glue sniffing, or with gaseous anesthetic agents. We recently reported several patients with ventricular tachycardia following therapeutic doses of psychotropic drugs, especially thioridazine (9).

DIAGNOSIS OF VENTRICULAR TACHYCARDIA

During the past several years the employment of special electrocardiographic lead techniques, such as esophageal leads, right atrial leads, and His bundle electrograms, have focused attention upon some of the problems in the diagnosis of ventricular tachycardia. The results of these studies have shed light upon the variability of ventriculoatrial relationships in ventricular tachycardia, and have focused attention upon the limitation of the conventional criteria employed for the diagnosis of ventricular tachycardia. Both at the bedside and from the conventional electrocardiogram, the diagnosis of ventricular tachycardia is difficult. In fact it is reasonable to conclude that ventricular tachycardia can be excluded by a response of the arrhythmia to carotid sinus pressure, or by the demonstration of a QRS complex of normal width on electrocardiogram. From the positive view, often only a presumptive diagnosis may be made. In many instances a diagnosis of ventricular tachycardia is suggested when the electrocardiogram shows a series of five or more broadened aberrant QRS complexes with a ventricular rate of 150–250/min and atrial activity is not discernible. However, there are several possible explanations of such an electrocardiographic pattern:

1. Ventricular tachycardia, with P waves obscured by the QRS complexes
2. Supraventricular tachycardia, such as atrial flutter or atrial or junctional paroxysmal tachycardia, with prior bundle branch block (Fig. 8–1)
3. Aberrant intraventricular conduction complicating supraventricular tachycardia including atrial fibrillation; the pattern is usually that of right bundle branch block (Fig. 8–2)

4. Preexcitation syndrome (Wolff–Parkinson–White syndrome) with supraventricular tachycardia (Fig. 8–3); more commonly the QRS complex is of normal form when paroxysmal supraventricular tachycardia complicates the preexcitation syndrome. The QRS is believed to be broad and aberrant during reentry proxysmal tachycardia when atrioventricular conduction takes place over the bypass tract, followed by ventriculoatrial conduction over the His bundle and AV node. Ventricular tachycardia is said to be virtually unknown in this disorder, but ventricular fibrillation may complicate atrial fibrillation with a rapid ventricular response.

CRITERIA FOR DIAGNOSIS

Criteria for the presumptive diagnosis of ventricular tachycardia:

1. Paroxysmal tachycardia is of sudden onset. The ventricular rate is usually 150–250/min, but may be as slow as 110/min. Ventricular paroxysmal tachycardia must be distinguished from a much slower ventricular arrhythmia

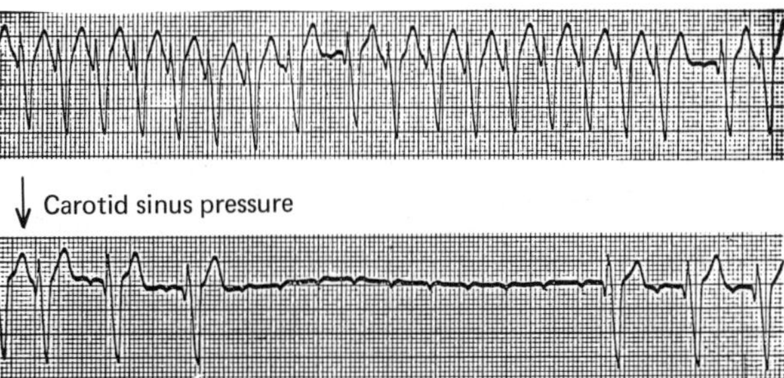

Fig. 8–1. **Paroxysmal atrial tachycardia, atrial rate 187/min, simulating ventricular tachycardia in a patient with bundle branch block. In lower strip, carotid sinus pressure produced almost complete AV block, and demonstrates the atrial tachycardia.**

Fig. 8–2. **Twenty-three-year-old female with rheumatic mitral insufficiency. Recording of Lead I and Lead V_1 in this patient with atrial fibrillation and rapid ventricular rate. In Lead I, second, third, fourth, and fifth QRS complexes, eleventh QRS complex, and thirteenth through the nineteenth QRS complexes represent aberrant intraventricular conduction. In Lead V_1, aberrant QRS complexes are demonstrated in third, fourth, and fifth, and in eighth, ninth, and tenth QRS complexes. These complexes are characteristic of aberrant intraventricular conduction showing an rSR′ pattern in Lead V_1. Runs of consecutive aberrantly conducted QRS complexes simulate ventricular tachycardia.**

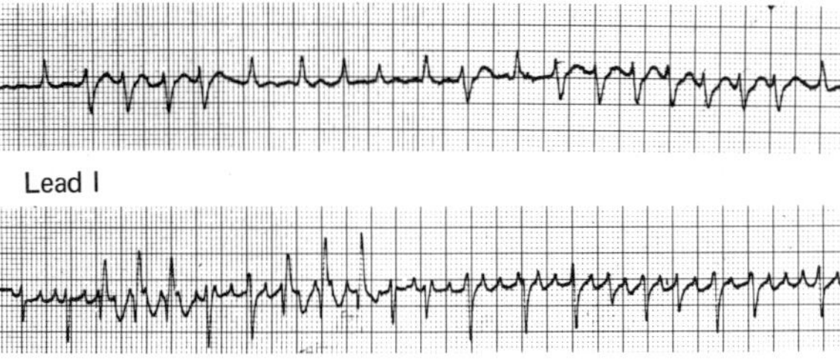

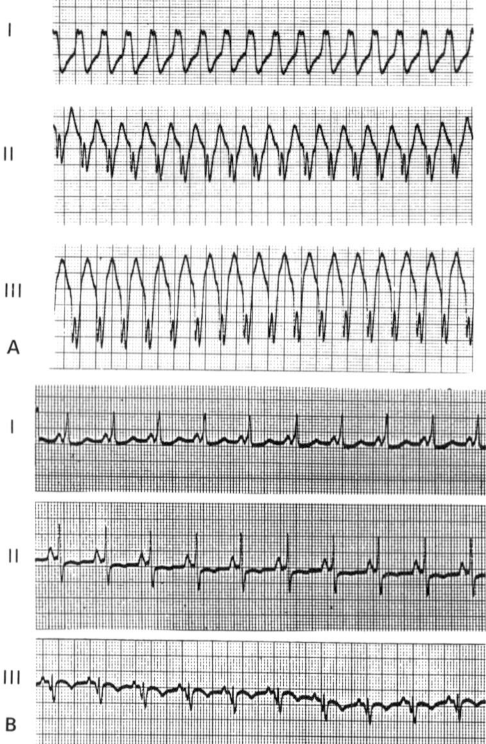

Fig. 8–3. **A. *Top*, Paroxysmal supraventricular tachycardia in 15-year-old patient with Wolff–Parkinson–White (or preexcitation) syndrome. Ventricular rate is 187 beats/min with regular rhythm. Atrial activity is not visualized. QRS complexes are broad, superficially suggesting the diagnosis of ventricular tachycardia. B. *Bottom*, Electrocardiogram of same patient showing sinus rhythm with a heart rate of 100 beats/min. Note the short PR interval and delta waves initiating QRS complex in Lead I. These findings are characteristic of Wolff–Parkinson–White syndrome. [From Fowler (8).]**

known as idioventricular tachycardia or nonparoxysmal ventricular tachycardia. In this latter arrhythmia there is a regular ventricular rhythm whose rate lies between 55–108/min (24) (Fig. 8–4). This arrhythmia most commonly is found in patients with acute cardiac infarction and does not usually produce a detectable hemodynamic perturbation, except for the change in the appearance of the electrocardiographic monitor strip. With idioventricular tachycardia, DC shock or drug therapy is not usually needed. In many cases digitalis intoxication is responsible and then digitalis should be withdrawn. Contrary to general belief the rhythm in ventricular tachycardia is usually regular unless the arrhythmia is multifocal, or there are fusion or captured beats (Fig. 8–5). 2. Isolated premature ventricular beats are of a form similar to those occurring during the paroxysm of ventricular tachycardia.

3. Dissociation occurs between ventricular and atrial mechanisms (Fig. 8–5). When this mechanism is present there is a beat-to-beat variation in systolic blood pressure. The higher systolic pressures occur when atrial systole pre-

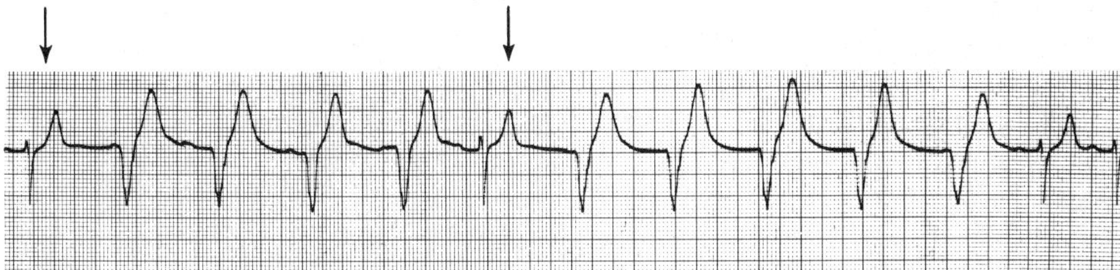

O.B. 65 Accelerated idioventricular rhythm

Fig. 8–4.   **Accelerated idioventricular rhythm (nonparoxysmal ventricular tachycardia). The ventricular rate is 70/min during the arrhythmia. The cycles indicated by the arrows and the two final cycles represent normal sinus beats. The arrhythmia most commonly arises when there is temporary slowing of the sinus rhythm. The most common clinical setting for this arrhythmia is that of acute cardiac infarction. Usually there are no severe hemodynamic consequences.**

Fig. 8–5.   *Upper strip,* **Ventricular tachycardia with captured beats in 54-year-old man with acute myocardial infarction. Ventricular rate, 105 beats/min; atrial rate, 86 beats/min. Arrows indicate cycles in which the ventricle is captured by conduction of atrial activation impulse. P waves are otherwise independent of QRS complexes. Note that QRS complexes of captured beats are narrower than QRS complexes of independent ventricular tachycardia, indicating that broad QRS complexes of ventricular tachycardia are not related to aberrant conduction with junctional tachycardia, but are broad because of abnormal site of impulse formation in ventricles.** *Lower strip,* **indicates P-QRS-T contour in same lead after normal sinus rhythm was established by DC countershock. [From Fowler (8).]**

Lead
V₁

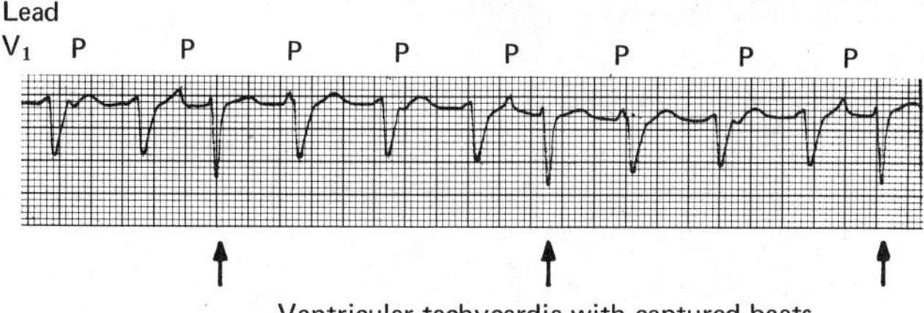

After DC countershock

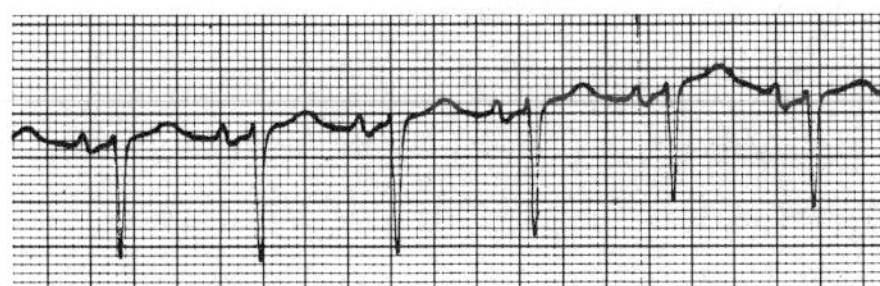

cedes ventricular systole by an optimum interval (30) (Fig. 8–6). The first heart sound may vary in intensity. Kistin showed that with paced ventricular tachycardia, retrograde conduction to the atria occurs in the majority of instances. Retrograde conduction to the atria also may occur during spontaneous ventricular tachycardia (Fig. 8–7). The demonstration of dissociated atrial and ventricular mechanisms does not absolutely disprove junctional tachycardia with aberrant ventricular conduction.

4. Ventricular captured beats occur. During ventricular tachycardia, when the atrial pacemaker activates the AV junction at a time outside the refractory period of the junction, conduction to the ventricle may take place with a more normal form of ventricular complex (Fig. 8–5). When this occurs the fact that the QRS complex is more nearly normal despite a shorter RR interval than that during the paroxysm militates against supraventricular tachycardia with aberrant ventricular conduction. If atrial capture of the ventricles does not occur spontaneously, pervenous electronic atrial pacing may be used to produce atrial capture (2). This procedure may also be useful therapeutically (Fig. 8–7).

5. Ventricular fusion beats appear on electrocardiogram during the paroxysmal arrhythmia. These represent a fusion of a QRS complex produced by supraventricular ventricular activation and a QRS produced by activation of the ventricle from the ectopic pacemaker. The ventricular complex of the electrocardiogram is preceded by a P wave, with a short PR interval. The QRS complex is of a form intermediate between the normal QRS and that of the paroxysmal tachycardia.

6. Although usually not practical in a hospital or clinical setting, His bundle electrograms may be used to identify the source of ventricular activation. When ventricular tachycardia is present, the QRS complexes are not preceded by A (atrial) or H (His) potentials (3,4).

TREATMENT OF VENTRICULAR TACHYCARDIA

Although electric DC shock is effective in terminating a paroxysm of ventricular tachycardia in better than 90% of instances (17), it should not be used in every instance. At times ventricular tachycardia may be reverted by a blow or thump administered to the precordium. When ventricular tachycardia is related to digitalis intoxication the use of electric shock may provoke fatal ventricular fibrillation (13). When ventricular tachycardia is repetitive, measures in addition to electric shock will be needed to prevent recurrences. In some instances electric shock achieves a normal sinus mechanism for only a few cardiac cycles, and then the arrhythmia recurs promptly. When ventricular tachycardia is accompanied by shock the blood pressure should be raised to 100–110 mm Hg systolic pressure by the infusion of metaraminol (Aramine) 100 mg/liter 5% dextrose in water or norepinephrine, 8 mg/liter 5% dextrose in water with 10 mg phentolamine (Regitine) added to the liter of 5% dextrose.

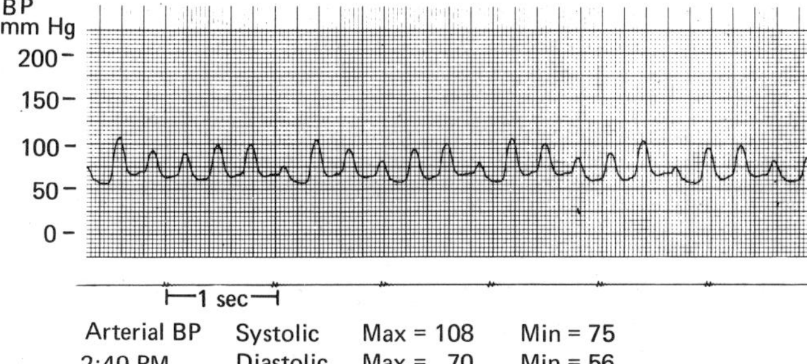

Fig. 8–6. Direct recording of brachial arterial pressure in a patient with ventricular paroxysmal tachycardia, showing beat-to-beat variation in peak systolic blood pressure. Varying pulse pressure is related to constantly changing relation between atrial and ventricular systole. As a rule ventricular premature beats in which P wave just precedes QRS complex have larger arterial pulse pressure because atrial systole then offers maximum aid to ventricular filling. [From Fowler (8).]

Fig. 8–7. Upper two strips show evidence of ventricular tachycardia with consistent retrograde conduction from ventricles to atria. Right atrial lead and Lead III are recorded simultaneously. Small positive QRS complexes in right atrial lead occur at same time as the negative QRS complexes in Lead III. Biphasic spike following QRS complexes in right atrial lead represents P waves. In lowest strip, right atrium is paced electronically at a rate of 140/min. The atrium is captured by fifth to eleventh pacing impulses. The ventricles are captured by paced atrial beats in these cycles, with a resulting narrower QRS complex. (By courtesy of John C. Fenton M.D.)

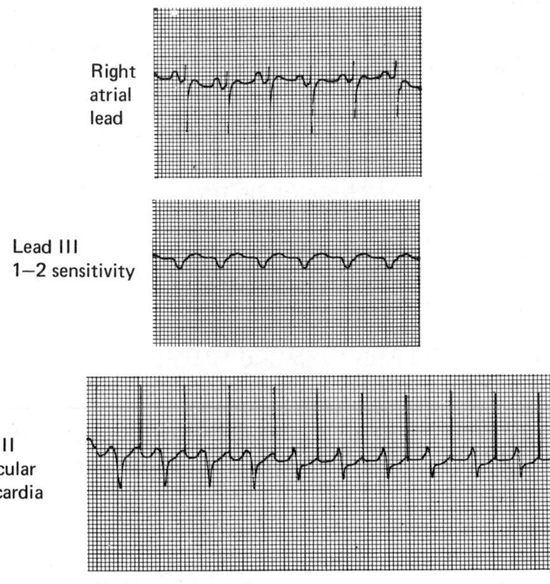

In some instances raising the blood pressure alone will suffice to restore a normal sinus mechanism. In others, restoration of normal blood pressure will render other methods more effective.

When ventricular tachycardia is not related to digitalis, I usually try 50–100 mg lidocaine (Xylocaine) as a single rapid intravenous dose (18). If this is ineffective I give 50 mg/min procaine amide intravenously for 5 or 6 minutes, while monitoring blood pressure and the electrocardiogram. If neither is effective I use DC electric shock, with the paddles applied anteroposteriorly; one placed over the precordium and one opposite this, over the back. Unless unconscious the patient is anesthetized with intravenous pentothal or with diazepam (Valium), 2.5–10 mg intravenously. Diazepam is best given in divided doses of 2.5 mg, waiting 5 minutes between doses to determine whether the needed effect has been obtained. Facilities for tracheal intubation and artificial respiration should be at hand. One begins with 50 w-sec capacitor discharge, increasing stepwise up to 400 w-sec, if necessary.

If the arrhythmia is successfully converted I usually give an intravenous infusion of lidocaine (Xylocaine), 50 ml of 2% solution in 500 ml 50% dextrose, at a rate of 2–3 mg/min. This is continued for a few days to prevent recurrences. The patient is usually placed in an intensive care or cardiac monitoring unit so that a cardiac monitoring system may be used to warn of frequent premature ventricular contractions, or a recurrence of ventricular tachycardia. When premature ventricular contractions occur in bursts of 2 or more, or are multifocal, or bigeminal, interrupt the T wave, or exceed 4–5/min, the dosage of prophylactic medication should usually be increased. When the dose of lidocaine is 4 mg/min or more, mental depression, convulsions, or cardiac asystole may result. One should be especially cautious with regard to the dosage of lidocaine when there is shock, hepatic failure, or severe congestive heart failure (29).

MEASURES OTHER THAN DC SHOCK

When DC electric shock fails or is not available for the treatment of ventricular tachycardia, there are a number of other potentially useful measures:

1. Lidocaine (Xylocaine), 50–100 mg is given rapidly intravenously, followed by 1–4 mg/min intravenously (14), (18) if conversion is successful with the bolus dose.
2. Procaine amide, 25–50 mg/min given intravenously. The total dose may be 1–3 g. The blood pressure and electrocardiogram should be monitored (14). Rarely 6–10 g/day is needed to prevent recurrences.
3. Diphenylhydantoin (Dilantin), 250 mg is given intravenously in 5 minutes (23).
4. Propranolol (Inderal) 0.1 mg/kg is given intravenously (25); a total dose of 3.0–5.0 mg may be given if necessary (28). There is danger of pulmonary

edema, cardiac arrest, or a hypotensive reaction. A commonly employed regimen is the injection of 1.0 mg diluted to 100 ml infused in 15 minutes. We usually reserve this as a last resort. It should not ordinarily be used in the presence of cardiac enlargement or heart failure.

5. Bretylium, 2–5 mg/kg every 8 hours, is given intramuscularly or intravenously. Bretylium is an investigational drug not as yet approved for the treatment of cardiac arrhythmias by the Food and Drug Administration. This agent may cause a fall of blood pressure. It is a positive inotropic agent and usually increases cardiac output (22). The usual initial dose is 300 mg, intravenously or intramuscularly. When given intramuscularly, no more than 150 mg should be given into one site. When given intravenously, the dosage is diluted into 20–30 ml 5% dextrose and infused slowly over a 5 minute period. The antiarrhythmic effect may be maintained by giving 300 mg bretylium every 6 hours for the first 24 hours and then every 8 hours thereafter, as long as needed. The intramuscular route is preferred since vomiting is more likely with the intravenous route.

6. Quinidine gluconate (0.6 g) may be dissolved in 50–100 ml 5% dextrose and infused slowly in 30 minutes while the electrocardiogram and blood pressure are monitored. The agent should be stopped promptly if the QRS complex begins to increase in width. This agent is seldom administered for this purpose at the present time. I have observed fatal ventricular fibrillation from its use.

7. Rarely, digitalis is used in the treatment of ventricular tachycardia when the arrhythmia does not result from digitalis (20).

When ventricular tachycardia results from digitalis intoxication, DC electric shock should probably not be used (17). One may infuse potassium chloride, 40 mEq in 500 ml 5% dextrose in a period of 2 hours. When there is uremia, oliguria, or increased serum potassium values, one is reluctant to employ this treatment. Lidocaine has been reported effective in experimental digitalis-induced ventricular tachycardia (13). One may use diphenylhydantoin, 50 mg/min intravenously for 5 minutes, or propranolol, 0.1 mg/kg body weight intravenously. Digitalis is to be discontinued for several days, and if needed, is to be resumed in reduced dosage.

A patient may have ventricular tachycardia or fibrillation in association with attacks of acute unstable angina pectoris. In such patients drug therapy may be completely ineffective and coronary bypass graft surgery is then required to control the arrhythmia.

PREVENTION OF RECURRENT ATTACKS

Following successful reversion in most patients with ventricular tachycardia, measures are indicated to prevent recurrent attacks. These may be divided into immediate intensive measures and less intensive measures to be employed after several days.

Immediate Preventive Measures

The patient should have a cardiac monitoring system to warn of frequent premature ventricular beats or a recurrence of ventricular tachycardia. I usually employ an intravenous drip of lidocaine (Xylocaine), 50 ml of 2% solution in 500 ml 5% dextrose in water. This is infused at a rate of 2–3 mg/min for several days after an attack of ventricular tachycardia. If this fails one may use procaine amide intravenously, 1–4 mg/min, or 500–750 mg intramuscularly every 6 hours. If this too fails we use bretylium, 2–5 mg intravenously or intramuscularly every 8 hours. In some patients pervenous electronic pacing of the right atrium or ventricle at a rate of 100–120 min is needed to prevent recurrences. Pacing may be combined with the above antiarrhythmic agents (6). Rarely, coupled pacing may be needed (10).

Less Intensive Preventive Measures

When the patient has been free of attacks of ventricular tachycardia for several days or a week, the antiarrhythmic agents are given in lower dosage. The lidocaine infusion is reduced to 1 mg/min for a day or so, and then discontinued to be replaced by another agent. Most commonly we use procaine amide, 500 mg every 6 hours, by mouth. Koch–Weser and Klein (16) suggested total doses of 50 mg/kg/day in divided doses at intervals of 3 hours. Less often we use quinidine gluconate, 300 mg every 6 hours, by mouth. Procaine amide therapy may be complicated by a lupus erythematosuslike reaction, with arthritis, pleuritis, pericarditis, fever, and rarely, arteritis (28a). After 6 months of continuous therapy as many as 50% of patients have positive lupus erythematosus cell tests, but only a few have symptoms (28a). These abnormalities are usually reversible. Oral quinidine therapy, in addition to causing tinnitus, impaired hearing, nausea, vomiting, diarrhea, fever, skin rash, and purpura, may also cause syncope related to ventricular fibrillation in perhaps 1–2% of patients (27). After oral quinidine for 3 days at a fixed dose the blood levels should be reasonably stable. I then obtain a blood level 30 minutes prior to 1 oral dose to determine whether or not the blood level lies within the desired therapeutic range of 3–6 mg/liter.

When procaine amide or quinidine are ineffective in preventing ventricular tachycardia, one may use oral propranolol (Inderal), 10–40 mg 4 times per day. This agent should not be used if there is AV block, heart failure, sinus bradycardia, or bronchial asthma. As a general rule the oral antiarrhythmic agent is discontinued after 4–6 weeks if there have been no recurrences of ventricular tachycardia and ventricular premature beats have not been frequent. If there have been additional previous attacks of ventricular tachycardia, the oral prophylactic antiarrhythmic agents are usually continued indefinitely. In some patients permanent atrial or ventricular electronic pacing is needed to prevent recurrences of ventricular tachycardia. Cardiac pacing may be used in combination with such oral antiarrhythmic agents as procaine amide or propranolol (6, 12). In some patients prevention of recurrent ventricular tachycardia has been achieved with pervenous right ventricular pacing at rates of 90–100/min. Often the initial pacing rate must be 120/min. Pacing is likely to be most effective when employed in combination with propranolol, 80–160 mg/day, or quinidine, 1.2 g/day, or procaine amide, 4 g/day. Finally mention should be made of the occasional instance of ventricular tachycardia which is associated with a ventricular aneurysm. Surgical resection of the aneurysm may be effective in preventing ventricular tachycardia (5). Ventricular tachycardia in eight patients with coronary disease was successfully treated with aortocoronary vein grafting, with resection of a ventricular aneurysm or a poorly contracting area in six (11). The treatment of difficult recurrent ventricular tachycardia was recently reviewed (31).

REFERENCES

1. Armbrust CA Jr, Levine SA: Paroxysmal ventricular tachycardia. A study of one hundred and seven cases. Circulation 1:28, 1950
2. Basley RM Jr, Goldstein S: Differentiation of ventricular tachycardia from junctional tachycardia with aberrant conduction: the use of competitive atrial pacing. Circulation 37:1015, 1968
3. Castellanos A, Castillo CA, Agba AS: Contribution of His bundle recordings to the understanding of clinical arrhythmias. Am J Cardiol 28:449, 1971
4. Chapman JH, Schrank JP, Crampton RS: Idiopathic ventricular tachycardia. An intracardiac electrical hemodynamic and angiographic assessment of six patients. Am J Med 59:470, 1975
5. DeSanctis RW, Block P, Hutter AM: Tachyarrhythmias in myocardial infarction. Circulation 45:681, 1972
6. DeSanctis RW, Kastor JA: Rapid intracardiac pacing for treatment of recurrent ventricular tachyarrhythmias in the absence of heart block. Am Heart J 76:168, 1969
7. Effler DB, Groves LK, Favaloro R: Surgical repair of ventricular aneurysm. Chest 48:37, 1965
8. Fowler NO: Cardiac Diagnosis and Treatment, 2nd ed. Hagerstown, Harper & Row, 1976
9. Fowler NO, McCall D, Chou T–C et al.: Electrocardiographic changes and cardiac arrhythmias in patients receiving psychotropic drugs. Am J Cardiol 37:223, 1976
10. Garcia R, Keyes JW: Recurrent ventricular tachycardia associated with complete heart block. Observations in a patient with the simultaneous use of a single stimulus implanted myocardial pacemaker and a "coupled-pulse generator". Am Heart J 71:533, 1966
11. Graham AF, Miller DC, Stinson EB et al.: Surgical treatment of refractory life-threatening ventricular tachycardia. Am J Cardiol 32:909, 1973
12. Hornbaker JH, Humphries JO, Ross RS: Permanent pacing in the absence of heart block. An approach to the management of intractable arrhythmias. Circulation 39:189, 1969
12a. Jeresaty RM: Editorial: Sudden death in the mitral valve prolapse-click syndrome. Am J Cardiol 37:317, 1976
13. Katz MJ, Zitnik RS: Direct current countershock and lidocaine in the treatment of digitalis induced ventricular tachycardia. Am J Cardiol 15:134, 1965
14. Kayden HJ, Brodie BB, Steele JM: Procaine amide. A review. Circulation 15:118, 1957
15. Kistin AD: Problems in the differentiation of ventricular arrhythmia from supraventricular arrhythmia with abnormal QRS. Prog Cardiovasc Dis 9:1, 1966
16. Koch–Weser J, Klein SW: Procainamide dosage schedules, plasma concentrations and clinical effects. JAMA 215:1454, 1971
17. Lown B: Electrical reversion of cardiac arrhythmias. Br Heart J 29:469, 1967
18. Lown B, Fakhro AM, Hood WB, Thorn GW: Coronary care unit; new perspectives and directions. JAMA 199:188, 1967
19. MacKenzie GJ, Pascual S: Paroxysmal ventricular tachycardia. Br Heart J 26:441, 1964

20. McGee RR, Tullis IF: Ventricular tachycardia with particular consideration of digitalis therapy. Am J Cardiol 3:300, 1959

21. Northfield TC: Cardiac complications of phaeochromocytoma. Br Heart J 29:588, 1967

22. Romhilt DW, Fowler NO: Bretylium tosylate. In Donoso E (ed): Drugs in Cardiology, Vol I. New York, Stratton, 1975, p 80

23. Rosen M, Lisak R, Rubin IL: Diphenylhydantoin in cardiac arrhythmia. Am J Cardiol 20:674, 1967

23a. Roy PR, Emanuel R, Ismail SA et al.: Hereditary prolongation of the Q-T interval. Am J Cardiol 37:237, 1976

24. Schamroth L: Immediate effects of intravenous propranolol on various cardiac arrhythmias. Am J Cardiol 18:438, 1966

25. Schamroth L: Idioventricular tachycardia. J Electrocardiol 1:205, 1968

26. Schlant RC, Dixon F, Elson SH, Rawls WJ, Williamson RJ Jr: Modification of the law of the heart: influence of early contracting areas. Circulation 30 (Supp. III):153, 1964

27. Selzer A, Wray HW: Quinidine syncope. Paroxysmal ventricular fibrillation occurring during treatment of chronic atrial arrhythmias. Circulation 30:17, 1964

28. Shand DG: Medical intelligence drug therapy. Propranolol. N Engl J Med 293:280, 1975

28a. Taylor J, Kosowsky B, Lown B: Complications of procaine amide in a prospective anti-arrhythmic study. Circulation 44 (Supp. II):43, 1971

29. Thomson PD, Melmon KL, Richardson JA et al.: Lidocaine pharmacokinetics in advanced heart failure, liver disease, and renal failure in humans. Ann Intern Med 78:499, 1973

30. Wilson WS, Judge RD, Siegel JH: A simple diagnostic sign in ventricular tachycardia. N Engl J Med 270:446, 1964

31. Winkle RA, Alderman EL, Fitzgerald JW, Harrison DC: Treatment of recurrent symptomatic ventricular tachycardia. Ann Int Med 85:1, 1976

9 | Digitalis-Induced Arrhythmias

TE-CHUAN CHOU

In spite of the accumulated clinical experience the use of digitalis in the treatment of congestive heart failure and cardiac arrhythmias is still frequently associated with serious or even fatal complications. The high incidence of digitalis intoxication may be attributed to several causes. The therapeutic range of the drug is narrow. The average therapeutic dose of digitalis leaf and of the commonly used cardiac glycosides is about 60% of their toxic doses. The amount required for the individual patient to obtain clinical improvement cannot be predicted in advance, but is derived by trial and error. It is often necessary to administer additional doses of the drug until evidence of toxicity appears before one is satisfied that the maximum beneficial effect has been achieved. Several reports indicate that the incidence of digitalis intoxication has actually increased in recent years. The widespread use of potent oral diuretic agents and the increase in the aging population are believed to be responsible. In a recent prospective study among hospitalized patients it was found that 23% of those receiving the drug developed definite toxic manifestations (2).

COMPLICATIONS OF DIGITALIS TOXICITY

Among the toxic effects of digitalis the cardiac complications are the most serious. Unfortunately they are often the earliest manifestations. In the 148 cases reported by von Capeller and coworkers, they appeared as the first indication of toxicity in 37% (35). There is a considerable difference of opinion as to whether the type of the initial sign of toxicity varies with different digitalis preparations. Many believe that digitalis leaf is more likely to produce gastrointestinal symptoms before cardiac toxicity. Others have found no significant difference between the various agents. In a series of patients in whom digitalis intoxication was deliberately induced, Church and associates failed to demonstrate any significant alteration in the pattern of intoxication with the commonly used glycosides including digoxin, digitoxin, and gitalin (4). Furthermore, the same glycoside is as likely to produce different toxic manifestations when repeatedly administered to the same patient as are different glycosides.

Digitalis is known to be capable of producing almost all types of cardiac arrhythmias. They may be either the result of a disturbance of the impulse formation, or an impairment of its conduction. The only exception is bundle branch block which is rarely, if ever, caused by digitalis. Different types of arrhythmias are often encountered in the same patient within a relatively short time. It is to be emphasized that although some of the arrhythmias to be described are quite characteristic of digitalis toxicity, none of them is pathognomonic. An erroneous diagnosis of digitalis intoxication is often made when the other clinical findings are not taken into consideration. Other evidence which is suggestive of digitalis toxicity includes the gastrointestinal symptoms such as anorexia, nausea, and vomiting; and the less common neurologic manifestations such as headache, vertigo, drowsiness, restlessness, and irritability, weakness, convulsions, delusions, mood disturbances, disorientation, and visual disturbances. The electrocardiographic signs of digitalis effect (not toxicity), consisting of the sagging of the ST segment, shortening of the QT interval, and inversion of the first portion of the T wave, do not correlate well with the degree of digitalization. They are often absent in cases having obvious intoxication. Conversely, striking changes may be seen in patients without evidence of toxicity. The presence or absence of these findings is not helpful in the diagnosis of digitalis excess. As the same arrhythmia may be the result of the underlying heart disease for which the drug is administered, the etiology of the arrhythmia is often very difficult to determine even for the experienced clinician.

SERUM GLYCOSIDE LEVEL IN THE DIAGNOSIS OF DIGITALIS TOXICITY

The recent development of the radioimmunoassay method for the determination of the serum level of cardiac glycosides has contributed significantly to the early recognition of digitalis toxicity (30). The serum level should be obtained whenever digitalis excess is suspected or the degree of digitalization is uncertain from clinical assessment alone. With digoxin, a value above 2 ng/ml is generally considered to be consistent with digitalis intoxication. It has been shown that in patients receiving digoxin, 90% of those with no clinical evidence of toxicity had a serum level of 2.0 ng/ml or below, while 87% of the patients with toxicity had concentrations above 2.0 ng/ml. It is important to emphasize the considerable overlap of the serum glycoside concentration in the toxic and nontoxic patients. Toxic manifestations may be observed in some patients with a serum level of 1.6 ng/ml, but not in others with up to a concentration of 3.0 ng/ml (33). In many patients a definite conclusion as to the presence or absence of digitalis intoxication cannot be reached in spite of the availability of both the clinical information and serum glycoside value.

The average therapeutic level of serum digitoxin is more than 10 times that of digoxin (31). A level above 26 ng/ml is generally considered toxic. The degree of overlap in the level of toxic and nontoxic patients tends to be greater than that of digoxin. This has been attributed in part to the greater extent of plasma protein binding of digitoxin, which is more likely to affect the distribution of the drug in the body (24).

CLASSIFICATION OF DIGITALIS-INDUCED ARRHYTHMIAS

The relative frequency of the various types of digitalis-induced arrhythmias based on 10 large series in the literature has been summarized (16). Table 9–1 gives the incidence of the individual arrhythmia in the reported 688 cases.

PREMATURE VENTRICULAR CONTRACTIONS

Ectopic beats arising from the ventricles are the most common arrhythmia and frequently the earliest manifestation of digitalis excess. They account for almost one-half of the arrhythmias induced by digitalis. The ectopic beats may arise from a single focus but are often multifocal in origin, the latter being more suggestive of digitalis toxicity. Ectopic ventricular complexes of different configurations should be seen in the same electrocardiographic lead before they can be considered as coming from multiple focuses. The seriousness of the rhythm disturbance depends, to a certain extent, on the frequency of the premature beats. Although the appearance of occasional premature contractions is usually of little hemodynamic consequence, they should be regarded as a warning signal. A failure to recognize their presence may lead to the development of ventricular tachycardia or ventricular fibrillation if the drug is continued. In a patient with atrial fibrillation premature ventricular contractions are sometimes very difficult to clinically detect. Frequent electrocardiographic recordings are advisable when the dosage of digitalis is increased, or

Table 9–1. RELATIVE INCIDENCE OF DIGITALIS-INDUCED ARRHYTHMIAS*†

Rhythm		Number of patients	Percentage of total
Frequent PVCs	Total	327	48
	Multifocal	107	16
	Bigeminy	165	24
Junctional tachycardia		90	13
Junctional rhythm		30	4
AV dissociation		62	9
Heart block	1°	84	12
	2°	77	11
	3°	77	11
PAT	Total	91	13
	With block	70	10
Atrial fibrillation		72	10
Atrial flutter		11	1.6
Premature atrial contractions		34	5
Premature junctional contractions		4	0.6
Sinus arrest		11	1.6
Sinus bradycardia		16	2.3
Sinus tachycardia		30	4
Wandering pacemaker		16	2.3
Ventricular tachycardia		71	10
Ventricular fibrillation		8	1.2

*Irons GV Jr, Orgain ES: Digitalis-induced arrhythmias and their management. Prog Cardiovasc Dis 8:539, 1966
†Total number of patients–688

if there is reason to believe that the patient has become more sensitive to the drug. Bigeminal and trigeminal rhythm due to ventricular extrasystoles are particularly characteristic of digitalis toxicity. Although they are not pathognomonic, they should be considered as digitalis related and be treated as such until it is proven otherwise. It is pertinent to mention that premature ventricular contractions are also the most common arrhythmia in the absence of digitalis. In a patient who has not received an adequate amount of digitalis, additional doses of the drug may reduce or abolish the premature contractions, probably by improving the cardiac status.

ATRIOVENTRICULAR BLOCK

Various degrees of AV block are the next most common rhythm disturbances caused by digitalis. This is not surprising as conduction delay at the AV junction is one of its known pharmacologic effects. This property is utilized therapeutically to slow the ventricular rate in patients with atrial fibrillation or atrial flutter.

There is a difference of opinion as to whether first degree AV block alone represents a therapeutic or a toxic effect. For practical purposes the appearance of a definite prolongation of the PR interval after the administration of digitalis should be regarded as an early warning sign. The dosage of the drug should either be reduced or the drug should be temporarily discontinued. Second and third degree AV block, when caused by digitalis, are definite signs of intoxication. The Wenckebach phenomenon, with gradual prolongation of the PR interval until an atrial impulse fails to be conducted, is frequently observed. Mobitz type II second degree AV block, in which the PR interval remains unchanged before the blocked beats, is rarely the result of digitalis. Complete heart block due to digitalis often has a faster ventricular rate than that resulting from other causes. In patients with atrial fibrillation an advanced degree of AV block is manifested by an excessive slowing of the ventricular rate; and a regular ventricular rhythm under this circumstance suggests complete AV block (Fig. 9–1). A similar conclusion can be made in patients with atrial flutter, in which case the complete AV block is signaled not only by a slow and regular ventricular rhythm but also by a variation of the FR interval. In a patient who has preexisting complete heart block and who is given digitalis for the treatment of congestive heart failure, an acceleration of the idioventricular rhythm due to enhanced automaticity of the subsidiary pacemaker should be regarded as a sign of digitalis toxicity.

NONPAROXYSMAL JUNCTIONAL TACHYCARDIA, AV JUNCTIONAL RHYTHM, AND AV DISSOCIATION

Nonparoxysmal junctional tachycardia is the result of an abnormal enhancement of impulse formation at the AV junction. The rate of the junctional discharge is about 70–130/min. The rhythm is regular. It differs from the

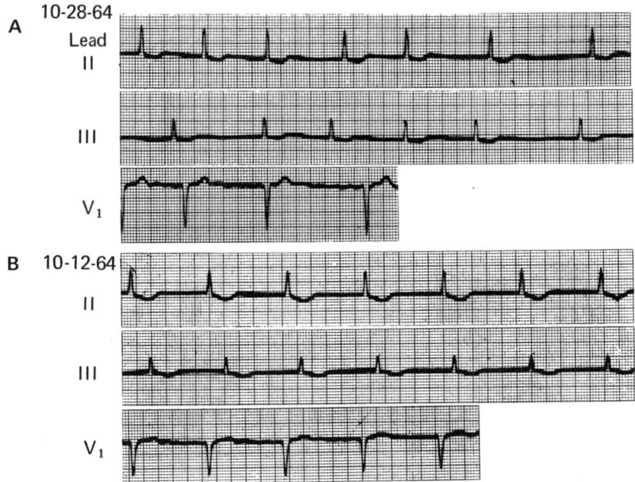

Fig. 9–1.   **Appearance of complete AV block in a patient with atrial fibrillation suggesting digitalis toxicity.** *A)* **Atrial fibrillation with slow ventricular response;** *B)* **Regularity of the ventricular rhythm indicates presence of complete AV block.**

paroxysmal variety of AV junctional tachycardia in that it lacks the sudden onset and termination, which is characteristically associated with the paroxysmal type. The latter usually has a rate of 150–220/min and is seen mostly in patients without demonstrable heart disease. If the enhanced automaticity of the AV junctional pacemaker leads to a retrograde activation of the atria, the junctional impulse will capture both the atria and the ventricles. In the electrocardiogram a constant PR or RP interval will be observed. If the retrograde conduction is impaired, the atria will remain under the control of the impulse arising either from the sinus node or an ectopic focus in the atrium. The atrial and ventricular rhythms are independent and the condition is called AV *dissociation.* The ventricular rate in AV dissociation is generally faster than the atrial rate except when atrial tachycardia coexists and results in a double tachycardia. When the atrial impulse occasionally captures the ventricles and "premature" conducted beat or beats are seen, it is called *interference dissociation* or AV dissociation with interference. This occurs if the atrial impulse arrives at the AV junction outside its refractory period and there is no antegrade AV block.

Nonparoxysmal junctional tachycardia and its variants are most commonly the result of digitalis intoxication. In a series of 30 cases studied by Pick and Dominguez digitalis was responsible for the arrhythmia in 16 patients. The rhythm may also be seen in patients with myocarditis, acute myocardial infarction, or after intracardiac surgery. In only a very few instances the etiology of the arrhythmia cannot be found.

Bidirectional tachycardia (28) is usually a supraventricular tachycardia, probably AV junctional in origin, with a regular alternation of two types of QRS complexes. There is a right bundle branch block pattern in every beat, but the mean QRS axes of the alternate ventricular complexes have opposite directions, probably due to alternate aberrant conduction in the two divisions of the left bundle branch. Bidirectional tachycardia usually occurs in subjects with advanced heart disease and is almost invariably related to digitalis.

AV junctional rhythm occurs when there is a suppression or failure of the pacemaker function of the SA node. When the rate of the sinus discharge becomes slower than the inherent rate of the AV junctional tissue the latter assumes the role of the dominant pacemaker. The ventricular rate varies between 40–60/min. The rhythm is usually regular although slight variation is occasionally observed. In the electrocardiogram the QRS complexes resemble those seen during normal sinus rhythm. Although junctional rhythm is often the result of digitalis intoxication, it may also be seen in patients with coronary artery disease, especially in association with myocardial infarction. It may also be encountered in healthy individuals with marked sinus bradycardia or in patients with sick sinus syndrome. As in the case of nonparoxysmal junctional tachycardia, the junctional impulse may either capture both the atria and the ventricles or the ventricles alone, leading to AV dissociation with or without interference (Fig. 9–2). A special form of junctional rhythm is *reciprocal rhythm.* When there is an unequal depression of the conductivity in the AV junction, the junctional impulse may spread to the atria through part of the junctional tissue, and after activating the atria, return through another portion of the AV junction to stimulate the ventricles. This phenomenon of reentry is especially favored by a slow retrograde conduction of the original impulse. In the electrocardiogram reciprocal rhythm can be diagnosed when there is a retrograde P wave with prolonged RP interval of greater than 0.20 sec which is followed by another premature ventricular complex. This form of junctional rhythm is most frequently seen in patients with digitalis intoxication.

VENTRICULAR TACHYCARDIA AND VENTRICULAR FIBRILLATION

Ventricular tachycardia is one of the most serious arrhythmias induced by digitalis. In the 30 cases reported by Dreifus and associates (6) the mortality rate was 68%. Although unifocal or multifocal premature ventricular contractions often precede the development of this rhythm, it may appear without

Fig. 9–2. **Interference dissociation due to digitalis. The AV junctional rhythm is interrupted by capture beats (fourth and eighth QRS complexes in Lead II, fourth complex in Lead V₁).**

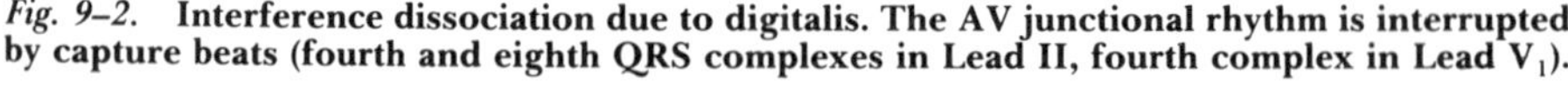

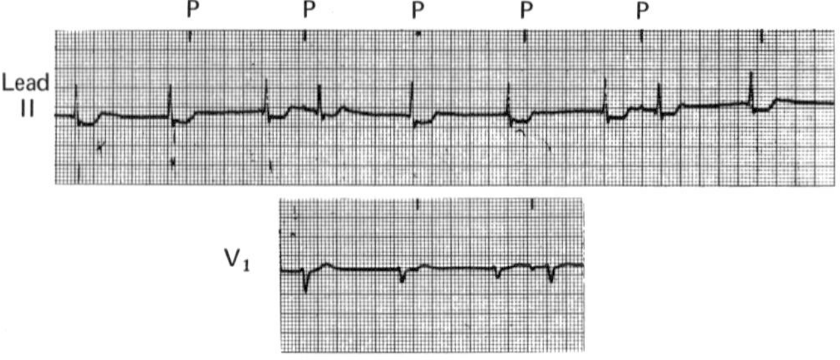

prior warning. It is often simulated by supraventricular tachycardia with aberrant ventricular conduction or bundle branch block, which may call for an increase in the dosage of digitalis. The differentiation is very important, even though not always possible. The presence of premature ventricular contractions with similar QRS complexes in the previous electrocardiograms, and the demonstration of independent atrial and ventricular activities with capture or fusion beats suggest strongly the ventricular origin of the arrhythmia. Ventricular fibrillation has been documented more frequently since continuous electrocardiographic monitoring has been employed. Unless it is recognized promptly, death is imminent.

PAROXYSMAL ATRIAL TACHYCARDIA WITH BLOCK

The role of digitalis in the production of paroxysmal atrial tachycardia with block (PAT with block) has been emphasized by Lown and associates (23). It has been estimated that in about 73% of hospitalized patients this arrhythmia is induced by digitalis. When the arrhythmia is unrelated to digitalis it is usually seen in patients with rheumatic heart disease, coronary artery disease, or when there is severe hypokalemia. It has also been observed in normal, young subjects. Loss of potassium may be responsible for the precipitation of PAT with block in many digitalized patients. In Lown's series of PAT with block due to digitalis, alteration in the balance of body potassium was the key factor in 60% of cases.

The electrocardiogram shows that the atrial rate is usually between 150–200/min. The P waves are often small and there is an isoelectric segment between the succeeding P waves. The degree of AV block varies with second degree block, including the Wenckebach phenomenon, which is the most common (Fig. 9–3). Occasionally there is a 1:1 conduction and the PR interval is normal. The AV block is demonstrated only during carotid sinus stimulation. This particular variant is called PAT with latent block, which may mimic the classical PAT until carotid sinus stimulation is applied (Fig. 9–4).

It is very important to differentiate PAT with block from atrial flutter, as the latter is rarely a sign of digitalis intoxication and usually calls for an additional amount of the drug. In atrial flutter the atrial rate is usually above 250/min. The baseline presents a saw-tooth appearance in some leads. When the atrial rate is between 200–250 and the atrial activities do not present a typical wave form, the separation of the two may be very difficult and a decision has to be based on the clinical setting with which the arrhythmia is associated and on the serum glycoside level.

ATRIAL FIBRILLATION

Although the literature indicates that atrial fibrillation accounts for approximately 10% of the arrhythmias induced by digitalis, it is less common in the author's experience. Their association should be suspected when the arrhythmia develops suddenly in a digitalized patient who previously had a normal sinus rhythm.

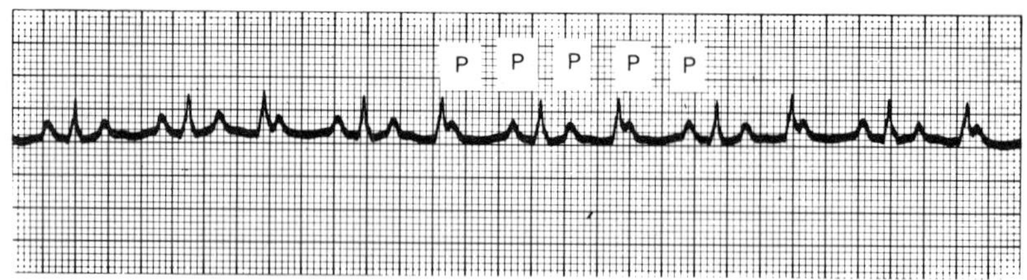

Fig. 9–3. Paroxysmal atrial tachycardia with block due to digitalis. There is a 3:2 conduction with Wenckebach phenomenon.

Fig. 9–4. Paroxysmal atrial tachycardia with latent block due to digitalis in a patient with chronic cor pulmonale. A. Normal sinus rhythm before the administration of digoxin; B. Supraventricular tachycardia developed after 1.0 mg of digoxin was given intramuscularly; C. AV block was induced by carotid sinus massage, confirming the diagnosis of PAT with latent block. Normal sinus rhythm returned later but a similar sequence of events recurred after another dose of digoxin was administered.

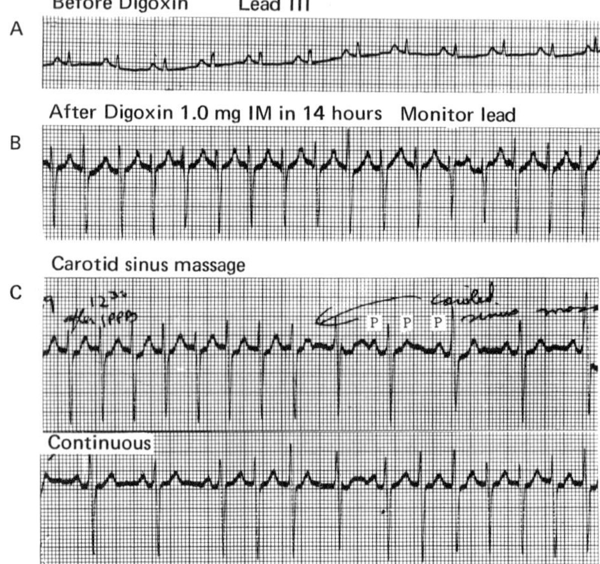

SINUS BRADYCARDIA, SINUS TACHYCARDIA, SINUS ARREST AND SINOATRIAL BLOCK

Electrocardiographic diagnosis of the disturbed sinus mechanism can usually be made without difficulty. However, the association of digitalis excess and sinus tachycardia is often not realized. Sinoatrial block is recognized by the presence of a prolonged PP cycle length which is usually 2 or more times the length of the normal PP interval. Frequently the PP interval is slightly less than the multiple of the normal cycle because of the presence of Wenckebach periods.

PREVENTION OF DIGITALIS-INDUCED ARRHYTHMIAS

PREDISPOSING FACTORS TO DIGITALIS INTOXICATION

Various factors are known to increase the susceptibility of the myocardium to digitalis. The recognition of these predisposing factors is essential to avoid the administration of an "average" amount of the drug which is excessive for the patient in question. The dosage to be used is naturally also dependent on the method of administration.

ROUTE OF ADMINISTRATION AND BIOLOGIC AVAILABILITY

It has been shown recently that oral administration of an equal dose of digoxin tablets from different manufacturers may result in a 4–7 times difference in the resulting peak serum digoxin levels (20). The variation was observed not only between the products of different companies but also between different lots from the same company. The clinical importance of this finding is obvious, although the incidence of digitalis toxicity due to changes in the source of the drug is unknown.

The average amount of digoxin absorbed from the oral tablet is about 50–75% of that given intravenously (12, 15). Therefore, when oral administration of digoxin has to be substituted by the intravenous route, the dosage should be reduced by one-half to avoid the development of toxicity. Intramuscularly given digoxin is about 80% absorbed, with considerable individual variations. It also causes severe pain. The intravenous route is preferred if the drug has to be given parentally. Oral absorption of digitoxin has generally been considered nearly 100% effective. The oral and intravenous dosage of this glycoside are therefore the same.

RAPID DIGITALIZATION

Marcus and associates confirmed the clinical observation that therapeutic levels of digitalization may be obtained by using a "maintenance dose" alone. Administering tritiated digoxin at the rate of 0.5 mg daily they demonstrated that the levels after 6 days were similar to those obtained in patients who had received an initial 2.0 mg loading dose in addition to the same maintenance dose. Their findings suggest that when rapid digitalization is not required, the large initial loading dose may be omitted and thereby reduce the possibility of intoxication.

AGE, BODY WEIGHT AND ADVANCED HEART DISEASE

The sensitivity to digitalis is increased with advanced age. In addition, the blood concentrations of digoxin are significantly higher in the elderly than in younger persons after the administration of the same dosage. The higher value has been attributed to the decrease of glomerular filtration rate and renal clearance of the glycoside. A comparatively smaller amount of the drug should be given to elderly patients (8).

Body weight is an important factor in the determination of the dosage of digitalis. However, it has been shown that in obese patients the resultant blood level of the glycoside is related to the lean body weight rather than the total body weight. In these individuals the dosage may be erroneously high if it is calculated according to the total body weight (7).

An individual with a normal heart is usually able to tolerate a large amount of the drug, but a patient with severe heart disease may develop serious arrhythmias with less than an average therapeutic dose. Evidence of toxicity often appears before any beneficial effect can be obtained. A patient who receives the same maintenance dose of digitalis for many years without complication may become toxic when his myocardium begins to deteriorate.

ELECTROLYTE IMBALANCE

The importance of electrolyte imbalance in the development of digitalis intoxication cannot be overemphasized. The use of various potent diuretics without an adequate supplement of potassium often leads to hypokalemia-one of the most common contributing factors in digitalis intoxication. A large amount of potassium may be lost through the gastrointestinal tract because of diarrhea or vomiting. Excessive urinary excretion may occur secondary to certain renal diseases. The close relationship between potassium and myocardial sensitivity to digitalis is clearly demonstrated in patients undergoing hemodialysis. Patients who have been on a maintenance dose of digitalis may not show any sign of digitalis toxicity until the serum potassium is brought from a high to a relatively low or normal level. It is to be emphasized that the loss of potassium may be entirely intracellular and the determination of the serum potassium level may not reveal its deficit. Conversely an intracellular shift of potassium as the result of glucose infusion may also precipitate digitalis intoxication. The synergistic action of calcium and digitalis is well known. Death has occurred when digitalized patients were given calcium gluconate intravenously. Alkalosis has been observed to intensify manifestation of digitalis intoxication, whereas acidosis increases digitalis tolerance. It has been suggested that the arrhythmias may be related to the accompanying hypokalemia rather than to the alkalosis *per se.* Hypomagnesemia may occasionally contribute to the development of digitalis toxicity (29). Such a possibility should be considered, especially in patients receiving diuretics but who have no evidence of potassium deficiency.

CHRONIC COR PULMONALE, RENAL INSUFFICIENCY AND THYROTOXICOSIS

A high incidence of digitalis intoxication has been observed in patients with chronic cor pulmonale. The increased sensitivity to the drug is probably related to arterial hypoxemia. In the presence of renal insufficiency the rate of digitalis excretion is impaired. In patients with normal renal function the daily loss of digoxin is about 35% of that in the body. In an anuric patient this is only 14%. With digitoxin, which is metabolized mostly in the liver, the daily loss is about 11% when both the renal and liver functions are normal. This is reduced to 7.6% in an anuric patient. Jelliffe and associates have suggested the proper daily maintenance dose of digoxin and digitoxin according to the patient's creatinine clearance (17,18). Patients with hypothyroidism are more sensitive to digitalis; the reverse is true in hyperthyroid subjects. Furthermore, the rate of excretion of digoxin is decreased in the former and increased in the latter. In atrial fibrillation caused by thyrotoxicosis a large amount of digitalis is required for the control of the ventricular rate. If the ventricular rate is taken as the sole criterion of a satisfactory response, the risk of intoxication will undoubtedly increase.

ACUTE MYOCARDIAL INFARCTION

The question of whether patients with acute myocardial infarction are more sensitive to cardiac glycosides remains unanswered (22). In clinical practice in patients with acute myocardial infarction and mild congestive heart failure, diuretics alone are employed first. If the failure is severe and if arrhythmias, which usually respond to digitalis therapy appear, the drug is used. A smaller dose and slower rate of digitalization is preferred.

WOLFF–PARKINSON–WHITE SYNDROME

In patients with the Wolff–Parkinson–White syndrome and atrial fibrillation, the accessory pathway is frequently utilized for the AV conduction. The wide QRS complexes and rapid ventricular rate often mimic ventricular tachycardia. Since digitalis does not impair the conduction through the accessory bundle, attempt to control the ventricular rate by increasing amount of the glycoside may result in toxicity. Under this circumstance other antiarrhythmic agents such as quinidine and procaine amide should be used in place of or in conjunction with digitalis (9).

FOLLOWING DC COUNTERSHOCK CONVERSION OF SINUS RHYTHM

With the introduction of direct current countershock for the treatment of cardiac arrhythmia, it has been observed that digitalis intoxication often appears following conversion of sinus rhythm when no indication of such was present before the conversion. In a series of 28 successful conversions of arrhythmias to normal sinus rhythm in patients receiving digitalis, 72% of the patients were found to demonstrate some electrocardiographic abnormalities compatible with digitalis intoxication (11). Two of these patients died as a result of ventricular fibrillation. Although the mechanism has not been well elucidated, the most likely explanation is that the electric discharge affects myocardial cellular membranes resulting in a leakage of intracellular potassium. When a critical loss has occurred, toxic effects from the myocardial-bound glycoside ensue (19). In support of this hypothesis is the experimental observation that administration of potassium prevents postshock arrhythmias, while infusion of glucose and insulin, which lower the concentration of extracellular potassium, potentiates and prolongs this phenomenon. It is, therefore, desirable that digitalis should be discontinued for a few days before attempting conversion by direct current countershock. The length of withdrawal depends on the type of digitalis preparation received by the patient. As the occurrence of postconversion arrhythmias is also directly related to the energy of the electric discharge, the latter should be kept at a low level in patients who have received digitalis recently.

TREATMENT

Once the diagnosis of digitalis intoxication is suspected or made, the drug should obviously be discontinued immediately. Even when toxicity is only suspected, it is generally safer to stop the drug temporarily and the subsequent course is followed. The possible beneficial effect of continuing the medication usually does not justify the risk of the serious complications it may cause if toxicity should exist. When the intoxication is simply the result of overdose and the diagnosis is made early, usually no other medication is necessary. If the arrhythmia is represented by occasional premature ventricular contractions, moderate degree of sinus bradycardia, supraventricular tachycardia with relatively slow ventricular rate or a mild degree of AV block and the patient is asymptomatic, active drug treatment is usually not required. The patient should be monitored closely with the electrocardiogram and the clinical course closely assessed. The time required for the signs of toxicity to subside depends on the rate of dissipation of the individual digitalis preparation. Arrhythmias in patients receiving long-acting cardiac glycosides (for example, digitoxin) may persist for more than 1 week after the drug is discontinued.

If the arrhythmia is of the more serious type, such as ventricular tachycardia and fibrillation, marked sinus bradycardia, supraventricular tachycardia with rapid ventricular rate, advanced AV block with slow ventricular rate, or if the patient becomes symptomatic, more aggressive approach is necessary. The appropriate therapy depends to a large extent on the mechanism of the arrhythmia, whether there is an increase in the automaticity of the ectopic pacemaker (tachycardia), or a depression of impulse formation or conduction (bradycardia).

POTASSIUM THERAPY

The usefulness of potassium therapy in the treatment of tachyarrhythmias and frequent premature ventricular contractions due to digitalis is well established. Any conditions which may be responsible for the loss of body potassium, such as gastrointestinal disturbances and excessive diuresis, should be corrected. Even if the serum potassium level is normal, administration of the cation may be useful. Digitalis-induced arrhythmias appear to be related to the intracellular loss of potassium from the myocardium and the cation reduces the diastolic depolarization of the ectopic pacemakers. Oral or intravenous administration of potassium is used, depending on the seriousness and the urgency of the complication. One g of potassium chloride in 10% solution, which contains 13 mEq of potassium, may be given by mouth every 4 hours. For intravenous use 40–60 mEq. of potassium chloride in 500 ml of 5% glucose in water may be administered over a period of 2–4 hours. When the intravenous route is used, constant electrocardiographic monitoring is required. The agent is most effective in the treatment of paroxysmal atrial tachycardia with block. Usually there is a gradual slowing of the atrial rate followed by 1:1 AV conduction before the rhythm is converted to a sinus mechanism. When the renal function is impaired the administration of potassium should be carried out under extreme caution even if hypokalemia is present. Although potassium therapy may be beneficial in the presence of a normal serum level, it is contraindicated when the serum potassium level is above the normal range. It is also contraindicated in patients with bradycardia, especially those with advanced AV block unless a definite deficiency can be demonstrated. In the absence of hypokalemia the effects of potassium and digitalis on the AV conduction are additive and severe conduction impairment may occur. Cardiac arrest has been reported as the result of depression of the ventricular responsiveness.

DIPHENYLHYDANTOIN

Diphenylhydantoin sodium (Dilantin) is perhaps one of the most effective drugs currently available for the treatment of arrhythmias caused by digitalis. It is useful in tachyarrhythmias of either supraventricular or ventricular origin, especially the latter. In the experimental animal it has been shown to depress ventricular automaticity and to enhance AV conduction, while having little or no effect on intraventricular conduction or sinus node. In the series of patients reported by Rosen and associates (27) diphenylhydantoin was successful in the conversion of supraventricular arrhythmia related to digitalis in 52.9%. The majority of the unsuccessful cases were those having atrial flutter or atrial fibrillation. The rate of success in those with ventricular arrhythmia was 92.3%. Similar results were obtained by Helfant and coworkers (14). The drug may be administered either parenterally or orally. The intravenous route is preferred where prompt conversion of the arrhythmia is desired. The initial dose is usually 250 mg in an infusion of 5% dextrose in water. The rate of administration is about 25–50 mg/min. Continuous electrocardiographic monitoring and blood pressure recording should be done. Any response will usually be observed within 5 minutes after the dose. An additional 100 mg may be given if the electrocardiogram demonstrates a favorable although incomplete response to the initial dose. If the rhythm is converted to a sinus mechanism or there is a significant slowing of the ventricular rate to suggest a favorable response, an additional 100 mg is given intramuscularly. Thereafter the patient is given 400 mg/day of the drug in divided doses, either intramuscularly or orally. The latter schedule may be adopted without the initial intravenous administration if the control of the arrhythmia is not urgently required. Bigger and associates demonstrated that in most of the cases which have responded to the treatment, the plasma level of diphenylhydantoin was from 10–18 μg/ml (3).

Side Effects

The side effects of Dilantin include light-headedness and transient pain at the site of infusion. Drowsiness, nystagmus, vertigo, and nausea may appear, especially when large doses are used and the plasma level of the drug is high. As the drug is a vasodilator as well as a myocardial depressant, transient hypotension of a minor degree is very common and occasionally severe hypotension may occur. Transient sinus arrest and asystole have been observed. The drug is contraindicated in patients with a high degree of AV block or marked bradycardia.

LIDOCAINE

Lidocaine (Xylocaine) given intravenously has been used extensively in recent years for the treatment of ventricular tachycardia and ventricular fibrillation in general, as well as those related to digitalis (13). The results from animal experiments suggest that except for diphenylhydantoin, lidocaine is probably the most effective antiarrhythmic drug available for the treatment of digitalis-induced ventricular tachycardia. Although its chemical structure is quite similar to that of procaine amide, the drug is much more rapidly metabolized after its administration. After an intravenous injection, lidocaine disappears rapidly from the blood with a halftime of 15–20 minutes. For the control of ventricular arrhythmias, an initial dose of 1 mg/kg of body weight is usually given intravenously as a single injection, which can be repeated every 3–5 minutes if necessary. The total amount given should usually be kept below 300 mg. After the arrhythmia has been controlled a maintenance infusion is immediately started, as the suppression of the ectopic focus usually lasts for only 4–15 minutes. The rate of the infusion may vary between 2–4 mg/min. Because of the rapid onset and the short duration of action of the drug, the infusion rate should be very accurately controlled. The toxic manifestations related to lidocaine are mostly from the central nervous system. They include drowsiness, paresthesias, decreased hearing, and convulsions. The convulsions are usually seen when large amounts of the drug are given, or when the rate of administration is very rapid. A direct cardiac toxic effect resulting in ventricular tachycardia or fibrillation has occasionally been observed. Depression of the sinus mechanism is a more common toxic effect.

QUINIDINE AND PROCAINE AMIDE

Quinidine has been used with success in both supraventricular and ventricular tachyarrhythmias caused by digitalis. The drug may be administered every 6 hours at the dosage of 0.3–0.4 g. The use of the drug is sometimes hazardous, especially when an AV conduction defect is present. Quinidine may cause depression of the sinus node, impairment of intraatrial, atrioventricular and intraventricular conduction, as well as the development of ventricular premature contractions, ventricular tachycardia, and fibrillation. Some of the arrhythmias due to quinidine have been found responsible for syncope in some patients receiving the drug. Frequent electrocardiographic monitoring is, therefore, indicated and should be repeated, especially before each additional dose is given. A widening of the QRS complex of 0.02 sec or more is an indication for reducing the dosage or stopping the drug. Quinidine blood plasma levels should be obtained, and a value between 4–6 mg/liter is desired. A level above 8 mg/liter is considered dangerous. Quinidine is probably less desirable than diphenylhydantoin, lidocaine, potassium infusion or procaine amide in the treatment of serious digitalis-induced tachyarrhythmias.

Procaine amide (Pronestyl) is effective in the treatment of premature ventricular contractions, ventricular tachycardia, AV junctional tachycardia, or paroxysmal atrial tachycardia with block. It is much less effective in the other types of atrial arrhythmias, such as atrial fibrillation induced by digitalis. The drug may be given intravenously with a rate not faster than 100 mg/min. The total amount should not exceed 1000 mg. It may also be administered intramuscularly in a dose of 500 mg, and repeated in 2 hours, if necessary. Its oral dose is from 250–500 mg every 3–4 hours. The toxic effects of procaine amide include hypotension, widening of the QRS complex, ventricular tachycardia, or fibrillation. Electrocardiographic and blood pressure monitoring are necessary.

PROPRANOLOL

The β-adrenergic blocking agents have been found effective in the treatment of frequent ventricular premature beats, ventricular tachycardia, and atrial tachycardia with block due to digitalis excess (10). Although their antiarrhythmic property depends mostly on the blocking of β-adrenergic receptors, a quinidinelike action is also believed to exist. Propranolol (Inderal) may be given orally or intravenously. For oral administration the usual dosage is 40–160 mg daily in 4 divided doses. The intravenous dose for the treatment of arrhythmias is 1–3 mg. A second dose may be repeated after 2 minutes, if necessary; but the total amount of the drug administered at one time should not exceed 0.1 mg/kg of body weight. Additional medication should not be given in less than 4 hours. When the drug is administered intravenously, it should be under constant electrocardiographic monitoring and the rate of administration should not exceed 1 mg/3 min period. The drug is contraindicated in patients with bradycardia, congestive heart failure, hypotension, allergic rhinitis during the pollen season, asthma, diabetes (if receiving insulin), and patients on adrenergic augmenting psychotropic drugs. Since most patients with digitalis toxicity have had congestive heart failure (for which the drug is used) this agent has a rather limited application.

BRETYLIUM TOSYLATE

Bretylium tosylate has been employed for the treatment of various types of arrhythmias, mostly ventricular in origin, some of which were due to digitalis (1). It was successful in the termination of digitalis-induced ventricular fibrillation, ventricular tachycardia, and bigeminal or multifocal premature ventricular contractions. The drug blocks postganglionic sympathetic transmission. It lowers the peripheral vascular resistance and produces orthostatic hypotension, which is its most important side effect. In contrast to most of the other antiarrhythmic drugs it has a positive inotropic action, probably because it increases the sensitivity of the heart to the endogenous catecholamines, similar to the effect seen after an anatomic sympathectomy. The drug may be given either intramuscularly or intravenously. The recommended initial dose is 5 mg/kg of body weight. The conversion of the arrhythmia occurs from within 5 minutes to several hours after administration. When given intravenously bretylium should be diluted in 50 ml of 5% dextrose in water, and given slowly over a 5 minute period. If the single dose is not effective, the drug may be repeated after 1 or 2 hours. The maintenance dose is 2–3 mg/kg of body weight, and is given at 8–12 hour intervals. The total experience with this drug is thus far quite limited. Its clinical use is still in the investigative stage. The drug has not yet been approved by the Food and Drug Administration and is not available commercially at the time of this writing.

DC COUNTERSHOCK AND RAPID INTRACARDIAC PACING

As a rule direct current countershock is contraindicated in patients with digitalis-induced arrhythmias. Serious ventricular arrhythmias may occur after the procedure in patients receiving digitalis, even when no evidence of digitalis excess was present before the shock. Vassaux and Lown (34) suggested that cardioversion may be used as a last resort in the treatment of paroxysmal atrial tachycardia with block due to digitalis excess when all of the antiarrhythmic drugs have failed. Low energy shock is used, accompanied by intravenous lidocaine to suppress ventricular ectopic beats. Because of the potential danger it is questionable whether this method will be adopted generally, and paroxysmal atrial tachycardia with block seldom presents as such an emergency to justify this highly risky procedure.

Rapid intracardiac pacing has been found useful in the treatment of supraventricular and ventricular tachycardia related to digitalis (21). If the arrhythmia is supraventricular, right atrial pacing is used. The tachycardia may be terminated because of overdrive and suppression of the ectopic pacemaker, alteration in the type of supraventricular arrhythmia which is not self-perpetuating, or interruption of a fixed circus movement. If the arrhythmia is ventricular in origin the heart may be paced from either the right atrium or the right ventricle, depending on whether AV block is present (5). If the heart can be captured successfully pacing can be continued until the effect of the excessive digitalis has subsided, at which point the pacing may be stopped.

Cardiac pacing may also be a useful adjuvant when the arrhythmia is treated with antiarrhythmic drugs. Quinidine, procaine amide, lidocaine, and diphenylhydantoin are potent myocardial depressants. Asystole may occur, especially when large doses of the drug are used. This is particularly true in patients with digitalis toxicity, as impairment of the AV conduction often coexists. A demand pacemaker is preferred and the pacemaker electrode is placed in the right ventricle. This device may serve as a valuable safeguard during the course of the drug therapy.

TREATMENT OF BRADYCARDIAS

The therapeutic approach for bradycardias due to digitalis is quite different from that for the tachycardias. The various cardiac depressants such as diphenylhydantoin, procaine amide, lidocaine, propranolol, and quinidine are obviously contraindicated. Potassium should not be used unless a definite deficiency can be demonstrated.

If the bradycardia is sinus in origin–sinus bradycardia, sinus arrest, or sinoatrial block–active treatment is usually indicated when the heart rate is less than 50/min. The decision as to the need of active therapy should not be based on the rate alone. Treatment is required if symptoms suggestive of decreased cerebral blood flow, angina pectoris, or congestive heart failure appear, or when ventricular ectopic beats are noted. Atropine is generally the drug of choice. The dosage is 0.4–1.0 mg every 3–4 hours, given either intravenously or hypodermically. Attention should be given for the possible development of acute glaucoma or urinary retention, especially in older individuals.

Similar treatment may be applied to slow AV junctional rhythm. Atropine may enhance the automaticity of the SA node, which may resume its role of the dominant pacemaker.

If the drug fails cardiac pacing is indicated. A transvenous demand pacemaker is preferred and the pacing may be accomplished through the right atrium if the AV conduction is normal. The pacing rate is usually 70/min or faster, depending on its effect in the relief of symptoms and suppression of the ventricular ectopic focus.

If the slow heart rate is the result of second or third degree AV block, atropine may also be used, but is usually not very effective in the improvement of the AV conduction. Isoproterenol (Isuprel), sometimes used in the treatment of complete AV block unrelated to digitalis, should be avoided when the AV block is digitalis-induced. In animal experiments serious arrhythmias often occur when isoproterenol is administered to digitalized animals. When active therapy is required temporary transvenous pacing from the right ventricle is most reliable and a demand pacemaker is employed. A fixed-rate pacemaker should not be used to avoid competition between the artificial pacemaker and the patient's own impulse when his AV conduction improves.

In patients with digitalis-induced bradycardia, whether related to sinus slowing or AV block, continuous electrocardiographic monitoring is desirable until the cardiac rhythm has returned to normal.

REFERENCES

1. Bacaner MB: Treatment of ventricular fibrillation and other acute arrhythmias with bretylium tosylate. Am J Cardiol 21:530, 1968
2. Beller GA, Smith TW, Abelmann WH, Haber E, Hood WB Jr: Digitalis intoxication. A prospective clinical study with serum level correlations. N Engl J Med 284:989, 1971
3. Bigger JT Jr, Schmidt DH, Kutt H: Relationship between the plasma level of diphenylhydantoin sodium and its cardiac antiarrhythmic effects. Circulation 38:363, 1968
4. Church G, Schamroth L, Schwartz NL, Marriott HJL: Deliberate digitalis intoxication. A comparison of the toxic effects of four glycoside preparations. Ann Intern Med 57:946, 1962
5. DeSanctis RW, Kastor JA: Rapid intracardiac pacing for treatment of recurrent ventricular tachyarrhythmias in the absence of heart block. Am Heart J 76:168, 1968
6. Dreifus LS, McKnight EH, Katz M, Likoff W: Digitalis intolerance. Geriatrics 18:494, 1963
7. Ewy GA, Groves BM, Ball MF, Nimmo L, Jackson B, Marcus FI: Digoxin metabolism in obesity. Circulation 44:810, 1971
8. Ewy GA, Kapadia GG, Yao L, Lullin M, Marcus FI: Digoxin metabolism in the elderly. Circulation 39:449, 1969
9. Gallagher JJ, Gilbert M, Svenson RH, Sealy WC, Kasell J, Wallace AG: Wolff–Parkinson–White syndrome. The problem, evaluation and surgical correction. Circulation 51:767, 1975
10. Gibson D, Sowton E: The use of beta-adrenergic receptor blocking drugs in dysrhythmias. Prog Cardiovasc Dis 12:16, 1969
11. Gilbert R, Cuddy RP: Digitalis intoxication following conversion to sinus rhythm. Circulation 32:58, 1965
12. Greenblatt DJ, Duhme DW, Koch–Weser J, Smith TW: Evaluation of digoxin bioavailability in single-dose studies. N Engl J Med 289:651, 1973
13. Grossman JI, Lubow LA, Frieden J, Rubin IL: Lidocaine in cardiac arrhythmias. Arch Intern Med 121:396, 1968
14. Helfant RH, Seuffert GW, Patton RD, Stein E, Damato AN: Clinical use of diphenylhydantoin (dilantin) in the treatment and prevention of cardiac arrhythmias. Am Heart J 77:315, 1969
15. Huffman DH, Azarnoff DL: Absorption of orally given digoxin preparations. JAMA 222:957, 1972
16. Irons GV Jr, Orgain ES: Digitalis-induced arrhythmias and their management. Prog Cardiovasc Dis 8:539, 1966
17. Jelliffe RW: An improved method of digoxin therapy. Ann Intern Med 69:703, 1968
18. Jelliffe RW, Buell J, Kalaba R, Sridhar R, Rockwell R, Wagner JG: An improved method of digitoxin therapy. Ann Intern Med 72:453, 1970
19. Kleiger R, Lown B: Cardioversion and digitalis. II. Clinical studies. Circulation 33:878, 1966
20. Lindenbaum J, Mellow MH, Blackstone MO, Butler VP Jr: Variation in biologic availability of digoxin from four preparations. N Engl J Med 285:1344, 1971
21. Lister JW, Cohen LS, Bernstein WH, Samet P: Treatment of supraventricular tachycardias by rapid atrial stimulation. Circulation 38:1044, 1968
22. Lown B, Klein MD, Barr I, Hagemeijer F, Kosowsky BO, Garrison H: Sensitivity to digitalis drugs in acute myocardial infarction. Am J Cardiol 30:388, 1972
23. Lown B, Wyatt NF, Levine HD: Paroxysmal atrial tachycardia with block. Circulation 21:129, 1960

24. Lukas DS, DeMartino AG: Binding of digitoxin and some related cardenolides to human plasma proteins. J Clin Invest 48:1041, 1969

25. Marcus FI, Burkhalter L, Lucchi C, Pavlovich J, Kopadia GG: Administration of tritiated digoxin with and without a loading dose. Circulation 34:865, 1966

26. Pick A, Dominguez P: Nonparoxysmal A–V nodal tachycardia. Circulation 16:1022, 1957

27. Rosen M, Lisak R, Rubin IL: Diphenylhydantoin in cardiac arrhythmias. Am J Cardiol 20:674, 1967

28. Rosenbaum MB, Elizari MV, Lazzari JO: Mechanism of bidirectional tachycardia. Am Heart J 78:4, 1969

29. Seller RH, Cangiano J, Kim KE, Mendelssohn S, Brest AN, Swartz C: Digitalis toxicity and hypomagnesemia. Am Heart J 79:57, 1970

30. Smith TW: Radioimmunoassay for serum digitoxin concentration: methodology and clinical experience. J Pharmacol Exp Ther 175:352, 1970

31. Smith TW: Contribution of quantitative assay technics to the understanding of the clinical pharmacology of digitalis. Circulation 46:188, 1972

32. Smith TW, Butler VP Jr, Haber E: Determination of serum digotin concentrations by radioimmunoassay. N Engl J Med 281:1212, 1969

33. Smith TW, Haber E: Digoxin intoxication: the relationship of clinical presentation to serum digoxin concentration. J Clin Invest 49:2377, 1970

34. Vassaux C, Lown B: Cardioversion of supraventricular tachycardias. Circulation 39:791, 1969

35. Von Capeller D, Copeland GD, Stern TN: Digitalis intoxication: a clinical report of 148 cases. Ann Intern Med 50:869, 1959

10 | # Treatment of Atrioventricular Block

JOHN A. KASTOR
MARK E. JOSEPHSON

The fundamental treatment for permanent symptomatic atrioventricular (AV) block is ventricular pacemaking. Drugs occasionally are useful, but pacemaking remains our principal mode of therapy. The application of pacemaking has become so routine and the complications so infrequent that the physician's principal task in treating patients with AV block is to recognize the condition and then to select those patients for whom pacemaking is indicated.

In recent years our approach to the patient with AV block has been increasingly influenced by developments in clinical cardiac electrophysiology brought about by the introduction of His bundle electrocardiography and the concept of the hemiblocks. In this discussion of the treatment of AV block these developments and their relevance to the clinical setting of AV block will be described in some detail. (24)

HIS BUNDLE RECORDINGS

Although the His bundle (H) electrogram had been recorded previously in man, the technique was not popularized in this country until 1969 (15, 59, 65). The electrode catheter is usually inserted percutaneously through the femoral vein and positioned near the tricuspid valve under fluoroscopic control. An arm vein approach has also been developed (13, 43). Fluoroscopy is not essential if a balloon-type electrode catheter is employed (38).

In patients with a normal conduction system, three deflections are usually recorded (Fig. 10–1). The atrial (A) wave, which reflects depolarization of the low right atrium, appears within the P wave after its onset. The other high amplitude spike is the ventricular (V) deflection produced by depolarization of ventricular myocardium near the catheter. The His bundle record is a low amplitude deflection appearing between the A and V waves and produced by rapid transmission of the electric impulse through that structure.

Two intervals have particular clinical importance. The AH interval reflects the time of conduction from low right atrium to bundle of His. The principal structure lying in this path is the AV node, and prolongation beyond normal of the AH interval indicates, for the most part, abnormally slow AV nodal conduction. The most widely accepted normal AH interval range for adults in sinus rhythm is 60–140 msec.

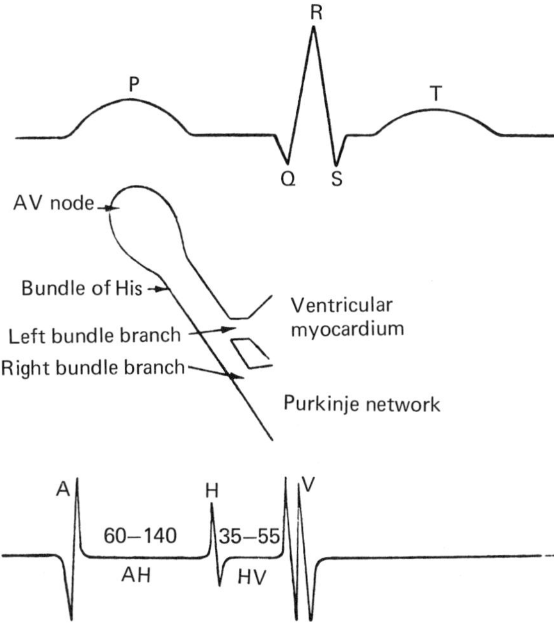

Fig. 10–1.   **A diagrammatic presentation of the bundle of His electrogram and its relation- ships. One beat of the surface electrogram is shown above and the His bundle electrogram (HBE) below. In the middle is a drawing of the AV junction aligned to correspond spacially with the temporal events of AV conduction. The atrial depolarization (A) wave detected in the HBE at the floor of the right atrium occurs after onset of the P wave, and just before the activation front enters the AV node. Notice that transmission across the AV node begins during atrial activation. If conduction within the AV node is normal the AH interval measures 60–140 msec. The activation signal enters the bundle of His later in the PR segment, and the His bundle deflection usually is seen between the P wave and the beginning of QRS. Conduc- tion within the His bundle, bundle branches, and Purkinje network is reflected by the HV interval, which terminates with the onset of ventricular activation detected from the surface ECG or V wave of the HBE. The most commonly accepted normal range for the HV interval is 35–55 msec.**

The HV interval (normal 35–55 msec in adults) corresponds, albeit somewhat imprecisely, to the conduction time from depolarization of the bundle of His to the beginning of ventricular myocardial activation. Prolon- gation of the HV interval implies that conduction from His bundle to the ventricles is delayed, an abnormality usually called infranodal block. Inves- tigators have suggested different normal values, due in part to variations in catheter position and deflection measurement (16). Consequently, at cer- tain ranges what is normal to some may be pathologic to others, and *vice versa.*

Finally, in addition to block in the AV node and the bundle-branch-Purkinje system, conduction within the bundle of His can also be estimated, with the His deflection itself used as the indicator of malfunction. The bundle of His is assumed to be functioning normally when the width of the His deflection is 25 msec or less. When His conduction is impaired the deflection becomes wider or split (19,41,48,60).

HEMIBLOCKS (FASCICULAR BLOCKS)

The infra-AV nodal specialized conducting system can be visualized as consisting of the bundle of His plus three intraventricular fascicles: 1) the right bundle branch, 2) the anterior (superior) division of the left bundle branch, and 3) the posterior (inferior) division of the left bundle branch. Whether or not the left bundle really parts into two discrete anatomic divisions in man has not been settled, but functionally this separation is a useful concept.

Left anterior hemiblock (LAH), a term introduced by Rosenbaum, (or fascicular block as preferred by others) describes a physiologic block in the anterior division of the left bundle branch (47,54). This abnormality is recognized in the electrocardiogram by the presence of abnormal left axis deviation (LAD) in the frontal plane. The electrocardiographic diagnosis of the hemiblocks may require the presence of additional features other than just abnormal axis deviation, but in most cases this will suffice. Rosenbaum suggests that the deviation be greater than $-45°$ for the diagnosis of LAH, although he concedes this to be an arbitrary recommendation. (54) One must be cautious in making the diagnosis of LAH when LAD appears with inferior myocardial infarction, or lung disease, either of which may produce LAD without block apparently being present in the anterior division.

Left posterior hemiblock (LPH), or fascicular block, is recognized by abnormal axis deviation to the right of about $+120°$ in the frontal plane, and indicates impairment of conduction in the posterior division of the left bundle branch (54). Left posterior hemiblock should be assigned with caution in the presence of anterolateral myocardial infarction, right ventricular hypertrophy, or a slender body build. The diagnosis of LPH can be made with greater certainty if the finding is recorded intermittently, and in most instances requires careful clinical-electocardiographic correlation.

Right bundle branch block (RBBB) can be produced in many normal people by the introduction of early atrial premature depolarizations. If such beats do not block in the AV node, they may find the right bundle branch partially or wholly refractory and a beat with RBBB will appear. The higher frequency of right bundle branch aberration with such testing suggests that the right branch has a longer refractory period than the left. Within the left bundle branch itself the anterior division conducts less readily than the posterior division, an observation which correlates with the more frequent finding of LAH than LPH when the conduction system is stressed with coupled atrial premature depolarizations (5).

BIFASCICULAR AND TRIFASCICULAR BLOCK

RIGHT BUNDLE BRANCH BLOCK

The concept of the hemiblocks has helped to explain why some patients with obstruction of two fascicles develop complete AV block. Thus when a patient has RBBB and LAH, complete AV block may be anticipated if the bundle of

His and/or posterior division in addition to the anterior division also fail to conduct. The incidence of RBBB and LAD has been reported to be 1% of patients in a large New York hospital. The progression to AV block in such patients was 10%, and may be as high as 6%/year according to a more recent study (29, 31). In the New York series, RBBB and LAD was the most common QRS morphology (59%) in the conducted beats of patients with a high degree of heart block.

Much of the recent electrophysiologic work in patients with RBBB and LAH has been conducted to answer the question: Who will develop atrioventricular block? Although data from different investigators are in conflict, information from two series could lead one to conclude that patients with HV intervals of 75 msec or more, and who have RBBB plus LAH or even just RBBB alone, are at particular risk of dying suddenly, presumably from an episode of complete block (42, 58). How often ventricular fibrillation rather than block is the cause of death in such patients is not known (7).

Even more potentially dangerous though much less common, is the combination of RBBB and LPH. The posterior division is the more stable fascicle and consequently less likely to fail. Thus, when it is blocked, conduction will be maintained over the more vulnerable anterior division which usually in time will also block. Rosenbaum has concluded that, "*Every* case of RBBB with LPH can be considered as a forerunner of complete heart block" (Italics added) (54). Other investigators have suggested that the likelihood of this progression has been exaggerated (8).

LEFT BUNDLE BRANCH BLOCK

Left bundle branch block implies more conduction system disease than right bundle branch block alone, in that patients with LBBB have abnormal conduction in both the anterior and posterior division of the left bundle, or in the short common left bundle itself. Many patients with LBBB may also have impaired conduction in the right bundle branch, although the incidence has not yet been fully established (3). The HV interval in patients with left bundle branch block is usually at least slightly prolonged (3, 49, 53).

CATEGORIES OF AV BLOCK

The amount of AV block is still subdivided into three degrees: First degree, identified by a prolonged PR interval; second degree, with intermittently dropped ventricular beats; and third degree, in which AV conduction is entirely absent and the ventricles are driven independently by a nonatrial pacemaker. With the information supplied by His bundle electrocardiography, AV block has been separated into that which is caused by pathology of 1) the AV node (AV nodal block) and 2) the His-bundle-branch-Purkinje system (infranodal block).

Mobitz first called attention to two types of second degree atrioventricular block on the electrocardiogram (39). His type I block usually reflects disease in the AV node, whereas Mobitz type II block is associated with disease of the His-bundle-branch-Purkinje tissues. This separation has physiologic, pathologic, and clinical relevance, and is useful in clarifying many aspects of AV block (2, 14).

AV NODAL BLOCK

FIRST DEGREE AV BLOCK

First degree AV block on the electrocardiogram usually signifies delay in AV nodal conduction, with a prolonged AH interval (Fig. 10–2). This is almost always the case when the QRS is normal, or when unifascicular block of the right bundle or of the anterior division of the left bundle is present (45, 53).

The AV node has the property of decremental conduction and produces delay when impulses try to cross it (22). In health this delay accounts for a large portion of the PR interval. When the AV node is diseased the transit time of an impulse originating in the sinus node may be sizable, resulting in the familiar prolonged PR interval of first degree AV block. The infranodal tissues are not able to sustain much prolongation of conduction without blocking. Thus except in unusual circumstances, the PR interval increases only slightly if at all when conduction disease develops in the His-bundle-branch-Purkinje system.

SECOND DEGREE AV NODAL BLOCK

When second degree AV nodal block develops, the Wenckebach phenomenon is frequently seen (67). This familiar pattern is recognized by the ap-

Fig. 10–2.   **First degree AV nodal block. In Leads I, II, III, and V$_1$, the PR interval is long (320 msec) and the QRS duration is normal (90 msec). The high right atrial electrogram (HRA) shows that P waves are not hidden within QRS (as found, for example, in atrial tachycardia with 2:1 AV nodal block), a finding frequently overlooked when first degree block is present. Conduction within the AV node is prolonged (AH interval of 250 msec). Infranodal conduction is normal (intraventricular block is absent and the HV interval is 45 msec).**

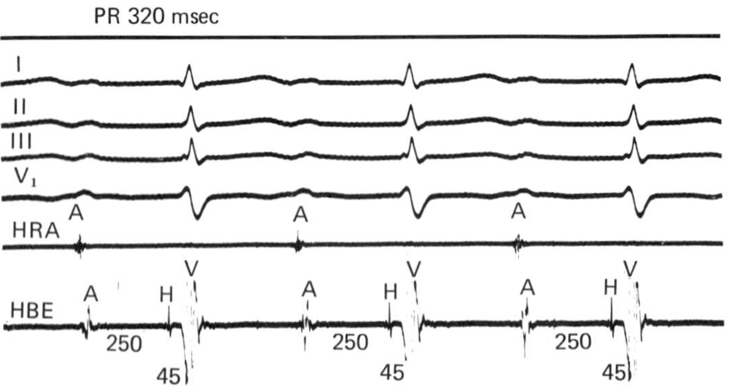

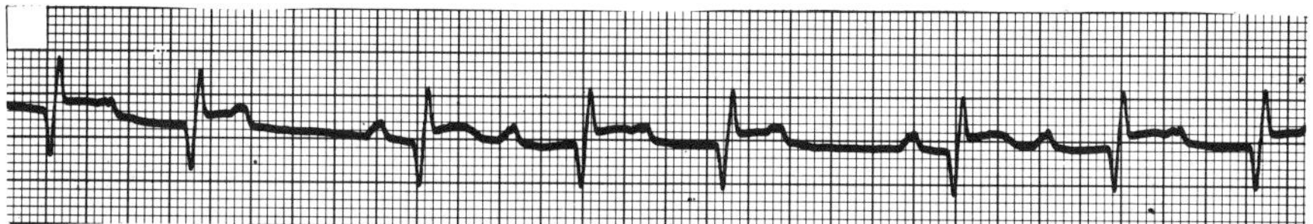

Fig. 10–3.   Second degree AV nodal (type I) block with Wenckebach periods in a patient with an inferior myocardial infarction. The PR intervals progressively prolong until a P wave is dropped. The block is located in the AV node.

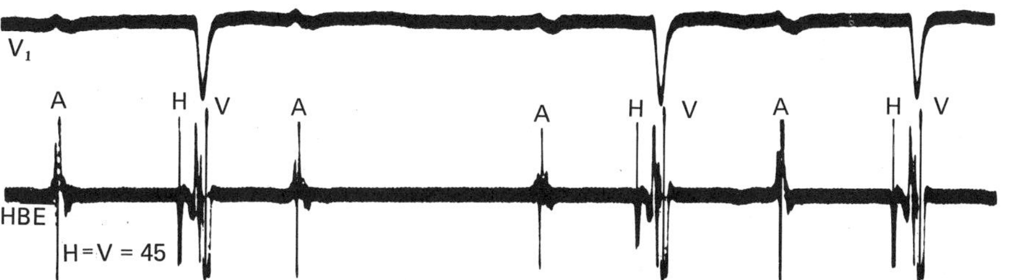

Fig. 10–4.   His bundle electrogram of second degree type I AV nodal block with Wenckebach periods. Lead V$_1$ and the HBE are shown. Notice that the PR interval progressively prolongs until a P wave and A deflection stand alone without conduction to the bundle of His and ventricles. Infranodal conduction is normal (HV interval equals 45 msec).

Fig. 10–5.   Two-to-one second degree AV nodal block is illustrated. Note that unifascicular block in the form of left anterior hemiblock is present (S wave greater than R wave in Lead II), but that bundle branch block is absent (QRS width equals 100 msec). In the His bundle electrogram the impulse from the atrium (A wave) blocks before reaching the bundle of His for every second beat.

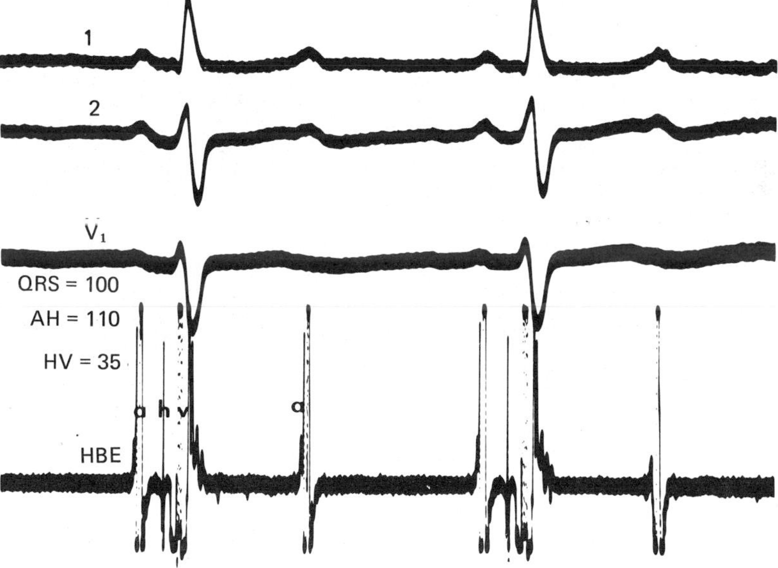

pearance of progressively longer PR intervals, followed by a dropped ventricular beat (Fig. 10–3). Sometimes the PR interval changes relatively little before the dropped beat, but careful examination will reveal that the last PR interval before the pause is longer than the first PR interval after the pause. A His bundle electrogram can almost always settle the question by the demonstration of prolonged AH intervals and a lone A wave without a bundle of His deflection when the ventricular beat is dropped (Fig. 10–4). Second degree type I block may also present as fixed 2:1 block (Fig. 10–5). Although QRS width is usually less than 110 msec when AV nodal block develops, bundle branch or fascicular block may coexist and complicate the diagnosis (8, 35).

Whereas Wenckebach periodicity has been observed occasionally in infranodal tissues, it is the AV node which characteristically responds in this manner when stressed pathologically by disease or electrically by rapid atrial pacing.

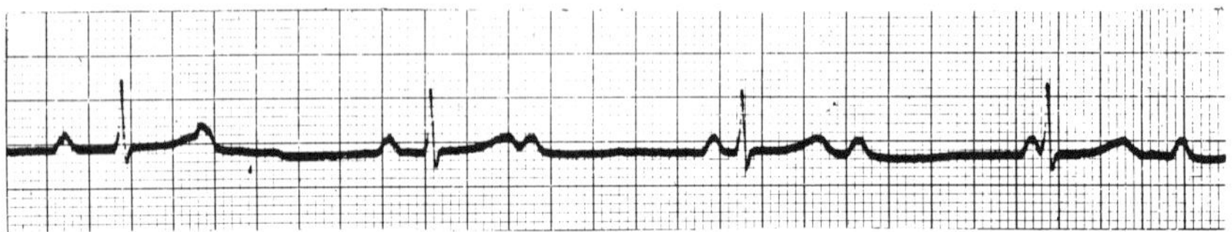

Fig. 10–6.   ECG of congenital third degree AV nodal block. The ventricular rate of 41/min is typical when this condition is present in adults. The atria are in sinus rhythm at 70/min. Complete AV dissociation due to the block is present. The QRS duration of 70 msec identifies a "supraventricular", probably His bundle, origin for ventricular activation.

Fig. 10–7.   Third degree congenital AV nodal block. Shown are Leads 1, Avᴇ, V₁ and electrograms from the high right atrium (HRA) and the bundle of His (HBE). Block in the AV node is revealed by: 1) supraventricular QRS morphology, 2) narrow QRS duration of 100 msec, 3) dissociation between depolarizations of the atria (A) and bundle of His (H), 4) each QRS complex preceded by a His depolarization. Infranodal block is not present in view of the normal QRS and HV interval (40 msec). The ventricular rate is 40/min. The time markers (T) are 10 msec apart.

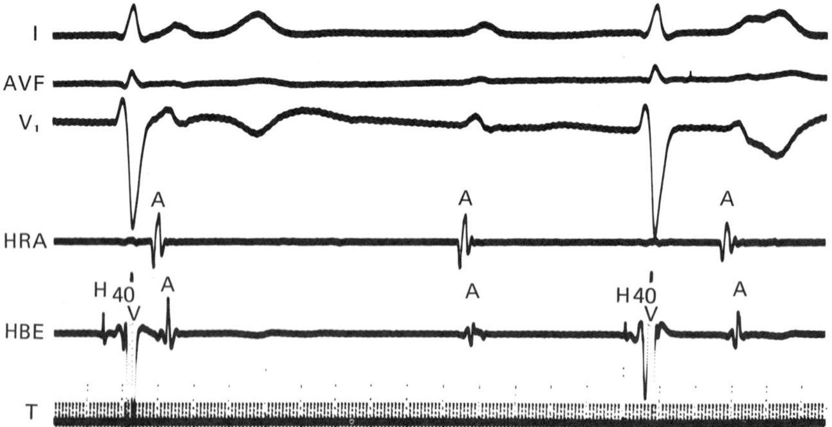

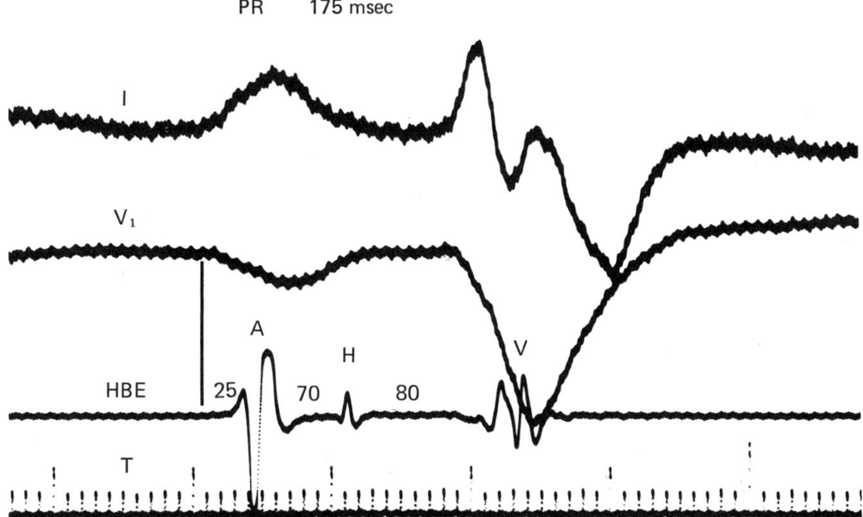

Fig. 10–8.   First degree infranodal block with a normal PR interval. In surface Leads 1 and V₁ an unusual left bundle branch block-like pattern is seen with QRS duration of 180 msec. (The very rapid recording speed has greatly expanded all horizontal measurements; note time line (T) separation of 10 msec). The HV interval reflecting infranodal conduction is markedly prolonged (80 msec). Since conduction from high right atrium to AV node (25 msec) and through the AV node (AH interval=70 msec) are normal, the total PR interval is only 175 msec, "normal" by traditional criteria.

Fig. 10–9.   First degree infranodal atrioventricular and bifascicular intraventricular block. In Leads I, II, and V₁ first degree AV block (PR interval of 245 msec), right bundle branch block (QRS duration 160 msec), and left anterior hemiblock are seen. From the surface ECG the location of the first degree AV block cannot be determined with certainty. The His bundle electrogram (HBE) reveals the block to be infranodal (HV interval of 100 msec). Conduction within the AV node (AH interval of 105 msec) is normal. This patient is at relatively high risk of developing second and third degree infranodal AV block.

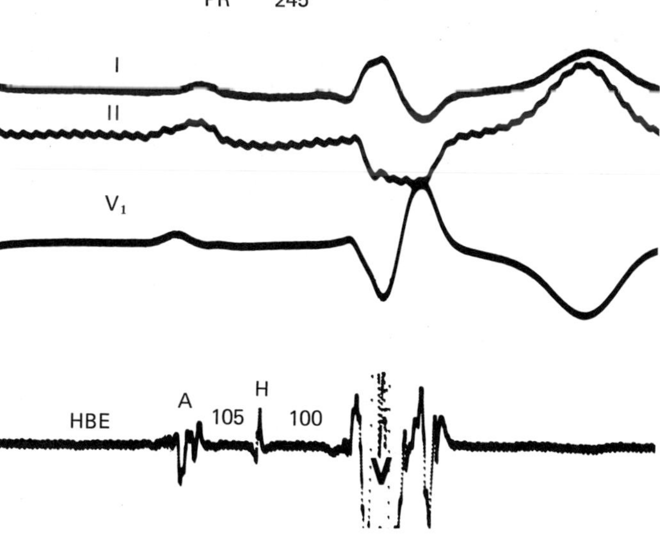

Fig. 10–10

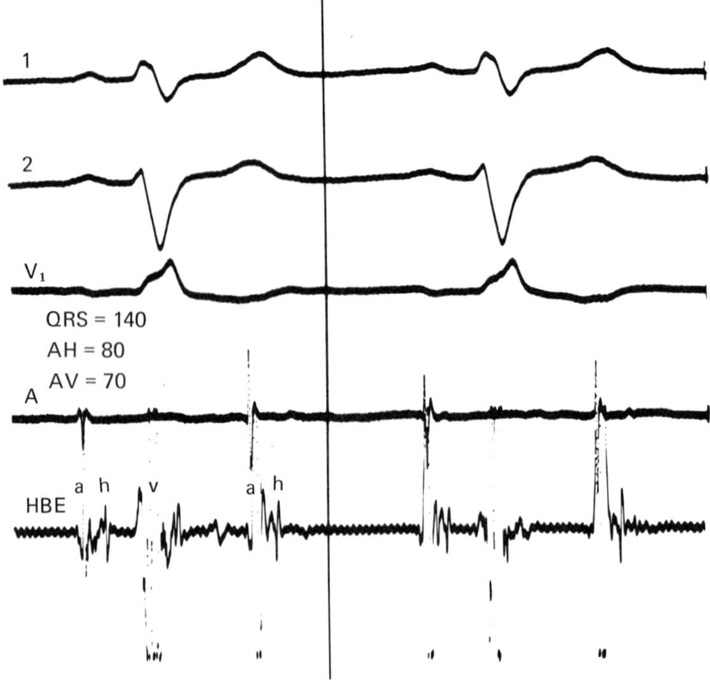

Fig. 10–11

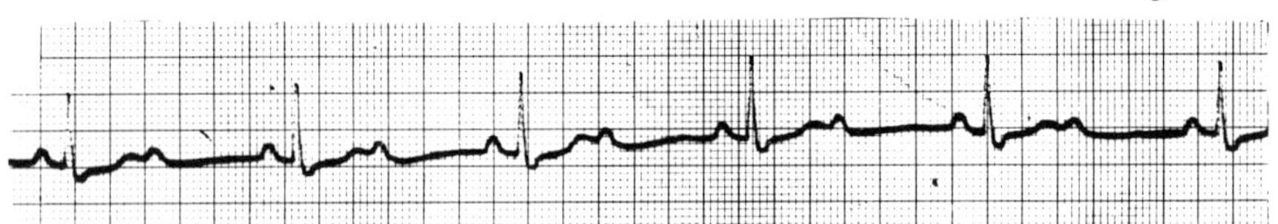

Fig. 10–12

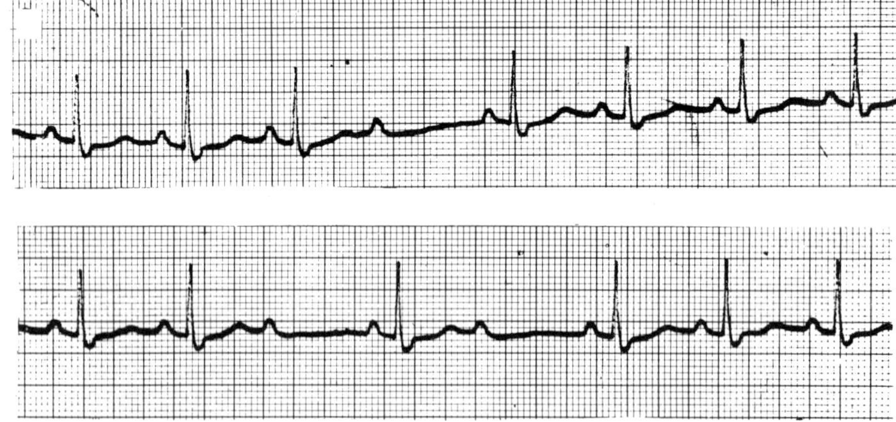

◀ *Fig. 10–10.* **Two-to-one infranodal AV block. From Leads I, II, and V$_1$ right bundle branch block and left anterior hemiblock can be observed. In the His bundle electrogram a prolonged HV interval (70 msec) is seen in the conducted beats. Following the second and fourth P waves, block occurs below the location where the His bundle electrogram is recorded. The blocked P waves, buried in the T waves, are identified on the atrial electrogram. The 2:1 block is located in either the posterior division of the left bundle branch or possibly the bundle of His. The right bundle branch and the anterior division of the left bundle branch are continuously blocked.**

THIRD DEGREE AV NODAL BLOCK

The most easily recognized example of this abnormality is complete congenital AV block when atria and ventricles are totally dissociated (Fig. 10–6) (27). The QRS morphology is usually "supraventricular" since the escape focus is either in the lower AV node (NH region) or His bundle. This "higher" escape focus dominates, rather than one in the ventricles, because of the inherently more rapid discharge rate of AV junctional pacemaking tissue. On the His bundle electrogram the A deflections are not followed by His deflections, which are seen preceding the V deflections (Fig. 10–7). With complete AV nodal block in adults, the ventricular escape rate averages 44/min (52). Although bundle branch or fascicular block may be present because of associated infranodal pathology, QRS width is usually less than 110 msec (52).

Atrioventricular nodal block is often a reversible lesion. It commonly occurs in digitalis intoxication, inferior myocardial infarction, myocarditis (including rheumatic fever), and following cardiac surgery. Most of the inciting causes of transient AV nodal block have inflammatory components, which in addition to delaying conduction in the node, also accelerate the escape focus lower within the node or the His bundle. Under such circumstances the regular ventricular rate may be in the normal range of 60–90, despite complete atrioventricular dissociation.

INFRA-NODAL BLOCK

FIRST DEGREE INFRANODAL BLOCK

First degree infranodal block may not be recognized on the electrocardiogram since slight but important HV prolongation alone may still leave the PR interval within the normal range (Fig. 10–8)(45). The HV interval does not, as a rule, prolong as much as the AH interval before the QRS is dropped. HV

◀ *Fig. 10–11.* **Two-to-one AV block is shown on this Lead II electrocardiogram. Identification of the site of block cannot be determined with certainty unless a sequence of conducted beats can be seen (see Fig. 10–12). Right bundle branch block suggests the presence of some infranodal disease, but unifascicular block may also be coincidentally found with AV nodal block.**

◀ *Fig. 10–12.* **Infranodal (type II) second degree AV block can now be identified since the PR intervals, which are normal, do not change before and after the dropped P wave.**

prolongation is likely to be found when bifascicular disease is present, as in: RBBB and LAH (over 50%); RBBB and LPH (nearly always); or LBBB (nearly always) (Fig. 10–9) (3, 44, 49, 53).

SECOND DEGREE INFRANODAL BLOCK

This variety of block, called Mobitz type II second degree AV block, is identified on the His bundle electrogram by an AH interval which does not change. In the dropped beat the AH combination is not followed by the V deflection of QRS. The HV interval of the conducted beats is usually prolonged (Fig.–10).

The electrocardiogram in the patient with second degree infranodal block usually has characteristics which guide one in localizing the region of block (2,30). The PR intervals are either normal or slightly prolonged, but do not measurably change in the conducted beats both before and after the dropped beats. If 2.1 block is present, a differentiation between AV nodal and infranodal block cannot be made (Fig. 10–11). At least two consecutive conducted beats must be seen in order to properly evaluate the status of the PR intervals (Fig. 10–12). In QRS morphology, fascicular and/or bundle branch block is usually present since infranodal block commonly occurs within the bundle branches (Fig. 10–12). The general rule usually applies: narrow QRS suggests AV nodal block; wide QRS suggests infranodal block (plus possible AV nodal block if the PR interval is prolonged in the conducted beats).

Mobitz type II second degree infranodal block is usually progressive. Most patients with this finding eventually develop higher degrees of AV block. This course stands in contrast to many patients with Mobitz type I second degree AV nodal block, in whom the abnormality is reversible (30).

THIRD DEGREE INFRANODAL BLOCK

Patients who die with third degree infranodal block have severe pathologic lesions in all three fascicles, and/or the His bundle itself (6,45,52,61). The cause of this process is unknown in many cases, although sometimes coronary artery disease is found. When myocardial infarction produces infranodal block, the anterior surface is more commonly involved. The bundle branches and fascicles themselves undergo ischemic destruction following occlusion, usually of the left anterior descending coronary artery.

In complete infranodal block the ventricles are driven by an intrinsic pacemaker, usually located in the bundle-branch-Purkinje system below the site of block. Therefore, the QRS will have a wide configuration as the ventricles are depolarized in an abnormal sequence (Fig. 10–13). The rate of such ventricular escape focuses is relatively slow, ranging from 15–47/min, with an average of 35/min according to one series (52). Such intrinsic pacemakers are also relatively unstable and may fail to discharge, giving rise to Morgagni-Adams-Stokes attacks. When a His bundle recording is made in a patient with third degree infranodal AV block, the A spike is followed by a His deflection, but this AH couplet is unrelated to the slower V deflections (Fig. 10–14).

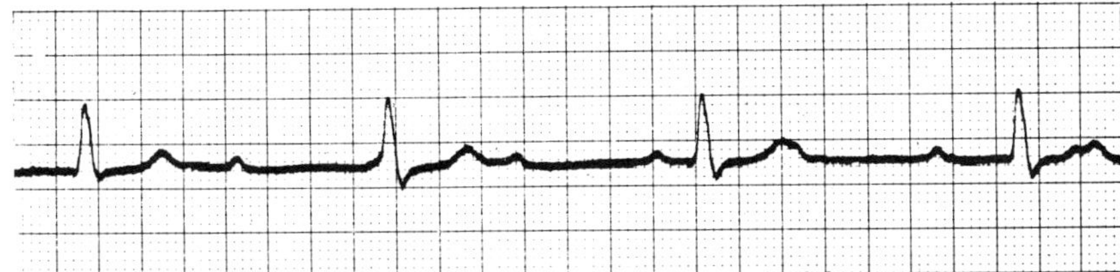

Fig. 10–13.   **ECG of third degree infranodal AV block in a 63-year-old man whose previous electrocardiograms had shown left bundle branch block. Presumably right bundle branch block then developed, producing complete trifascicular AV block. Note that the QRS duration is 160 msec and the ventricular rate is 40. His bundle study revealed normal AV nodal function (AH interval 100 msec), but complete dissociation between the AH couplets and the V waves. (Compare with Fig. 10–6)**

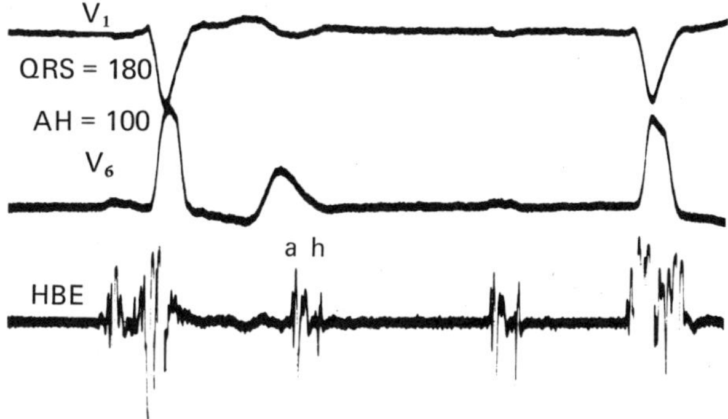

Fig. 10–14.   **Third degree infranodal AV block. There is no relation between the P waves and QRS complexes. Each A wave is followed by a His deflection with block occurring below the bundle of His. The ventricles are driven by an intrinsic pacemaker in the right ventricle, as shown by the presence of a "left bundle branchlike" QRS complex in leads V_1 and V_6.**

Fig. 10–15.   **Type II second degree block within the bundle of His. Shown are Lead V_1 and a His bundle electrogram. Within the AV interval the H deflection is split into two parts (H and H′), a sign of delayed conduction within the bundle of His. The second P wave is followed by the first of the His deflections, and the impulse then blocks within the bundle. Note that in addition to the intraHis block, right bundle branch block is present. The HV interval is slightly prolonged at 60 msec.**

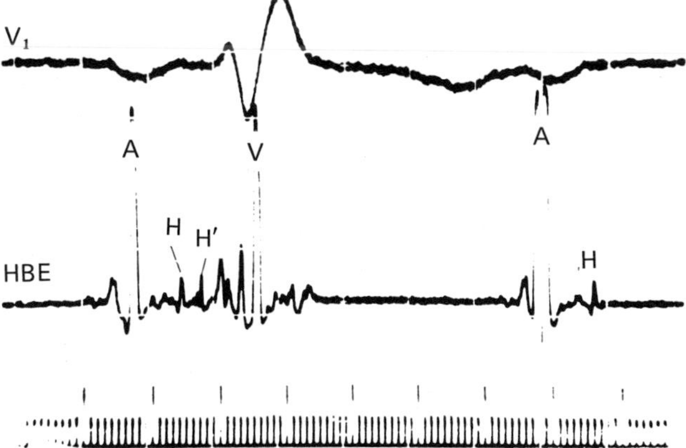

INTRA-HIS BLOCK

Although infrequently identified on the electrocardiogram, block within the bundle of His itself (intra-His block) is not rare (52). It usually appears as Mobitz type II second degree block or complete infranodal block. The principal distinguishing electrocardiographic feature is that the QRS may be narrow or supraventricular in form, and bundle branch or fascicular block need not be present (19,41,48,60). This is so because the block occurs above the bifurcation into the bundle branches. Wenckebach periods are seldom seen because the bundle of His functions like bundle-branch-Purkinje tissue rather than like the AV node. However, since the intrinsic pacemaker may be low in the His bundle and relatively high in the specialized conduction tissue, the escape rate in patients with third degree intra-His block is faster than when the block is lower within the bundle-branch-Purkinje tissues. An average rate of 45/min has been reported (52).

Intra-His block is infrequently recognized on the electrocardiogram because bundle branch, unifascicular, or bifascicular block may be present along with the abnormality within the His bundle itself. Only with an intracardiac record can the diagnosis then be made with the demonstration of a wide or split bundle of His deflection (Fig. 10–15). For clinical purposes the differentiation between intra-His block and bundle-branch-Purkinje block is not critical, since their clinical course appears to be similar. Most, if not all, patients with second degree infranodal block will develop complete AV block, and are at risk of Morgagni-Adams-Stokes attacks and sudden cardiac death.

EXCEPTIONS TO THE GENERAL RULES

A few cases have been reported of type II block within the AV node. Additional observations and review of published data suggest that many, if not all of these patients, actually had type I block as expected (2,48). Type I block has been conclusively demonstrated in the bundle branches, but this finding is uncommon (45). For practical purposes it can be stated that in humans type I block is produced in the AV node and type II block, below the AV node, either within the bundle of His or the bundle branches. Furthermore, when the QRS is narrow (less than 110 msec), the block will be AV nodal, or less frequently within the bundle of His, and when the QRS is wide the block is more likely to be infranodal (10,52).

For the sake of precision and in view of recent data, it must be added that some of the distinctions between type I and type II block may be more apparent than real. Small prolongations in the PR interval have been detected in typical Mobitz type II block with rapid recording speed of the ECG record and careful measurement (11). It appears that the infranodal structures, like the AV node, function with progressive delay, although special techniques are required to demonstrate this property (25). For clinical purposes the differentiation of Mobitz remains extremely useful.

AV BLOCK IN ACUTE MYOCARDIAL INFARCTION-ANATOMIC CORRELATIONS

It has long been thought that the AV node is usually involved when heart block complicates inferior myocardial infarction, and the His-Bundle-Branch-Purkinje tissues suffer when the block develops in patients with anterior infarction. His bundle electrograms have confirmed these assumptions. The explanation can be found in a review of the pertinent coronary anatomy.

INFERIOR MYOCARDIAL INFARCTION

Inferior myocardial infarction is usually caused by occlusion of the right coronary artery (85–90% of patients), or the left circumflex coronary artery (10–15% of patients) (23). The AV node itself is supplied by whichever of these two vessels perfuses the posterior portion of the interventricular septum and left ventricle. Thus the AV node perfusing artery will often be occluded during the course of an inferior myocardial infarction. Whether or not block develops depends upon collateral blood supply to the AV node, among other factors.

Histopathologic studies have shown that conduction defects in this setting are usually due to ischemia rather than necrosis of the atrium, AV node, and proximal His bundle (32,62). This helps explain the clinical observation that conduction defects in inferior myocardial infarction are often transient (55).

ANTERIOR MYOCARDIAL INFARCTION

Since the mortality is high it is fortunate that heart block uncommonly complicates anterior myocardial infarction. Even with the ventricular rate controlled by pacemaking, most patients will die from cardiogenic shock because of the large amount of ventricular myocardium which has been destroyed (4,46). The coronary artery usually involved is the left anterior descending, with or without the left circumflex. The His bundle, bundle branches and Purkinje tissues malfunction because septal, and right and left ventricular tissues in which they lie are infarcted. For complete AV block to develop, in most cases both bundle branches must cease to conduct, and this usually requires rather widespread destruction. Thus even when ventricular rhythm is maintained by pacing, power failure or irreversible ventricular fibrillation may seal the patient's fate (4).

INDICATIONS FOR PACEMAKER TREATMENT

The loss of normal atrioventricular conduction in heart block may produce: 1) decreased cardiac output with inadequate perfusion and congestive failure; 2) ventricular asystole with abrupt loss of central nervous system function; 3) myocardial ischemia in patients with concurrent coronary artery disease; and 4) ventricular irritability with the appearance of premature beats, ventricular tachycardia, or ventricular fibrillation. Clearly when any of these developments result from AV block, ventricular pacing is indicated either temporarily or permanently (Table 10–1).

AV NODAL BLOCK

First degree AV nodal block almost never requires pacemaker treatment. Even when the block is permanent regular evaluation is sufficient to observe when and if the block progresses to a higher degree. The decision regarding treatment of patients with second and third degree AV nodal block requires a careful evaluation of the clinical condition of the patient and an estimate regarding the temporary or permanent character of the block. As a general rule pacing is required infrequently because the abnormality usually passes in time and the ventricular rate, thanks to AV junctional acceleration, may be sufficiently rapid to maintain relatively normal cardiac function at rest.

The dilemma about treatment when AV nodal block is present arises most frequently when heart block complicates inferior myocardial infarction. The following approach has been found helpful. First eliminate the possibility that the block results from vagotonia by careful intravenous administration of atro-

Table 10–1. PACEMAKER THERAPY OF ATRIOVENTRICULAR CONDUCTION DEFECTS*

Conduction defect	Temporary pacing recommended during acute myocardial infarction	Permanent pacing recommended
First degree AV nodal block alone	No	No
Second degree AV Nodal block alone	No**	No
Third degree AV nodal block alone	No**	No
First degree infra nodal block alone	Yes†	No
Second degree infra nodal block alone	Yes	Yes
Third degree infra nodal block alone	Yes	Yes
RBBB alone	No	No
RBBB and LAH‡	Yes	No§
RBBB and LPH‡	Yes	No†
LAH alone	No	No
LPH alone‡	Yes†	No†
LBBB alone‡	Yes†	No

* In general pacing is indicated if symptoms due to block are documented or strongly suspected.
** Temporary pacemaking indicated in the presence of a) ventricular rate less than 50/min, b) persistent or recurring chest pain, c) ventricular irritability, d) congestive heart failure or, e) cardiogenic shock.
† Tentative recommendation, data available currently are incomplete.
‡ If present before infarction, pacing not indicated.
§ HV prolongation greater than 75 msec documented by His bundle electrogram is probably an indication for permanent pacing.

pine in up to three 0.5 mg doses (Fig. 10–16 and 10–17). Insert a temporary pacemaker if the following should develop: 1) congestive failure or the earliest signs of cardiogenic shock; 2) a ventricular rate of less than 50/min; 3) persistent or recurring chest pains; 4) ventricular irritability. In contrast to the course in anterior infarction, bundle branch block is not a dangerous development when it appears in the setting of inferior infarction (35). Permanent pacing after recovery from heart block with inferior infarction is rarely needed (21).

When AV nodal block temporarily appears after cardiac surgery (an uncommon problem) the same criteria may be applied in deciding whether ventricular pacing is needed. Most bradycardias in this setting are due to electrophysiologic malfunction of the sinoatrial node and/or atria. When AV nodal block occurs from digitalis toxicity or myocarditis, temporary pacemaking is also seldom needed.

Patients with permanent third degree congenital AV nodal block uncommonly require pacemaking, since the escape rate is sufficiently rapid to provide adequate cardiac output for most normal activities. However, permanent acquired AV nodal block is less benign. Many of these patients have associated myocardial disease, and the slow ventricular rate may not be well tolerated (52).

Fig. 10–16. Effects of atropine on type I second degree AV nodal block. This 60-year-old man has had an inferior myocardial infarction (elevated ST segments in Lead II) and was admitted with 3:2 AV block. Two and one half hours later complete AV dissociation had appeared due to progression of the AV block (middle strip). Despite the slow ventricular rate the sinus rate had not increased, which suggests a relatively high degree of vagal tone. Atropine was given (bottom strip), and with partial relief of vagotonia 2:1 block appeared. (See Fig. 10–17)

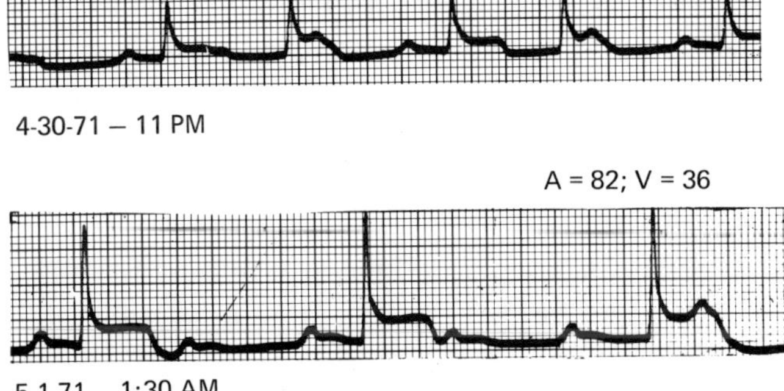

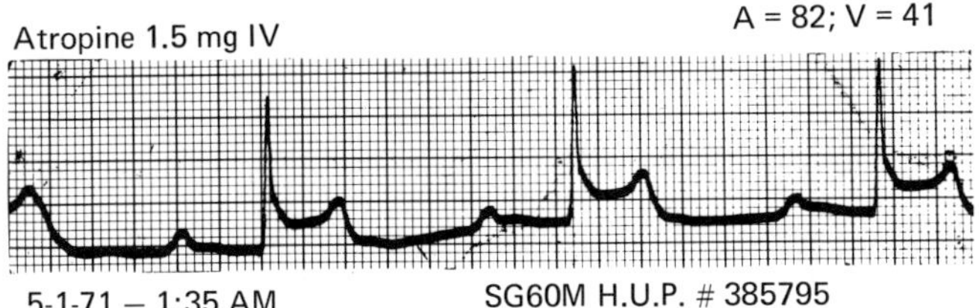

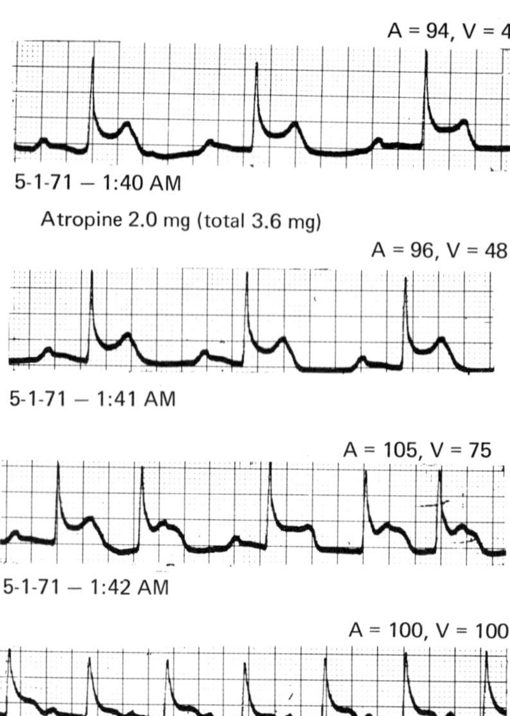

Fig. 10–17.   **Effects of atropine on type I second degree AV block, (continuation of Fig. 10–16). With additional atropine, the sinus rate speeded and the degree of block decreased until only PR prolongation remained (bottom strip). Usually only 0.5–1.0 mg, much less than 3.6 mg, is required to achieve this result. Use of atropine to relieve vagal tone as a cause of type I block will occasionally be effective, and should be tried in appropriate patients with myocardial infarction.**

INFRANODAL BLOCK

Since infranodal block is usually progressive, permanent pacemaker treatment is indicated when symptomatic second degree (Mobitz type II) and third degree infranodal block are detected. One has no hesitation in advising such treatment when patients have decreased cardiac output, congestive failure, syncope, angina, or ventricular irritability associated with the slow heart rate. In fact such decisions are quite properly made whatever may appear on an intracardiac electrogram.

ASYMPTOMATIC INFRANODAL BLOCK

The criteria for pacing are less well established for asymptomatic patients with first degree AV block plus fascicular block, or second or third degree infranodal block.

Asymptomatic patients with first degree AV block need not be paced because the PR prolongation usually reflects block within the AV node, but those with bifascicular disease should, in particular, be followed closely. If HV prolongation has been documented, especially careful observation is indicated. Syncopal or presyncopal symptoms must be evaluated promptly, since the progression to second and third degree infranodal block may be imminent.

Are there reliable methods available to predict which asymptomatic patients with fascicular disease will progress to high degrees of AV block? Opinion is divided on this point, but data are becoming available which suggest that patients with prolonged HV intervals of more than 75 msec are at greater risk of sudden death than those with normal or only slightly long HV intervals. In one series mortality was lower when pacers had been inserted in patients with bifascicular disease and long HV intervals (42). Rapid atrial pacing and programmed premature atrial stimulation have not provided much additional information other than just the HV intervals. These techniques occasionally reveal fragile infranodal conduction for which prophylactic demand pacemaker insertion might be advisable. However, patients who have normal response to such testing may develop AV block shortly thereafter (17).

The asymptomatic patient with type II second degree AV block, who only drops an occasional ventricular beat, may present the most controversial problem among all the categories of AV block. First, the diagnosis must be correctly made and confirmed by intracardiac records, if possible. It is the general experience that such patients develop third degree atrioventricular block with high regularity. It is our current belief that such patients are better served by having ventricular demand pacemakers as protection against the possibility of syncope or death. However, conclusive data in this regard are not yet available.

The conflict about pacing patients with asymptomatic third degree infranodal AV block may never be settled because pacemaking is usually established routinely. The authors and others have observed that patients who thought they were asymptomatic often find, surprisingly, that they feel much better once a faster heart rate had been established. Furthermore, the possibility of death from the first episode of ventricular asystole is prevented.

INFRANODAL AV AND FASCICULAR BLOCK IN MYOCARDIAL INFARCTION

The usual, but not exclusive, setting for this development is anterior infarction with widespread destruction of myocardium and underlying conduction tissues (20,62). Temporary pacemakers are always inserted when type II second or third degree block is recognized. Control of the ventricular rate must be obtained in these patients, who have a very high mortality and commonly die in pump failure.

When fascicular block develops acutely, the question of temporary pacing arises because type II second or third degree AV block may follow. Indications for pacing still vary among institutions, but on the basis of the data currently available, we favor the following approach. A temporary right ventricular pacemaker is inserted when intraventricular block appears in the form of: 1) **RBBB**

On admission

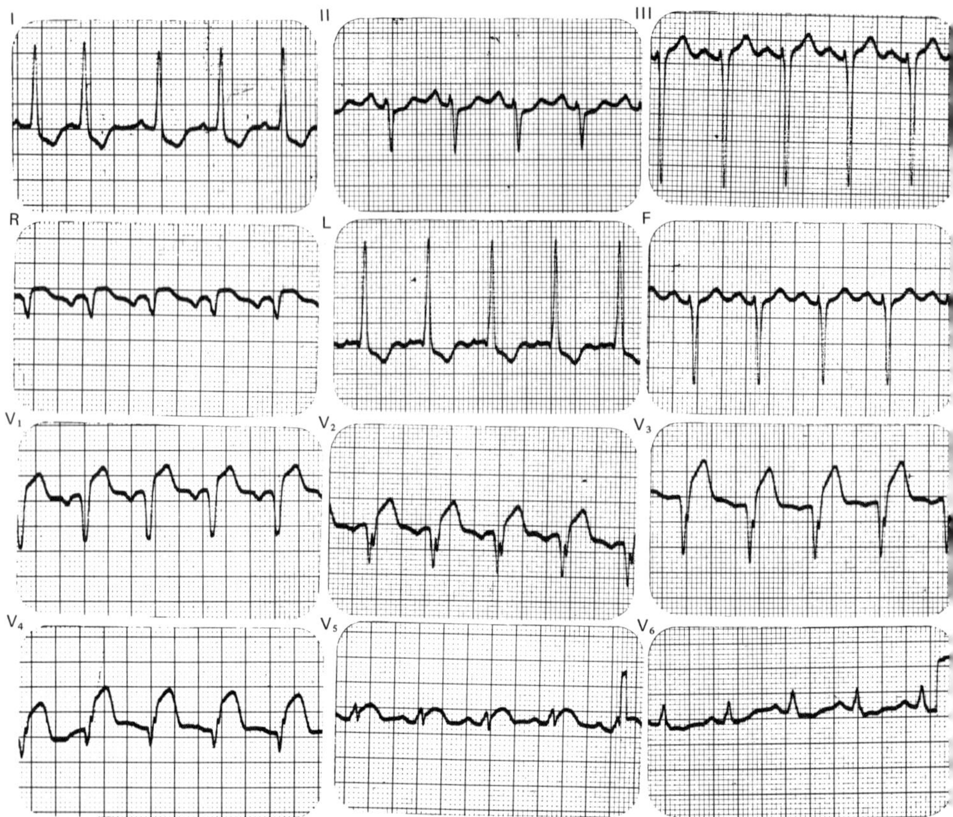

Fig. 10–18.   **ECG of left anterior hemiblock which has developed acutely in a patient with an anterior myocardial infarction.**

plu LAH (Fig. 10–18 and 10–19), 2) RBBB plus LPH (Fig. 10–20), 3) LPH alone, or 4) possibly LBBB (1,18,21,36,37,50,51,56,66). One recent study has suggested that acquired LBBB may not be a harbinger of AV block in this setting (36). The likelihood that complete infranodal block will follow is highest in those patients whose fascicular block: 1) develops within 24 hours after onset of the infarction, 2) persists for more than 6 hours, 3) is associated with a prolonged HV interval on the bundle of His electrogram (36,37). If the fascicular or bundle branch block was present before the infarction, progression to AV block is unlikely (36,37).

The prognostic importance of a prolonged PR interval in cases of myocardial infarction is uncertain and probably of lesser significance than an abnormal HV interval (1,37,57,66). This seems reasonable since much of PR interval lengthening occurs in the AV node, whereas HV prolongation, which reflects infranodal disease, may be slight, though significant, and little affect the PR interval (Fig. 10–8).

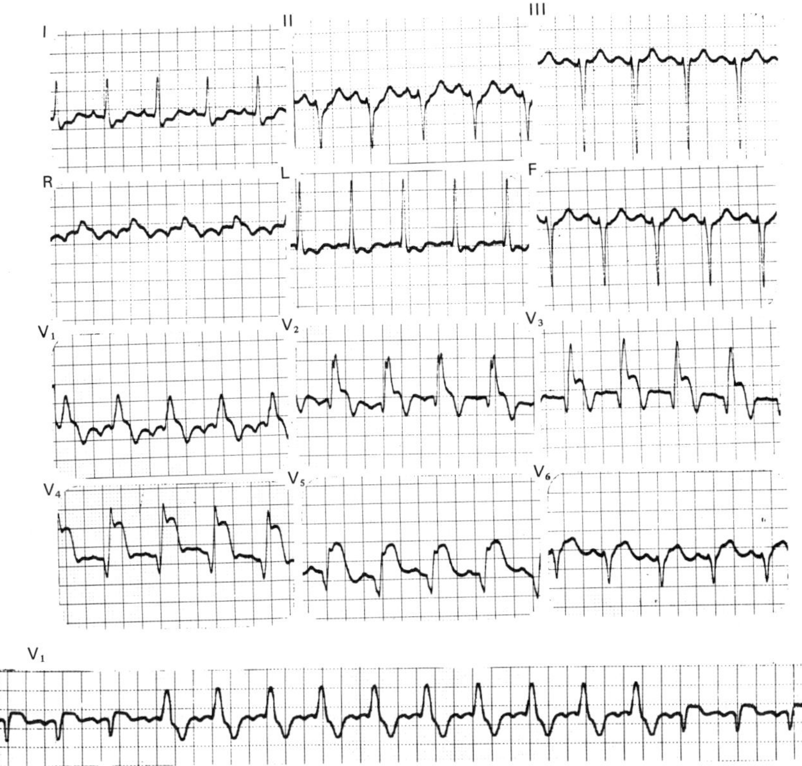

Fig. 10–19.   **Intermittent right bundle branch block (RBBB) has also appeared in the patient whose admission ECG is shown in Fig. 10–18. Note inconstant RBBB in the rhythm strip. Such a patient is at risk of developing second and third degree infranodal block, and a temporary ventricular pacemaker should be inserted.**

At this point an important, although infrequently mentioned, exception to the plan already outlined must be discussed. Patients who have had a previous myocardial infarction may not "follow the rules," because coronary artery perfusion has already been distorted. A particularly dramatic example is illustrated in Figure 10–21.

Who, among the few patients who recover from an anterior myocardial infarction complicated by second or third degree infranodal block and regain 1:1 AV conduction, should receive a permanent pacemaker in order to prevent sudden cardiac death from a future episode of heart block? Data concerning such patients are now becoming available, and as we interpret the reports, patients are more likely to live longer if they are paced (1,40,66), although some investigators are not so certain (64).

Presently we are not sure whether permanent pacing will be helpful in patients with myocardial infarction who have developed persistent fascicular disease without AV block. One group has reported a high post discharge mortality in patients with persistent bifascicular or incomplete trifascicular block, particularly when RBBB persisted and the HV interval was prolonged

On admission, prior to arrest

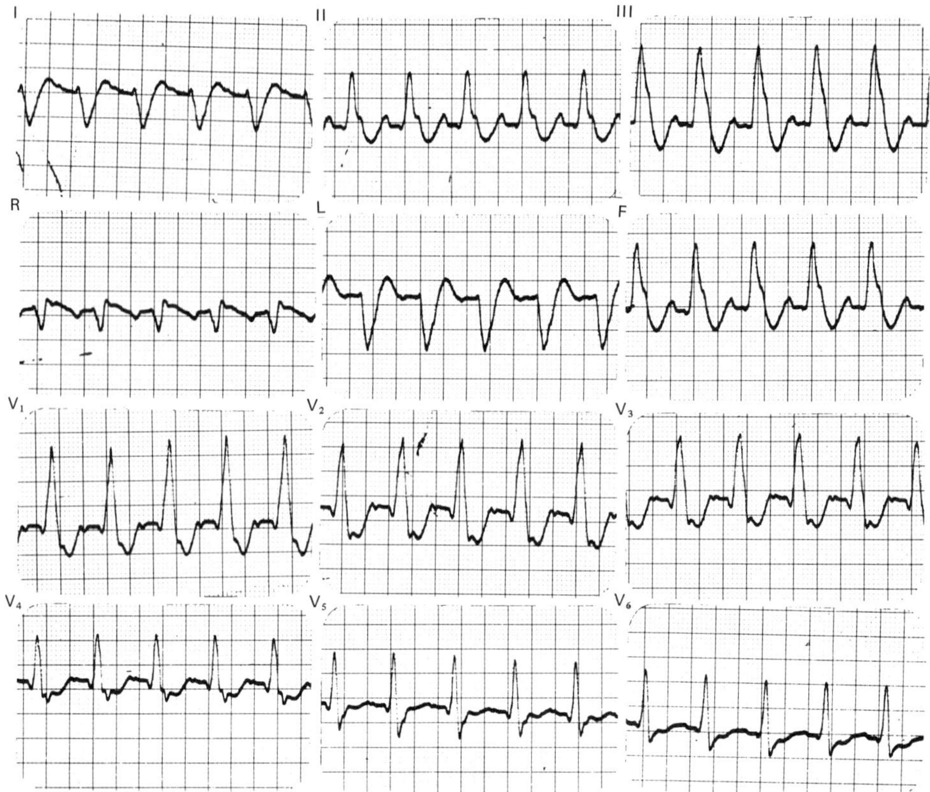

Fig. 10–20. **ECG of complete right bundle branch block and left posterior hemiblock in a patient with acute anterior myocardial infarction. The sinus tachycardia was produced by congestive heart failure from the widespread myocardial damage present. Although the PR interval was normal (180 msec), the HV interval was prolonged (70 msec). Thus first degree infranodal AV block due to partial trifascicular disease was present. A temporary ventricular electrode should be inserted in such cases.**

(33, 34). Some of these deaths may have been caused by complete infranodal block. Ventricular fibrillation rather than heart block may have been the terminal event, and this possibility must temper our enthusiasm about permanently pacing patients with bifascicular block, whether or not myocardial infarction has occurred (7).

TECHNIQUES OF PACING

The methods, types of equipment, and complications in pacemaking will not be reviewed in this discussion. The reader is referred to articles and books which are specifically addressed to these important topics (12, 26, 28, 63).

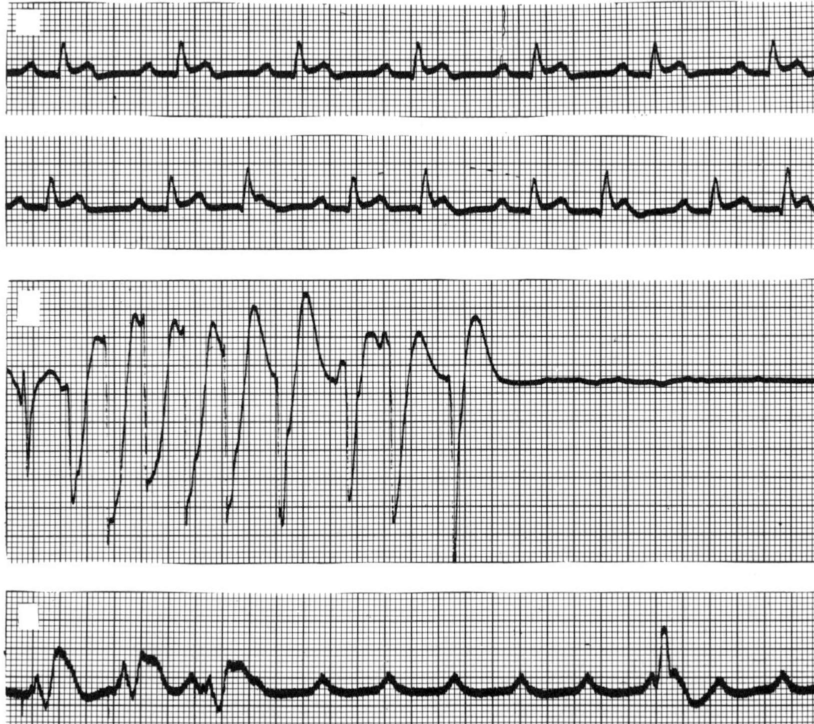

Fig. 10–21.   **ECGs of infranodal complete AV block in a man who was admitted with an acute *inferior* myocardial infarction. 2:1 block with narrow supraventricular QRS is seen in the top panel and 3:2 AV block with Wenckebach periods in the second panel. These tracings were interpreted as showing Mobitz type I block in the AV node, and an electrode was not inserted. Later on the day of admission he developed ventricular tachycardia (third panel) and complete, apparently, infranodal AV block (bottom panel). It was then discovered that the patient had previously had an anterior myocardial infarction, but the ECG findings were masked by "regrowth" of R waves in the precordial leads. This case emphasizes the point that previous myocardial damage may dramatically affect the expected course of conduction disturbances which complicate myocardial infarction.**

DRUGS IN THE TREATMENT OF AV BLOCK

Vagolytic or β-adrenergic drugs may be useful following the acute development of atrioventricular block, either to relieve a transient block or to sustain a patient until a pacemaker electrode can be introduced. Atropine sulfate should first be tried. Sometimes one, two, or three 0.5 mg injections, given intravenously, will decrease or relieve heart block when it is due to increased vagal tone, as in acute inferior myocardial infarction (Fig. 10–16 and 10–17).

Drugs which stimulate the β-adrenergic receptor site, such as isoproterenol or epinephrine, may be infused by intravenous drip to facilitate AV conduction or increase the discharge rate of subsidiary pacemakers. One to four or more μg/min may be necessary. Such drugs may arouse dangerous ventricular irrita-

irritability and may increase myocardial oxygen consumption to unacceptable levels in patients with acute ischemic injury, so care must be taken when they are used.

The prescription of drugs for the chronic treatment of atrioventricular block is no longer appropriate when permanent ventricular pacemaking is available.

Acknowledgement

The authors want to acknowledge the collaboration of James G. Kitchen III, who participated in the preparation of a previous publication on this subject (28). The continued encouragement, support, and critical advice of Joseph K. Perloff, Chief, Cardiovascular Section, are much appreciated.

REFERENCES

1. Atkins JM, Leshin SJ, Blomqvist O et al.: Ventricular conduction blocks and sudden death in acute myocardial infarction. Potential indications for pacing. N Engl J Med 288:281, 1973
2. Barold SS, Friedberg HD: Second degree atrioventricular block. Am J Cardiol 33:311, 1974
3. Cannom DS, Goldreyer BN, Damato AN: Atrioventricular conduction system in left bundle-branch block with normal QRS axis. Circulation 46:129, 1972
4. Chamberlain DA, Leinbach RC, Vassaux CE et al.: Sequential atrioventricular pacing in heart block complicating acute myocardial infarction. N Engl J Med 282:577, 1970
5. Cohen SI, Lau SH, Stein E et al.: Variations of aberrant ventricular conduction in man: evidence of isolated and combined block within the specialized conduction system. Circulation 38:899, 1968
6. Davies M, Harris A: Pathological basis of primary heart block. Br Heart J 31:219, 1969
7. Denes P, Dhingra R, Wu D et al.: Sudden cardiac death in patients with chronic bifascicular block (abstr). Circulation 51–52 (Supp. II) II–113, 1975
8. Dhingra RC, Denes P, Wu D et al.: The significance of second degree atrioventricular block and bundle branch block. Observations regarding site and type of block. Circulation 49:638, 1974
9. Dhingra RC, Denes P, Wu D et al.: Chronic right bundle branch block and left posterior hemiblock. Clinical, electrophysiologic and prognostic observations. Am J Cardiol 36:867, 1975
10. Dreifus LS, Watanabe Y, Haiat R et al.: Atrioventricular block. Am J Cardiol 28:371, 1971
11. El Sherif N, Scherlag BJ, Samet P: Analysis of second degree A–V block following acute myocardial ischemia of the canine His–Purkinje system. Clin Res 21:417, 1973
12. Furman S, Escher DJW: Principles and Techniques of Cardiac Pacing. New York, Harper & Row, 1970
13. Gallagher JJ, Damato AN, Lau SH et al.: Antecubital vein approach for recording His bundle activity in man. Am Heart J 85:199, 1973
14. Gilchrist AR: Clinical aspects of high-grade heart-block. Scott Med J 3:53, 1958
15. Giraud G, Puech P, Latour H: The physiological electrical activity of Tawara's node and of His bundle in man. Endocavitary electrocardiographic registration. Bull Acad Natl Med (Paris) 144:363, 1960
16. Goldreyer BN, Kahl FR, Manchester JH et al.: Analysis of the H–V interval—conduction velocity within the human bundle of His (abstr). Circulation 47–48 (Supp. IV):IV–170, 1973
17. Goldreyer BN, Kastor JA, Manchester JH et al.: Posterior division refractoriness in patients with right bundle branch block and left anterior hemiblock. Am J Cardiol 31:135, 1973
18. Gould L, Riedel J, Reddy OVR, Comprecht RI: Prognosis of left anterior hemiblock in acute myocardial infarction. J Electrocardio 8:333, 1975

19. Gupta PK, Lichstein E, Chadda K: Electrophysiological features of complete AV block within the His bundle. Br Heart J 35:610, 1973
20. Harper JR, Harley A, Hackel DB, Estes EH Jr: Coronary artery disease and major conduction disturbances. Am Heart J 77:411, 1969
21. Harper R, Hunt D, Vohra J et al.: His bundle electrogram in patients with acute myocardial infarction complicated by atrioventricular or intraventricular conduction disturbances. Br Heart J 37:705, 1975
22. Hoffman BF, Cranefield PF: Electrophysiology of the Heart. New York, McGraw–Hill, 1960
23. James TN: The coronary circulation and conduction system in acute myocardial infarction. Prog Cardiovasc Dis 10:410, 1968
24. Kastor JA: Atrioventricular block. N Engl J Med 292:462, 572, 1975
25. Kastor JA, Josephson JE: Slow conduction—a constant feature of human His–Purkinje function. Am J Cardiol 37:147, 1976
26. Kastor JA, Leinbach RC: Pacemakers and their arrhythmias. Prog Cardiovasc Dis 13:240, 1974
27. Kelly DT, Brodsky SJ, Mirowski M et al.: Bundle of His recordings in congenital complete heart block. Circulation 45:277, 1972
28. Kitchen JG III, Kastor JA: Pacing in acute myocardial infarction—indications, methods, hazards and results. Cardiovasc Clin 7:219, 1975
29. Kulbertus HE: The magnitude of risk of developing complete heart block in patients with LAD–RBBB. Am Heart J 86:278, 1973
30. Langendorf R, Pick A: Atrioventricular block type II (Mobitz). Its nature and clinical significance. Circulation 38:819, 1968
31. Lasser RP, Haft JI, Friedberg CK: Relationship of right bundle-branch block and marked left axis deviation (with left parietal or peri-infarction block) to complete heart block and syncope. Circulation 37: 429, 1968
32. Lev M: The normal anatomy of the conduction system in man and its pathology in atrioventricular block. Ann NY Acad Sci 111:817, 1964
33. Lichstein E, Gupta PK, Chadda KD: Long term survival of patients with incomplete bundle-branch block complicating acute myocardial infarction. Br Heart J 83:924, 1975
34. Lichstein E, Gupta PK, Chadda KD et al.: Findings of prognostic value in patients with incomplete bilateral bundle branch block complicating acute myocardial infarction. Am J Cardiol 32:913, 1973
35. Lie KI, Wellens HJ, Schuilenburg RM, Durrer D: Mechanism and significance of widened QRS complexes during complete atrioventricular block in acute myocardial infarction. Am J Cardiol 33:833, 1974
36. Lie KI, Wellens HJ, Schuilenburg RM, Durrer D: Observations on acquired and chronic bundle branch block in myocardial infarction. Circulation 51–52 (Supp. II): II–113, 1975
37. Lie KI, Wellens HJ, Schuilenburg RM et al.: Factors influencing prognosis of bundle branch block complicating acute antero-septal infarction. The value of His bundle recordings. Circulation 50:935, 1974
38. Meister SG, Banka VS, Chadda KD et al.: A balloon-tipped catheter for obtaining His bundle electrograms without fluoroscopy. Circulation 49:42, 1974
39. Mobitz W: Uber den paielallen Herzblock. Z Klin Med 107:546, 1928
40. Mullens CB: Indications for pacing after acute myocardial infarction in patients with fascicular blocks. J Electrocardiol 8:297, 1975
41. Narula OS: Intraventricular conduction defects. In Narula OS (ed): His Bundle Electrocardiography and Clinical Electrophysiology. Philadelphia, FA Davis, 1975, pp 177–202
42. Narula OS, Gann D, Samet P: Prognostic value of H–V intervals. In Narula OS (ed): His Bundle Electrocardiography and Clinical Electrophysiology. Philadelphia, FA Davis, 1975, pp 437–449
43. Narula OS, Runge M, Samet P: A new catheter technique for His bundle recordings via the arm veins. Br Heart J 35:1226, 1973
44. Narula OS, Samet P: Right bundle branch block with normal, left or right axis deviation. Am J Med 51:432, 1971

45. Narula OS, Scherlag BJ, Samet P et al.: Atrioventricular block. Localization and classification by His bundle recordings. Am J Med 50:146, 1971
46. Page DL, Caulfield JB, Kastor JA et al.: Myocardial changes associated with cardiogenic shock. N Engl J Med 285:133, 1971
47. Pryor R: Fascicular blocks and the bilateral bundle branch block syndrome. Am Heart J 83:441, 1972
48. Puech P, Grolleau R: L'activite du faisceau de His normale and pathologique. Circulation 49:592, 1974
49. Ranganathan N, Dhurandhar R, Phillips JH et al.: His bundle electrogram in bundle-branch block. Circulation 45:282, 1972
50. Rizzon P, DiBiase M, Baissus C: Intraventricular conduction defects in acute myocardial infarction. Br Heart J 36:660, 1974
51. Rizzon P, Rossi L, Baissus C et al.: Left posterior hemiblock in acute myocardial infarction. Br Heart J 37:711, 1975
52. Rosen KM, Dhingra RC, Loeb HS et al.: Chronic heart block in adults. Clinical and electrophysiological observations. Arch Intern Med 131:663, 1973
53. Rosen KM, Rahimtoola SH, Chuquimia R et al.: Electrophysiological significance of first degree atrioventricular block with intraventricular conduction disturbance. Circulation 43:-491, 1971
54. Rosenbaum MB, Elizari MV, Lazzari JO: The Hemiblocks. Oldsmar, FL, Tampa Tracings, 1970
55. Rotman M, Wagner G, Waugh RA: Significance of high degree atrioventricular block in acute posterior myocardial infarction. Circulation 47:257, 1973
56. Scanlon PJ, Pryor R, Blount SG Jr: Right bundle-branch block—associated with left superior or inferior intraventricular block—associated with acute myocardial infarction. Circulation 42:1135, 1970
57. Scheinman M, Brenman B: Clinical and anatomic implications of intraventricular conduction blocks in acute myocardial infarction. Circulation 46:753, 1972
58. Scheinman MM, Brenman M, Moden G, Peters R: Cooperative prospective study of bundle branch block. Circulation 51–52: Supp. II–113, 1975
59. Scherlag BJ, Lau SH, Helfant RH et al.: Catheter technique for recording His bundle activity in man. Circulation 39:13, 1969
60. Schuilenburg RM, Durrer D: Problems in the recognition of conduction disturbances in the His bundle. Circulation 51:68, 1975
61. Steiner C, Lau SH, Stein E et al.: Electrophysiologic documentation of trifascicular block as the common cause of complete heart block. Am J Cardiol 28:436, 1971
62. Sutton R, Davies M: The conduction system in acute myocardial infarction complicated by heart block. Circulation 38:987, 1968
63. Thalen HJTh (ed): Cardiac Pacing. The Netherlands, Van Gorcum, 1973
64. Waters DD, Mizgala HF: Long term prognosis of patients with incomplete bilateral bundle branch block complicating acute myocardial infarction. Role of cardiac pacing. Am J Cardiol 34:1, 1974
65. Watson H, Emslie–Smith D, Lowe KG: The intracardiac electrogram of human atrioventricular conducting tissue. Am Heart J 74:66, 1967
66. Waugh RA, Wagner GS, Haney TL et al.: Immediate and remote prognostic significance of fascicular block during acute myocardial infarction. Circulation 47:765, 1973
67. Wenckebach KF: Arrhythmia of the Heart. A Physiological and Clinical Study. London, William Green & Sons, 1904

<table><tr><td>11</td><td>

The Use of β-Adrenergic Blocking Agents in the Treatment and Prevention of Cardiac Arrhythmias*

</td></tr></table>

ROGER A. WINKLE
DONALD C. HARRISON

The importance of the sympathetic nervous system in controlling the heart during health and disease has been appreciated for many years. Regulation of heart rate during rest and exercise, as well as the control of cardiac arrhythmias and their clinical manifestations, has been attributed in part to the level of sympathetic nervous system activity in the heart. The sympathetic nervous system exerts its influences on the heart by stimulation of the β-receptor system (2), and studies have shown that stimulation of β-adrenergic receptors alone can produce cardiac arrhythmias. Therefore, it was appropriate that propranolol, the first specific β-blocking drug available for widespread clinical use, should be used in the treatment of cardiac arrhythmias (6, 15, 29). Our experience with this and other β-blocking agents in the treatment and prevention of cardiac arrhythmias during the past 10 years has been extensive (11, 12, 15, 19, 33). It is the purpose of this article to review the use of β-blockers in the treatment of specific cardiac arrhythmias, and to illustrate their use in selected patients, present their proposed mechanisms of action, and describe their side effects and contraindications.

PHYSIOLOGIC ACTION OF THE SYMPATHETIC NERVOUS SYSTEM ON ELECTRIC EVENTS IN THE HEART

The physiologic basis for assuming that the sympathetic nervous system exerts a significant influence on cardiac rate and rhythm has been provided by studies demonstrating interrelationships between cardiovascular control and sympathetic nervous system activity (5, 16). Investigators have found that stimulation of cardiac sympathetic nerves and the administration of catecholamines increase the ventricular rate. An infusion of norepinephrine, the primary neurotransmitter substance, has been shown to produce ventricular extrasystoles in patients with and without heart disease. Definition of the electrophysiologic effects of sympathetic nervous stimulation in the heart has indicated that in-

*This work was supported in part by NIH Grants Nos. HL-5866, and Program Project Grant No. 1-P01-HL-15833; and a grant from the American Heart Association, No. 67–708.

creased sympathetic activity will increase automaticity (mediated by an increase in the slope of phase 4 of the intracellular action potential of sinoatrial nodal fibers). It will also increase the conduction velocity of impulses passing through atrial and ventricular tissue, decrease the functional refractory period of the atrioventricular node, and decrease the diastolic threshold for ventricular stimulation (16, 30). Electrocardiographic changes resulting from increased activity of the sympathetic nervous system include an increase in heart rate, a shortened PR interval, and a shortening of the QT interval (9).

THEORY OF SYMPATHETIC NERVOUS TRANSMISSION AND RECEPTOR MECHANISMS

The mechanism by which sympathetic activity in the heart is mediated is of considerable importance. The most widely accepted hypothesis is that norepinephrine, the primary transmitter substance, is released from the sympathetic nerve endings and attaches to a receptor. Since the initial work of Langley in 1905, the circulatory effects of catecholamines have been known to be both excitatory and inhibitory. Prior to 1948, this dichotomy was attributed to the existence of two neurotransmitter substances, epinephrine and norepinephrine, each having a different specific action. A clear demonstration by U.S. Von Euler in 1946, however, that norepinephrine represented the primary and possibly the only neurotransmitter substance for the sympathetic nerve, prompted the development of other theories to explain the dual neurocirculatory action of catecholamines. In 1948 Ahlquist proposed the existence of two adrenergic receptors, alpha (α) and beta (β), on the basis of neurocirculatory responses to injections of a number of sympathomimetic agents. This hypothesis was strengthened materially during the following decade by the introduction of several pharmacologic agents which blocked the neurocirculatory effects of α-adrenergic stimulation. General acceptance of the Ahlquist proposal followed the 1958 discovery by Powell and Slater of the first specific agent to block the neurocirculatory response attributed to β-stimulation. Dichloroisoproterenol, an analogue of the accepted specific β-stimulating drug isoproterenol, was found by Powell and Slater to competitively inhibit the β-adrenergic activity of sympathomimetic agents (25). This drug was not widely used in clinical practice, however, because it produced initial sympathomimetic stimulating effects before the onset of blockade. Pronethalol was the second competitive β-receptor antagonist to be introduced. After a limited clinical trial, it was found to produce carcinomatous changes in mice, and was withdrawn from use. In 1964 another β-blocking agent, propranolol, was synthesized and clinical trials were initiated (6, 9). In 1968 this drug was approved by the Federal Food and Drug Administration for use in cardiac arrhythmias and hypertrophic subaortic stenosis. Since that time numerous compounds with β-adrenergic blocking activities have been synthesized and submitted to clinical trial. The structural formulas of several compounds which have β-blocking activity are shown in Figure 11–1.

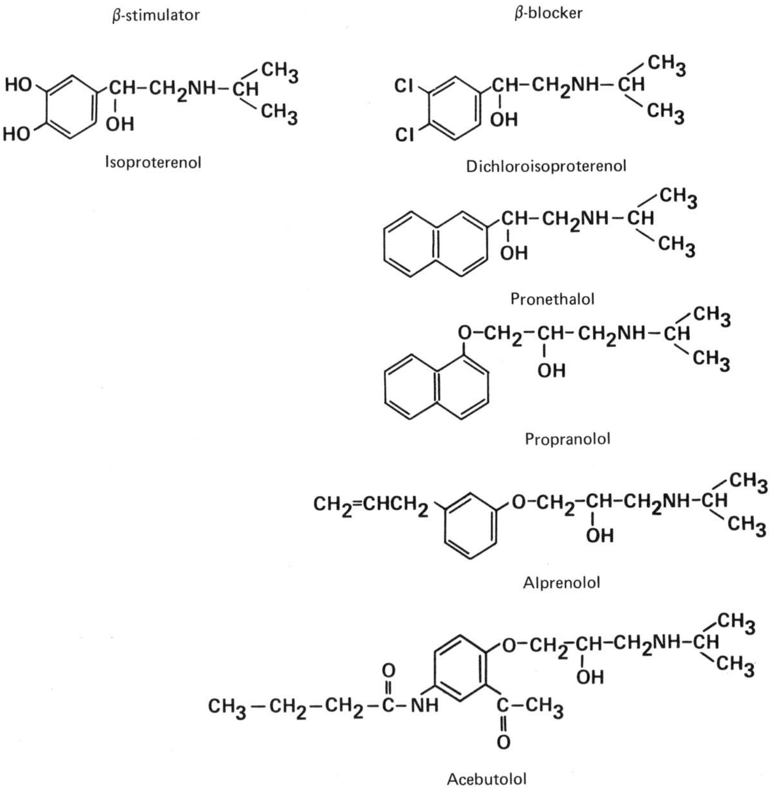

Fig. 11–1. **Structural formulas for β-adrenergic stimulator (isoproterenol) and several β-blockers.**

Investigations using these antiadrenergic drugs have indicated that all sympathetically mediated activities in the heart are due to stimulation of β-adrenergic receptors, in accord with the Ahlquist classification (2). Stimulation of β-adrenergic receptors produces an increase in heart rate, an increase in cardiac contractile force, a decrease in the functional refractory period of the atrioventricular node, and in specific instances, the occurrence of cardiac arrhythmias (22, 30). It is, therefore, apparent why cardiac arrhythmias were among the first clinical conditions to be treated with propranolol, the first widely available β-blocking drug.

PROPERTIES OF β-BLOCKING AGENTS

In order to understand the mechanism of action of β-blocking drugs as antiarrhythmic agents, and the similarities and differences among the various β-blocking agents, it is important to recognize four properties associated with these compounds. 1) β-blockade, 2) direct membrane properties, 3) differences in tissue specificity, and 4) β-stimulating properties.

β-blockade, the one property common to all β-blocking drugs, provides the majority, if not all, of their antiarrhythmic activity. These compounds competitively inhibit catecholamines at all β-receptor sites within the heart and decrease the automaticity of cardiac pacemaker cells, as evidenced by a reduction in the slope of phase 4 of the intracellular cardiac action potential. This effect on the sinoatrial nodal tissue results in a slowing of the normal cardiac pacemaker mechanism and is manifested as a decrease in the heart rate. The mechanism of action of β-blocking drugs for suppressing ectopic pacemaker activities is presumed to be through a reduction in phase 4 automaticity.

β-blockade also causes changes in atrioventricular conduction which are important for the management of supraventricular arrhythmias. Once again these agents directly oppose the effects of catecholamine stimulation of the atrioventricular conduction system, resulting in a decrease in conduction velocity and a prolongation of the functional refractory period of the atrioventricular node (27). This action accounts for propranolol's ability to interrupt reentrant paroxysmal supraventricular tachycardia and slow the ventricular response to atrial fibrillation and flutter. In contrast to the effect on the normal atrioventricular conduction pathway, propranolol exerts no effect on conduction through the accessory pathways seen in preexcitation syndromes (26).

Although the antiarrhythmic properties of β-blocking agents appear in all instances to result from direct opposition to the effect of catecholamine stimulation on the heart, there are certain clinical situations in which arrhythmias are specifically associated with excess circulating catecholamines. β-blocking agents provide specific protection against the arrhythmia in these settings. Arrhythmias may occur in patients undergoing general anesthesia and in patients with pheochromocytoma, especially during induction of anesthesia and manipulation of the adrenal tumor. It has also been suggested that many arrhythmias occurring in the early hours following myocardial infarction are aggravated by elevated levels of circulating catecholamines, and that β-blocking drugs can be useful in this situation.

Some β-adrenergic blocking agents also possess direct membrane activity, referred to as *quinidine-like* activity. This is characterized by changes in the intracellular cardiac action potential, including a reduction in the rate of rise and overshoot of phase 0 of the action potential, a decrease in conduction velocity, and a decrease in spontaneous phase 4 depolarization. Studies demonstrating direct membrane properties of β-blockers have been carried out in a variety of tissue preparations, including isolated rabbit and guinea pig atria and human papillary muscles. It was initially assumed that these effects were important for antiarrhythmic activity (21); however, a vast body of evidence has accumulated which contradicts this assumption: 1) the stabilizing effects of β-blocking agents on the membrane occurs only at concentrations 50–100 times greater than those achieved in man; 2) the dextroisomer of propranolol, which has membrane activity but lacks significant β-blocking properties, is unsuccessful for suppression of ventricular ectopic beats at concentrations several times higher than those required of the racemic form of propranolol (8); 3) practolol, which has no direct membrane activity, is effective as an antiarrhythmic agent (13, 17, 18). There is some experimental evidence to indicate that β-blocking agents which possess membrane activity may be more effective in treating digitalis-induced arrhythmias, but the clinical importance of this observation is unknown.

Although the antiarrhythmic effects of β-blocking agents result from cardiac activity, β-receptors are found in a variety of tissues in the body. Extracardiac receptors which are of clinical concern are those in the smooth muscle of the vascular bed and bronchi. Stimulation of β-receptors by catecholamines in these sites produces vasodilation and bronchodilation, thus, administration of a β-blocking drug will result in vasoconstriction and bronchoconstriction. Important differences in β-blocking compounds result in differences in tissue sensitivity of β-receptors to the action of β-blockers. The majority of β-blocking compounds act not only on the heart but also on the vascular bed and bronchi. There are some, however, which act only on the β-receptors of the heart, and have little or no effect on β-receptors in other tissues. Such compounds are termed *cardioselective* β-blocking agents. The prototype of these cardioselective agents is practolol, which is devoid of significant activity on the vascular bed and bronchi. Preliminary reports indicate that acebutolol is relatively cardioselective, producing less β-blockade in the vascular bed and bronchi than in cardiac sites.

In addition to their β-blocking properties, many of these compounds possess sympathomimetic or β-stimulating activity. Practolol's lack of myocardial depressant activity, when compared with propranolol's ability, has been in part attributed to its intrinsic sympathomimetic properties. Even β-blocking agents which are relatively free of β-stimulating activity, such as propranolol, may have metabolites with intrinsic sympathomimetic properties (24).

It is generally assumed that for equivalent degrees of β-blockade the antiarrhythmic activity of the various β-blocking agents should be equal. However, the subtle differences among β-blocking agents are important for determining the clinical setting for which each drug is appropriate and, to a large extent, influence the toxicity of each agent. It will be increasingly necessary to understand these subtle differences as more β-blocking agents become available for clinical use.

β-BLOCKING AGENTS FOR THE TREATMENT OF SPECIFIC ARRHYTHMIAS

The uses of β-blocking agents as antiarrhythmic drugs can be considered under two broad categories: 1) the treatment of acute arrhythmias, and 2) the prevention of recurrent arrhythmias. Acute arrhythmias are treated by intravenous drug administration, whereas chronic arrhythmias are treated orally. The average intravenous and oral doses of the commonly used β-blocking drugs are listed in Table 11–1. Certain general guidelines apply to the use of these agents. When administering the drugs intravenously the dose should be given slowly, not exceeding the rates listed in Table 11–1. The patient's blood pressure and electrocardiogram should be monitored continuously and the infusion terminated if adverse side effects occur. For long-term oral prophylaxis it is desirable to begin with smaller doses and gradually increase the dose until the desired clinical effect is achieved, or until toxicity prevents further increases in dose. Patients should be observed periodically for evidence of congestive failure or adverse effects of the drug on the cardiac conduction system.

During the initial evaluation of propranolol in this country this agent was given to 199 patients (age range 18–78 years) at Stanford Medical Center for the treatment of cardiac arrhythmias of various etiologies (Tables 11–2 and 11–3). The drug was given intravenously to 142 patients, the majority of whom received an initial dose of 100 μg/kg in a solution of 50 ml of 5% dextrose in water, administered over a 10 minute period. This dose has been shown to produce a moderate and safe degree of β-adrenergic blockade, as demonstrated experimentally by a decrease in resting heart rate and an inhibition of the heart rate response to isoproterenol infusion (13). In the postoperative patient and in patients with acute myocardial infarction in whom significant β-blockade might produce increasing congestive heart failure or excessive slowing of the heart rate, the dose of propranolol was reduced to 20–50 μg/kg, given over a period of 15 minutes. Patients with evidence of mild congestive heart failure, but with rapid heart rates, were treated with cautiously administered doses of propranolol, accompanied by frequent observations of the central venous pressure and frequent observation for pulmonary congestion. Except in the presence of digitalis toxicity, patients receiving digitalis glycosides continued this medication during treatment with propranolol.

Fifty-seven patients were given oral propranolol as prophylaxis against recurring arrhythmias. The initial dosage, 10 mg 4 times a day, was gradually

Table 11–1. SUMMARY OF DOSES OF β-BLOCKING DRUGS

	Intravenous dose		Oral dose
	Average maximum dose (mg/kg)	Average rate of administration (mg/min)	Average total daily dose (mg)
Propranolol (Inderal)	0.15	1.0	80–320
Oxyprenolol	0.2	1.0	160–320
Alprenolol (Aptine, H56/28)	0.2	1.0	400
Pindolol	0.015	0.1	20–40
Practolol (ICI 50172, AY 21–011)	0.4	2.5	400–1200
Acebutolol (Sectrol, M&B 17,803)	0.4	2.5	600–1200
Sotalol (MJ 1999)	0.4	2.5	80–320

Table 11–2. CARDIAC ARRHYTHMIAS TREATED WITH INTRAVENOUS PROPRANOLOL

Arrhythmia	Number	On digitalis	Favorable slowed or reverted	Unfavorable no response
Supraventricular tachycardia	22	2	16	6
Atrial fibrillation	61	49	57	4
Atrial flutter	17	11	15	2
Nodal tachycardia	5	4	3	2
Digitalis-induced Atrial	6	6	6	0
Ventricular	5	5	3	2
PO supraventricular*	16	16	12	4
PVCs or ventricular† tachycardia	10	4	3	7

*PO=postoperative
†PVCs=premature ventricular contractions

Table 11–3. CARDIAC ARRHYTHMIAS TREATED PROPHYLACTICALLY WITH PROPRANOLOL

Arrhythmia	Number	Favorable slowed or reverted	Unfavorable no response
Paroxysmal supraventricular tachycardia	26	14	12
Atrial fibrillation or flutter	14	10	4
PVCs*	8	2	6
Tachycardia with WPW†	5	5	0
Paroxysmal ventricular tachycardia	4	2	2

*PVCs=premature ventricular contractions
†WPW=Wolff–Parkinson–White syndrome

increased to a total dose of 240–320 mg/day (60–80 mg 4 times a day), depending on individual tolerance. Because of acute arrhythmias, 14 patients were first treated with intravenous propranolol; after initial control of their heart rate had been achieved, prophylactic treatment against recurrence was attempted with oral propranolol. All patients maintained on oral propranolol were seen in clinic at regular intervals. Thirty-six of the 57 patients with recurrent arrhythmias had been treated at some time with digitalis glycosides, and 27 of the 57 had been treated with quinidine. Whenever it appeared that digitalis or quinidine, or both, were ineffective in altering the frequency or severity of the arrhythmia, these drugs were discontinued. Only eight patients remained on digitalis, and four on quinidine. Propranolol was evaluated by means of reports prepared by the patient. Only those who experienced complete disappearance of the arrhythmia or marked reduction in its frequency or duration, or both, were considered to be benefited. Follow-up continued for more than 4 years in some patients.

The following sections discuss the use of β-adrenergic blocking agents for the treatment of specific cardiac arrhythmias in clinical settings. The immediate effect on each type of arrhythmia will be discussed and, where appropriate, information given concerning the long-term prophylaxis of recurrent arrhythmias. Although a vast literature exists concerning the efficacy of β-blocking agents for treating acute arrhythmias, there is virtually no information available to compare their efficacy with that of other antiarrhythmic drugs known to affect similar arrhythmias. Clinical experience and numerous reports suggest that β-blocking agents can be effective for prophylaxis in various types of arrhythmias, but in no instances have carefully controlled, double-blind studies been performed.

PAROXYSMAL SUPRAVENTRICULAR TACHYCARDIA

Paroxysmal supraventricular tachycardia (PSVT) is rarely life-threatening, however, in many patients it is recurrent and is associated with distressing symptomatology. Goldreyer and others have demonstrated that this rhythm is often explained by a reentrant pathway which involves the atrioventricular node (14). It can frequently be terminated by maneuvers such as carotid sinus massage, which increases vagal tone, slows atrioventricular conduction, and prolongs the functional refractory period of the atrioventricular node. β-blocking agents are frequently successful for terminating acute episodes of PSVT. The mechanism of action is assumed to be interruption of the reentrant circuit, which results from the known effects of these agents on atrioventricular nodal conduction. Patients with the Wolff-Parkinson-White syndrome may have episodes of PSVT which involve both the atrioventricular node and an accessory preexcitation pathway (31). The ability of propranolol to terminate PSVT in patients with the Wolff-Parkinson-White syndrome probably relates to its effect on atrioventricular nodal conduction, since it is ineffective in altering the conduction properties of the accessory pathway (26).

During the initial evaluation of propranolol at Stanford University Hospital 22 patients with PSVT were treated with intravenous propranlol after all vagotonic maneuvers were unsuccessful. Only two of these patients were on maintenance digoxin at the time of treatment. Sixteen of the 22 patients demonstrated slowing of the rate of tachycardia, and 9 of the 16 converted to sinus rhythm within 60 minutes after receiving intravenous propranolol (Fig. 11–2). The rate of the tachycardia in the remaining six patients did not change. Slowing of the rate of the tachycardia in some patients probably represents the effect of propranolol upon the reentrant pathway. When carotid sinus massage is unsuccessful before administration of propranolol it may be successful after propranolol administration. The effectiveness of propranolol and other β-blocking agents for the treatment of acute episodes of PSVT has been confirmed by numerous investigators.

The β-blocking agents are also successful for prophylaxis against recurrent

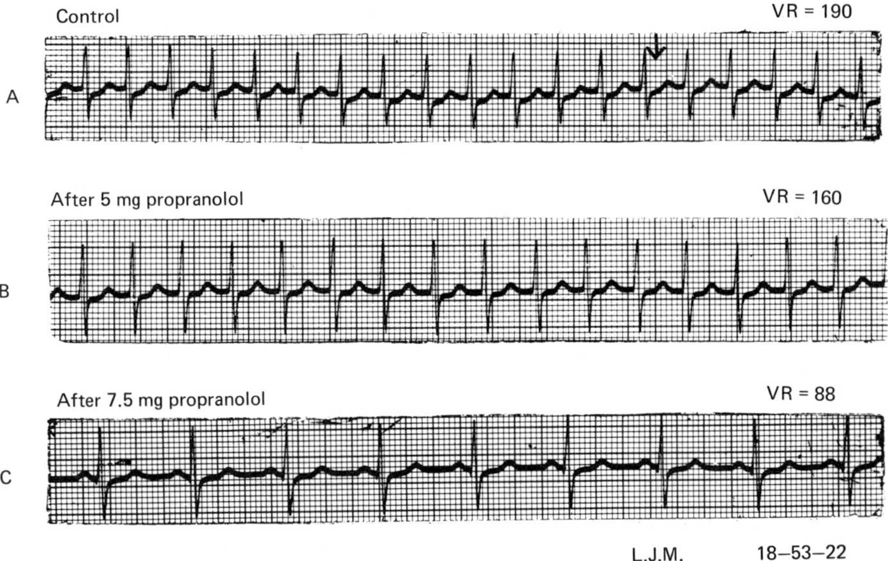

Fig. 11–2. **Electrocardiograms of patient with paroxysmal supraventricular tachycardia. A) Control rate of 190 beats/min; B) after 5 mg propranolol the heart rate slowed to 160 beats/ min; C) after 7.5 mg propranolol the tachycardia reverted to sinus rhythm at 88 beats/min. (VR–ventricular rate)**

episodes of PSVT. In our early experience 26 patients with recurrent PSVT were treated with propranolol in doses ranging from 60–320 mg/day. The attacks were abolished or reduced in frequency or severity in 14 patients. Frieden and coworkers reported the results of long-term therapy in 12 patients with PSVT (10). In their series 7 of 12 patients had a reduction in the frequency of attacks, and five were free of attacks, with follow-up ranging from 5–22 months. Propranolol is also successful for treatment of recurrences of PSVT associated with the Wolff–Parkinson–White syndrome. Some clinicians consider β-blockers to be the agents of choice for the treatment of recurrent PSVT in this condition. In the Stanford series propranolol markedly reduced the frequency of attacks in five of five patients (with the Wolff–Parkinson–White syndrome) in whom digitalis and/or quinidine had been unsuccessful.

ATRIAL FIBRILLATION

The β-blocking agents consistently slow the ventricular response to atrial fibrillation. This effect follows from their ability to alter the conduction properties of the atrioventricular node. Despite the consistent slowing of ventricular response patients rarely are converted to sinus rhythm following administration of β-blocking agents. It has been reported that concomitant administration of propranolol and quinidine increases the latter's ability to convert atrial fibrillation to sinus rhythm, and simultaneous administration of both drugs can aid in successful maintenance of sinus rhythm (20, 28).

In our experience with propranolol 37 patients with atrial fibrillation were given intravenous propranolol on 61 occasions. Twenty-nine of these patients were on digitalis preparations at the time propranolol was administered. The ventricular rate slowed in 57 of the 61 instances. The heart rate responses recorded on 25 consecutive occasions are illustrated in Figure 11–3. In six patients digitalis had produced only slight decreases in ventricular heart rate, despite doses which were sufficient to produce gastrointestinal side effects. In all of these patients the heart rate fell to 70–90 beats/min within 15–20 minutes of propranolol administration. The most pronounced slowing occurred in nondigitalized patients who had more rapid ventricular rates. The slowing persisted for 2–6 hours after a single intravenous dosing.

The current role of β-blocking agents in the treatment of acute atrial fibrillation is to slow the ventricular response in patients in whom digitalis preparations are either contraindicated or ineffective. Patient selection should be limited to those without depression of myocardial function, or in whom depression of myocardial function is caused by the rapid ventricular response. Patients with mitral stenosis are often ideal candidates for treatment with β-

Fig. 11–3. **Heart rate (beats/min) before and after the administration of 100 μg/kg pro-pranolol on 25 occasions in patients with atrial fibrillation.**

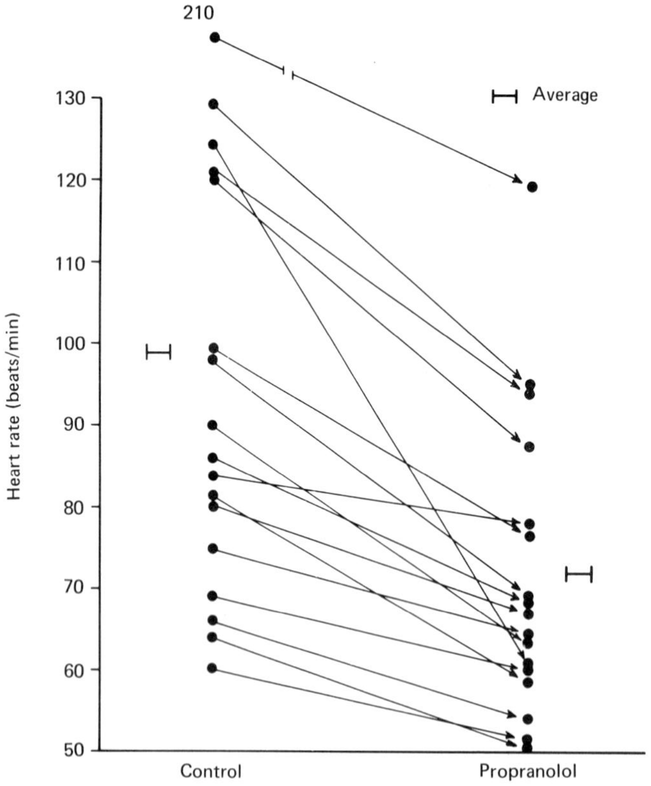

blocking agents. In our series four patients with mitral stenosis and evidence of mild pulmonary edema showed slowing in ventricular rate which was accompanied by a decrease in shortness of breath and other physical evidence of pulmonary congestion. This was a rapid response which occurred during or immediately after the administration of propranolol. Whenever doubt exists concerning the state of myocardial function, use of one of the β-blockers with less cardiac depressant action than propranolol's is preferable when such agents are available. The ability of β-blocking agents to control ventricular response in patients with atrial fibrillation and the Wolff–Parkinson–White syndrome is uncertain where the atrial impulses are conducted to the ventricle via the accessory pathways. Propranolol has no effect on the refractory period of this pathway and presumably is unsuccessful in controlling the ventricular response in this circumstance.

Long-term administration of propranolol is useful for patients with chronic atrial fibrillation, whose ventricular response is inadequately controlled by digitalis preparations. When digitalis fails to control the ventricular response despite the occurrence of side effects, addition of small doses of β-blocking agents can be of help in effecting control. For patients with paroxysmal atrial fibrillation, propranolol (with or without digitalis preparations) can be successful in controlling recurrences of the arrhythmia or in diminishing the symptoms associated with recurrences. In the Stanford series 10–14 patients with paroxysmal atrial fibrillation or flutter had fewer attacks, or slower ventricular rates during attacks, while receiving propranolol 60–200 mg/day. Several of these patients had received digitalis, with varying degrees of success. It is our impression that digitalis glycosides and propranolol are synergistic under these circumstances.

ATRIAL FLUTTER

The primary beneficial effect of β-blocking agents in the treatment of atrial flutter is a slowing of ventricular response, although a slightly higher rate of reversion to sinus rhythm has been reported for atrial flutter than has been observed for atrial fibrillation. Propranolol may also be given in conjunction with digitalis preparations for control of ventricular response in atrial flutter.

Seventeen patients with atrial flutter were treated with intravenous propranolol; significant slowing of the ventricular rate was observed in 15, and four patients reverted to sinus rhythm within 1 hour of treatment. The slowing of the ventricular rate was due primarily to an increase in atrioventricular block (Fig. 11–4); the atrial flutter rate increased transiently in several patients. At the time these studies were conducted, 11 of the 17 patients were on maintenance digitalis. Three patients with atrial flutter had been treated with large doses of digoxin, 1.25–1.75 mg, within 24 hours before treatment with propranolol. In one patient propranolol successfully slowed the ventricular rate after digitalis had been ineffective, and an elective cardioversion was later carried out. The increase in atrioventricular block produced by propranolol persisted from 2–8 hours in these patients. It was frequently our practice, therefore, to slow the ventricular rate by means of intravenous propranolol administration initially, and to maintain the slowing, when necessary, by means of a maintenance program of 30–40 mg four times per day, given orally.

VENTRICULAR ARRHYTHMIAS

The β-blocking agents are generally not utilized for immediate control of life-threatening ventricular arrhythmias. These arrhythmias often occur in patients with depressed ventricular function or in clinical circumstances which dictate the use of other antiarrhythmic agents, such as lidocaine, or immediate termination with dc countershock. When serious ventricular arrhythmias are resistant to other therapy or occur repeatedly despite administration of other antiarrhythmic drugs, they can occasionally be controlled by the addition of a β-blocking agent. Such resistant arrhythmias may be triggered by catecholamine excess during the early hours after acute myocardial infarction. When a β-blocker is used to treat these arrhythmias, one of the agents with less myocardial depressant effect than propranolol's is preferred.

Long-term administration of β-blocking agents can, in some patients, be successful for control of recurrent episodes of ventricular tachycardia or for suppression of isolated asymptomatic premature ventricular contractions. The overall efficacy of propranolol in suppressing these arrhythmias is unknown. Our impression is that propranolol is most successful for those patients whose arrhythmias are associated with exertion or are more frequent at faster heart rates.

We recently evaluated the effect of propranolol on ventricular arrhythmias in patients with mitral valve prolapse (33). Nine patients had frequent premature ventricular contractions (PVCs) on control ambulatory electrocardiograms; and five demonstrated an average of 90% reduction in PVC frequency

Fig. 11–4.   Effects of propranolol in atrial flutter. During control (top panel) the AV block was 2:1; 15 minutes after propranolol, 0.1 μg/kg was given, the AV block was 4:1 (center panel); and at 2 hours the AV block was still 4:1. AR–atrial rate, VR–ventricular rate. (beats/min). [From Harrison, *et al.* (15)].

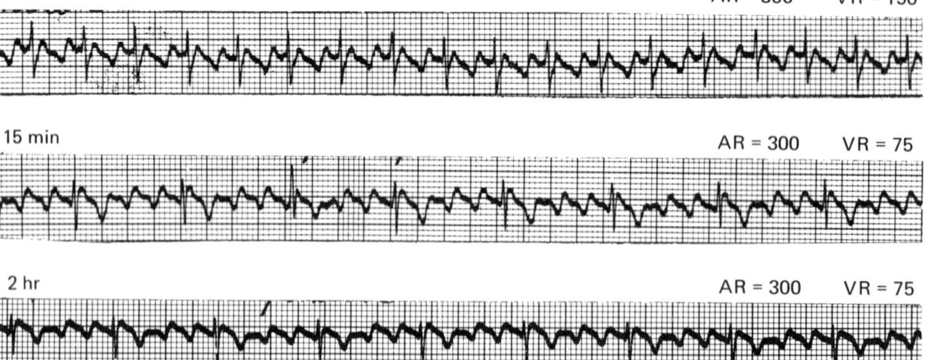

on ambulatory electrocardiograms obtained during the course of propranolol therapy. Ventricular tachycardia was eliminated in three of four patients. These patients noted a marked reduction in palpitation, and symptomatic improvement was maintained for periods averaging 1 year.

We recently evaluated the β-blocking agent acebutolol for suppression of isolated PVCs. Eleven patients with frequent PVCs on 24 hour control ambulatory electrocardiogram monitoring were treated for one week with 300 mg every 8 hours. Repeat 24 hour ambulatory electrocardiograms were obtained at the end of 1 week of therapy; all 11 patients demonstrated a reduction in

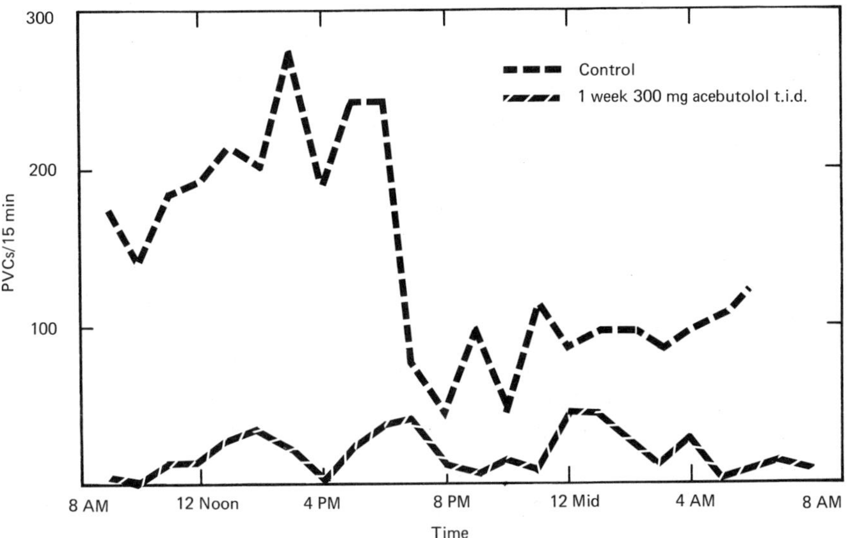

Fig. 11–5. **Premature ventricular contraction (PVC) frequency for one patient over 24 hours, as determined by ambulatory ECG before acebutolol (upper line), and at the end of one week of treatment with 300 mg acebutolol/8 hours (lower line). A marked reduction in PVC frequency was noted while the patient was taking acebutolol.**

Fig. 11–6. **Electrocardiograms showing the effects of propranolol in one patient with atrial tachycardia induced by digitalis excess. The arrhythmia is shown in the top panel and the response 2 minutes after completion of an infusion of propranolol, 100 μg/kg, in the lower panel. [From Gianelly, *et al.* (11)].**

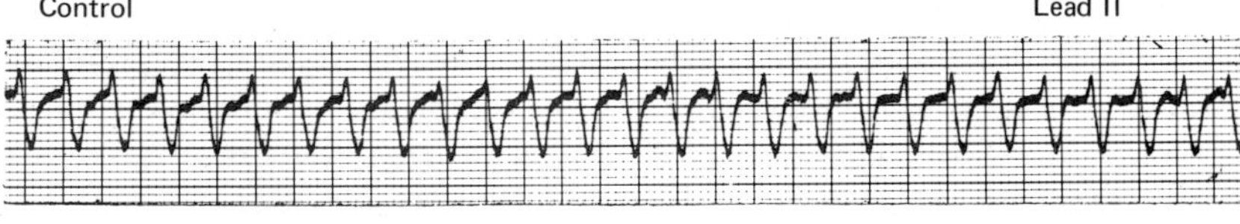

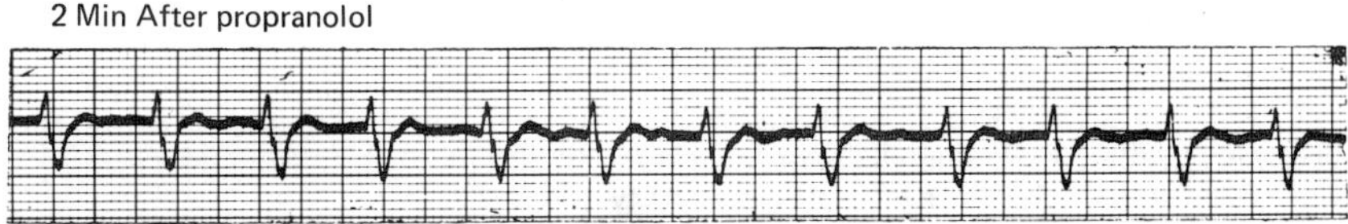

PVC frequency. This reduction was greater than 70% in 8 of the 11 patients (Fig. 11–5). We have found acebutolol safe and effective for long-term treatment of a small number of patients with extremely frequent ventricular ectopic activity and/or recurrences of ventricular tachycardia or fibrillation. The major advantage of acebutolol over propranolol appears to be that it is better tolerated by the patients in terms of noncardiac side effects.

DIGITALIS-INDUCED ARRHYTHMIAS

The usual treatment of digitalis-induced arrhythmias is careful electrocardiographic monitoring and withdrawal of the digitalis. Potassium may be administered when appropriate. When digitalis-induced arrhythmias require further therapy, diphenylhydantoin and lidocaine are probably the agents of choice. Propranolol and other β-blocking agents are extremely successful for the treatment of virtually all arrhythmias associated with digitalis toxicity. *

In the Stanford series digitalis toxicity was suspected in six patients with atrial tachycardia and varying atrioventricular block. Propranolol slowed the ectopic rhythm in all six patients, and appeared to revert it to sinus rhythm in two patients (Fig. 11–6).

Ventricular arrhythmias have also been treated in patients suspected of having digitalis intoxication. In five such patients propranolol decreased ventricular irritability in three, and produced no change in two patients. All of these patients had received digitalis in potentially toxic doses just prior to detection of ventricular irritability.

ARRHYTHMIAS IN HYPERTHYROIDISM

The β-blocking agents can be useful in controlling arrhythmias associated with hyperthyroidism. Specifically, they can slow sinus tachycardia or, alone or in combination with digitalis, can slow the ventricular response to atrial fibrillation when it is associated with hyperthyroidism. Immediate rate control may be obtained with either intravenous or oral therapy which may be continued while awaiting the effects of antithyroid therapy.

POSTOPERATIVE ARRHYTHMIAS

A variety of arrhythmias may occur after cardiac surgery. These are generally rapid supraventricular arrhythmias, many of which are responsive to propranolol and other β-blocking agents. In the Stanford series propranolol was administered to 16 patients with postoperative arrhythmias. Twelve of the 16 patients responded with a slowing of the supraventricular arrhythmia (Fig. 11–7). The majority of patients undergoing cardiac surgery are critically de-

---

*These agents, as a rule, would not be used when there is AV block with normal or slow ventricular rate resulting from digitalis toxicity.

pendent upon catecholamine stimulation of the heart to maintain cardiac function. Therefore, β-blocking agents should be used in this situation only when the arrhythmias are causing hemodynamic embarrassment and alternative forms of therapy fail to control the arrhythmia. Markedly reduced doses of β-blocking agents should be administered and should be discontinued if a worsening cardiac function occurs before control of the arrhythmia is obtained. When available, β-blocking agents without major myocardial depressant action, such as practolol (17), should be used in this clinical setting.

β-BLOCKING AGENTS FOR THE PREVENTION OF SUDDEN DEATH AFTER MYOCARDIAL INFARCTION

Several well controlled studies have indicated that prophylactic administration of propranolol affords no reduction in the in-hospital mortality after acute myocardial infarction (5, 7, 23). More recently attention has focused on preventing sudden death after hospital discharge. Patients are at increased risk of dying suddenly in the first year after myocardial infarction, probably as a result of episodes of ventricular tachycardia and/or ventricular fibrillation. In several studies, prophylactic antiarrhythmic agents have been administered to this group of patients. Three studies compared the results of administering β-blocking agents or placebo in this patient population (1, 3, 32), and all three studies demonstrated a small but significant reduction in the incidence of sudden death in the group who were given β-blocking drugs. These studies

Fig. 11–7. Electrocardiograms of a patient who developed a rapid supraventricular rate 2 hours after Starr–Edwards replacement of the mitral valve (top panel). The arrhythmia reverted to sinus rhythm with an intraventricular conduction defect after 3 mg propranolol (bottom panel). [From Gianelly and Harrison (12)].

Control

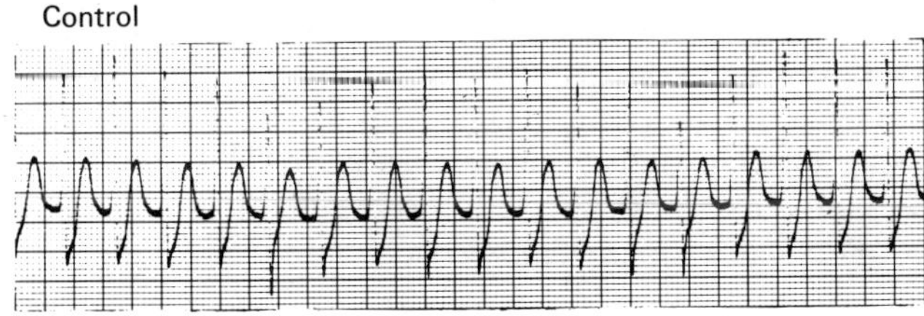

After 3 mg propranolol

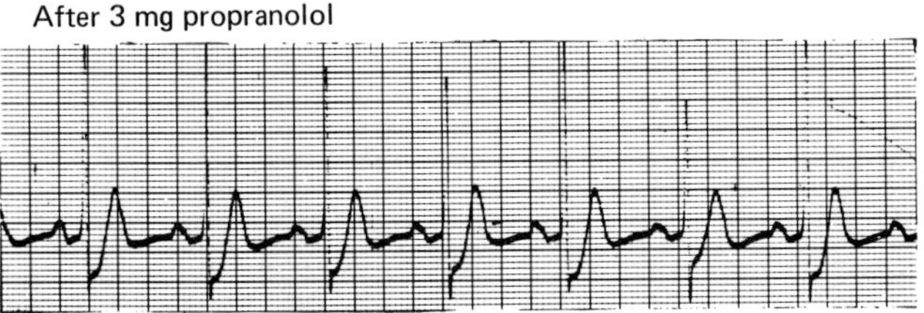

are promising and further work in this area may provide guidelines for prophylactic long-term treatment with β-blockade after myocardial infarction to reduce the risk of sudden death.

SIDE EFFECTS OF β-BLOCKING AGENTS

A number of major and minor side effects have been reported after the administration of β-blocking agents. All β-blocking agents possess the potential for myocardial depression. This generally assumes importance only in patients who are dependent upon catecholamine stimulation for preservation of myocardial function, such as patients with preexisting congestive heart failure, who have experienced acute myocardial infarction, or are in the early postoperative period. The hypotension or shock which can be precipitated by administering β-blocking agents to critically ill cardiac patients probably results from their myocardial depressant effect. Less myocardial depression is produced by agents with inherent β-stimulating properties, such as practolol, than by pure β-blocking agents, such as propranolol. Other adverse reactions from β-blocking drugs result from their effect on the cardiac conduction system. Patients may show excessive bradycardia, sinoatrial arrest, prolonged atrioventricular conduction, and complete heart block. The noncardioselective β-blocking agents can intensify the bronchoconstriction seen in patients with preexisting asthma or chronic obstructive pulmonary disease.

The most frequent side effects associated with chronic oral propranolol therapy are increased fatigue and depression. Other side effects include nausea, vomiting, peripheral vascular insufficiency in patients with existing peripheral vascular disease, and alterations in carboyhydrate metabolism (including hyper– and hypoglycemia). Abrupt withdrawal of chronic propranolol therapy in nonhospitalized patients with coronary artery disease and angina pectoris may occasionally result in increased angina, myocardial infarction and death. Gradual reduction of the drug is recommended in this clinical setting. Practolol has been associated with the development of drug-induced systemic lupus erythematosus in a small number of patients. It has recently been withdrawn from use for long-term treatment because a small number of patients on long-term treatment developed a psoriasis-like skin rash and irreversible ocular changes, including conjunctival and corneal scarring.

Many of the side effects of β-blocking drugs can be avoided by proper patient selection before the administration of these agents. The relative con-

Table 11–4. CONTRAINDICATIONS TO PROPRANOLOL

1. Overt or latent congestive heart failure
2. Acute depression of myocardial function, *e.g.*, shock following acute myocardial infarction
3. Second or third degree heart block
4. Asthma
5. Chronic obstructive lung disease

traindications to propranolol, the only available β-blocker in the United States, are given in Table 11–4. Those side effects which do occur and which are secondary to excessive β-blockade may possibly be reversed by administration of large doses of isoproterenol. In those patients with depressed myocardial function for whom no other antiarrhythmic therapy is successful, a β-blocker may occasionally be continued in conjunction with digitalis and diuretics.

SUMMARY AND CURRENT STATUS OF β-BLOCKING AGENTS AS ANTIARRHYTHMIC DRUGS

During the past 10 years a variety of β-blocking drugs have been introduced for clinical trials. These compounds all possess antiarrhythmic activity mediated primarily through their β-blocking properties. Differences in chemical structure among these compounds result in differences in tissue specificity and myocardial depression, both of which influence the toxicity of a given β-blocking drug.

The β-blocking drugs are effective for treating various types of acute arrhythmias and for the prevention of recurrent arrhythmias. These agents can slow the ventricular response in atrial fibrillation and flutter and terminate and prevent episodes of paroxysmal supraventricular tachycardia, especially those associated with the Wolff–Parkinson–White syndrome. The β-blocking drugs are effective for control of digitalis-induced arrhythmias and arrhythmias associated with hyperthyroidism, anesthesia, and pheochromocytoma. They are effective in selected patients who have recurrent ventricular arrhythmias. The recently demonstrated effectiveness of β-blocking drugs for the prevention of sudden death in patients with coronary artery disease may ultimately result in widespread use of these drugs for this purpose.

At the present time propranolol is the only generally available β-blocking drug. Practolol, which has several advantages over propranolol, will probably never become available for general clinical trials because of its serious long-term side effects. Acebutolol and other newer β-blockers are currently undergoing clinical trials. At present propranolol remains a second line drug for the treatment of acute arrhythmias. In most patients with rapid supraventricular arrhythmias the positive inotropic action of digitalis is preferred to the negative inotropic effects of propranolol. Further, since most acute ventricular tachyarrhythmias occur in patients with decreased ventricular function, propranolol is contraindicated.

As newer β-blocking drugs with more cardiospecificity and less myocardial depressant effects are developed, the spectrum of clinical settings for which β-blockers are the agents of choice may broaden.

Acknowledgment

The authors would like to thank Sherilyn C. Robison for her technical assistance in the early clinical trials of propranolol carried out at Stanford.

REFERENCES

1. Ahlmark G, Saetre H, Korsgren M: (Letter): Reduction of sudden deaths after myocardial infarction. Lancet 2:1563, 1974
2. Ahlquist RP: Study of adrenotropic receptors. Am J Physiol 153:586, 1948
3. A Multicentre International Study: Improvement in prognosis of myocardial infarction by long-term beta adrenoreceptor blockade using practolol. Br Med J 3: 735, 1975
4. Anzola J, Rushmer RF: Cardiac responses to sympathetic stimulation. Circ Res 4: 303, 1956
5. Balcon R, Jewitt DE, Davies JPH, Oram S: A controlled trial of propranolol in acute myocardial infarction. Lancet 2: 917, 1966
6. Black JW, Crowther AF, Shanks RG, Smith LH, Dornhorst AC: New adrenergic beta-receptor antagonist. Lancet 1: 1080, 1964
7. Clausen J, Jørgensen FS, Toin J, Felsby M, Nielsen BL, Strange B: Absence of prophylactic effect of propranolol in myocardial infarction. Lancet 2: 920, 1966
8. Coltart DJ, Gibson DG, Shand DG: Plasma propranolol levels associated with suppression of ventricular beats. Br Med J 1: 490, 1971
9. Epstein SE, Braunwald E: Beta-adrenergic receptor blocking drugs: mechanism of action and clinical applications. N Engl J Med 275: 1106, 1966
10. Frieden J, Rosenblum R, Enselberg CD, Rosenberg A: Propranolol treatment of chronic intractable supraventricular arrhythmias. Am J Cardiol 22: 711, 1968
11. Gianelly RE, Griffin JR, Harrison DC: Use of propranolol in the treatment and prevention of cardiac arrhythmias. Ann Intern Med 66: 667, 1967
12. Gianelly RE, Harrison DC: Drugs used in the treatment of cardiac arrhythmias. DM, January, 1967
13. Gibson DG, Balcon R, Sowton E: Clinical use of I.C.I. 50172 as an antidysrhythmic agent in heart failure. Br Med J 3: 161, 1968
14. Goldreyer BN, Damato AN: The essential role of atrioventricular conduction delay in the initiation of parosyxmal supraventricular tachycardia. Circulation 43: 679, 1971
15. Harrison DC, Griffin JR, Fiene TJ: Effects of beta adrenergic blockade with propranolol in patients with atrial arrhythmias. N Engl J Med 273: 410, 1964
16. Hoffman BF, Cranefield PF: Physiological basis for cardiac arrhythmias. Am J Med 37: 670, 1964
17. Jewitt DE, Croxson R: Practolol in the management of cardiac dysrhythmias following myocardial infarction and cardiac surgery. Postgrad Med (Suppl) 47: 25, 1971
18. Jewitt DE, Mercer CJ, Shillingford JP: Practolol in the treatment of cardiac dysrhythmias due to acute myocardial infarction. Lancet 2: 227, 1966
19. Kerber RE, Goldman RH, Gianelly RE, Harrison DC: Treatment of atrial arrhythmias with alprenolol. JAMA 214: 1849, 1970
20. Levi GF, Proto C: Combined treatment of atrial fibrillation with quinidine and beta-blockers. Br Heart J 34: 911, 1972
21. Lucchesi BR, Whitsitt LS: Pharmacology of beta-adrenergic blocking agents. Prog Cardiovasc Dis 11: 410, 1969
22. Mendez C, Aceves J, Mendez R: Anti-adrenergic action of digitalis on the refractory period of A–V transmission system. J Pharmacol Exp Ther 133: 199, 1961
23. Norris RM, Caughey DE, Scott PJ: Trial of propranolol in acute myocardial infarction. Br Med J 2: 398, 1968
24. Paterson JW, Conolly ME, Dollery CT, Hayes A, Cooper RG: The pharmacodynamics and metabolism of propranolol in man. Pharmacol Clin 2: 127, 1970

25. Powell CE, Slater IH: Blocking of inhibitory adrenergic receptors by a dichloro analog of isoproterenol. J Pharmacol Exp Ther 122: 480, 1958.

26. Rosen KM, Barwolf C, Ehsani A, Rahimtoola SH: Effects of lidocaine and propranolol on the normal and anomalous pathways in patients with prexcitation. Am J Cardiol 30: 801, 1972

27. Seides SF, Josephson ME, Batsford WP, Weisfogel GM, Lau SH, Damato AN: The electrophysiology of propranolol in man. Am Heart J 88: 733, 1974

28. Stern S: Conversion of chronic atrial fibrillation to sinus rhythm with combined propranolol and quinidine treatment. Am Heart J 74: 170, 1967

29. Stock JPP, Dale N: Beta-adrenergic blockade in cardiac arrhythmias. Br Med J 2: 1230, 1963

30. Wallace AG, Schall SF, Sugimoto T, Rozear M, Alexander JA: Electrophysiologic effects of beta blockade and cardiac denervation. Bull NY Acad Med 43: 1119, 1967

31. Wellens HJJ, Durrer D: The role of an accessory atrioventricular pathway in reciprocal tachycardia. Observations in patients with and without the Wolff–Parkinson–White syndrome. Circulation 52: 58, 1975

32. Wilhelmsson C, Wilhelmsen L, Vedin JA, Tibblin G, Werko L: Reduction of sudden deaths after myocardial infarction by treatment with alprenolol. Lancet 2:1157, 1974

33. Winkle RA, Lopes MG, Fitzgerald JW, Schroeder JS, Harrison DC: Propranolol for patients with mitral valve prolapse. Am Heart J (In press)

12 | Prevention and Treatment of Cardiac Arrhythmias Complicating Acute Myocardial Infarction

GENE F. CONWAY

Prevention and prompt, effective treatment of arrhythmias are necessary to minimize the morbidity and the mortality consequent to acute myocardial infarction. Sudden deaths are usually caused by ventricular arrhythmias; 45–50% of all deaths from myocardial infarction may be the direct or indirect result of cardiac arrhythmias (20). Serious arrhythmias occur most often in the first few hours and in patients having more severe infarctions. Although an arrhythmia may not itself cause death, tachyarrhythmias often cause hypotension and shorten coronary artery filling time, which may result in further myocardial damage, congestive heart failure or shock, thus indirectly causing death.

Continuous monitoring has shown that from 75–95% of all patients with acute myocardial infarction have cardiac arrhythmias (8, 23), many of which are transient or insignificant. Runs of two or more premature ventricular contractions (PVCs), multifocal PVCs, PVCs falling on the T-wave of the preceding QRS, or increasing frequency of PVCs were recognized as frequent antecedents of ventricular tachycardia or fibrillation (11). Multifocal premature atrial contractions (PACs) frequently were found to precede the development of atrial fibrillation or flutter. Serious arrhythmias occur more frequently in the presence of congestive heart failure, hypotension, anoxia, and acidosis. Consequently patients must also be closely observed for the development of these complications.

METHODS OF TREATMENT AND PREVENTION

Agents Which Suppress Myocardial Automaticity

The names, dosages, routes of administration, and side effects of the drugs generally used in the treatment of arrhythmias are given in Table 12–1.

LIDOCAINE

Of these drugs lidocaine (Xylocaine) has proven the most useful. Lidocaine appears not to impair intraventricular conduction (2, 5), but shares the negative inotropic effect common to practically all of the drugs which are effective in the treatment of ventricular automaticity (1, 4). Lidocaine may cause less depression of contractility at an effective therapeutic level than quinidine or procaine amide (Pronestyl) (25).

To suppress ventricular arrhythmias lidocaine is given intravenously as a bolus of 50–100 mg and repeated, if necessary, within 5–10 minutes to a total dosage of 5 mg/kg of body weight given within a span of 20–30 minutes. This is usually followed by a continuous intravenous infusion of from 1–3 mg/min, as necessary to suppress ventricular automaticity. We find a continuous infusion pump, (Ivac Corp., San Diego, CA. or Sigmamotor, Inc., Middleport, N.Y.), a valuable aid in maintaining a constant, slow infusion.

The most common side effects of lidocaine which we have encountered have been light-headedness and somnolence, or a fuguelike state. These are usually promptly reversed by temporarily discontinuing or decreasing the rate of infusion. Others have described tinnitus and visual disturbances (8). The most significant side effects have been hypotension, respiratory depression or apnea; however, these usually follow the administration of an excessive dose of lidocaine (7). Seizures appear to be relatively uncommon, and usually follow too rapid administration or an excessive total dose of lidocaine. Infusions of less than 3 mg/min have not caused side effects, except in patients with hepatic dysfunction, congestive heart failure or advanced age. Pacemaker depression (*e.g.*, sinoatrial arrest or marked sinus bradycardia) and depression of AV conduction may be seen with therapeutic doses of lidocaine (Fig 12–1). In such an event it may be necessary to pace the patients heart electrically while continuing the administration of lidocaine.

PROCAINE AMIDE

Procaine amide is an effective drug for the treatment of ventricular extrasystoles and ventricular tachycardia. However, it may produce significant hypotension when given intravenously, even in doses of less than 100 mg/min, as is often recommended for the treatment of ventricular tachycardia. Consequently, if given intravenously, it is advisable to give procaine amide at 50 mg/min or less (12) and to have norepinephrine (Levophed) readily available. Given as a slow, continuous intravenous infusion of 2–5 mg/min, procaine amide may suppress ventricular automaticity when other treatment has failed (28). Procaine amide may also be given intramuscularly at intervals of 4–6 hours in doses of 250–750 mg. Similar doses may be administered by mouth. Procaine amide is excreted through the kidneys, hence the patient with renal disease may develop toxic levels of procaine amide, as may patients with congestive heart failure.

DIPHENYLHYDANTOIN

Diphenylhydantoin (Dilantin) has been known for several years to be capable of suppressing myocardial automaticity and has been occasionally used in the

Table 12–1. DRUGS MOST USED FOR TREATMENT OF ARRHYTHMIAS

Drug	Treatment dosage			Maintenance dosage			Side effects or toxic effects
	IV	IM	PO	IV	IM	PO	
Lidocaine* (Xylocaine)	50–100 mg by direct injection, repeat in 5–10 min if needed, to a total dose no greater than 5 mg/kg within 30 min	Not given	Not given	Infusion of 1–3 mg/min	200 mg q 3 h (rarely given)	Not given	Somnolence, seizures, respiratory depression from overdosage
Procainamide* (Pronestyl)	50 mg/min to total of 1–1.5 gm	1 g stat and 0.5 g q 4–6 hr	1 g stat and 0.5 g q 4–6 hr	Infusion of 2–5 mg/min	0.25–0.5 g q 4–6 hr	0.25–0.75 g q 6 hr	Hypotension with IV administra-tion, intra-ventricular conduction defects, depressed AV conduction (rare)
Quinidine	Not given	0.4–0.6 g stat and 0.3–0.4 g	0.6 g, then 0.4 g q 3 hr	Not given	0.3–0.4 g q 4–6 hrs	0.2–0.4 g q 6 hr	Hypotension, ventricular

		q 4–6 hr (lactate or gluconate)			(rarely used)		arrythmias, thrombocytopenia, intra-ventricular conduction delay, impaired AV conduction, gastro-intestinal disturbances
Diphenyl-hydantoin* (Dilantin)	0.1 gm/5 min, may be repeated to total 0.3 gm/30 min	0.25–0.5 g	0.2–0.4 g q 4 hr	Not given	0.1 g q 6 hr	0.1 g q 6 hr	Hypotension, (?) impaired AV conduction
Digoxin (Lanoxin)**	0.25–0.5 mg and 0.125–0.25 mg q 2–4 hr usual total 0.5–1.0 mg within 24 hr	0.25–0.5 mg and 0.125–0.25 mg q 2–4 hr usual total 0.5–1.0 mg within 24 hr	0.5–0.75 mg and 0.25–0.5 mg q 4–6 hr usual total 1.0–1.5 mg in 24 hr	Rarely given	0.125–0.25 mg *q.d.* or *b.i.d.*	0.125–0.5 mg av 0.25 mg q.d.	Ventricular arrhythmias, impaired AV conduction, atrial tachycardia, junctional rhythm

*Lidocaine, procainamide, quinidine, and diphenylhydantoin should not be given to patients who have AV block unless the ventricular rate is controlled by artificial pacing. These drugs should be administered rarely and then with caution to patients who have preexisting intraventricular defects.

**Dosage of Lanoxin revised in accordance with recommendations of Burroughs Wellcome Co., Feb., 1976

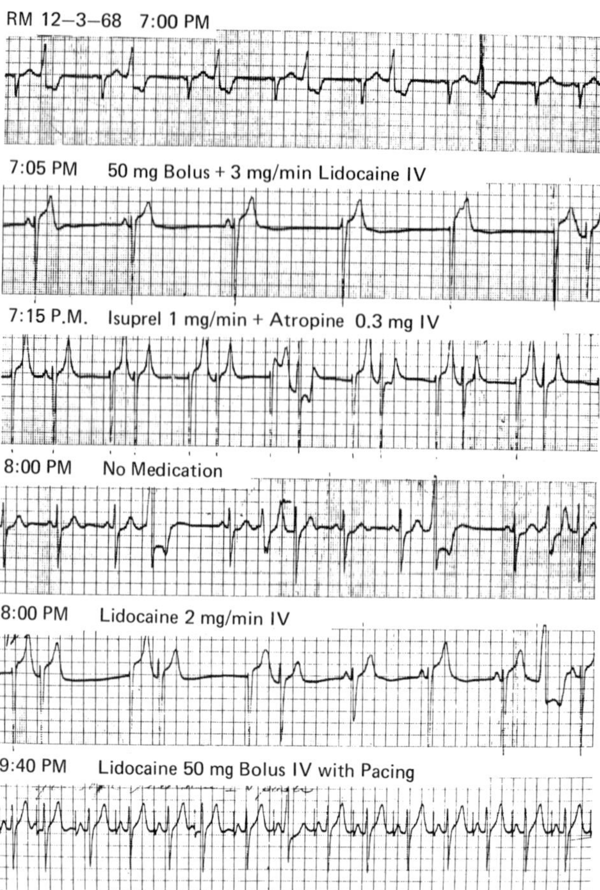

Fig. 12–1.   **A 68-year-old man with an acute inferior myocardial infarction was given lidocaine to suppress premature ventricular contractions shown in 7:00 PM strip. Marked sinus slowing with a junctional escape rhythm resulted (7:05 PM strip). Injection of atropine and infusion of Isuprel accelerated the junctional pacemaker and reciprocal beats appeared, some of which are aberrated (7:15 PM strip). After medication was discontinued multifocal premature ventricular contractions appear (8:00 PM strip). An infusion of lidocaine was started and sinus slowing with junctional escape beats resulted soon after (second 8:00 PM strip). Arrhythmia was finally controlled by atrial pacing at 90/min and lidocaine; a 50 mg bolus was given and followed by a continuous infusion of 2 mg/min After 36 hours no treatment was required. (Tracings from monitor.)**

treatment of cardiac arrhythmias. It appears to be effective both in ventricular and atrial arrhythmias, but experimental work indicates that dosages which are effective in controlling arrhythmias may cause significant depression of myocardial contractility (21). For this reason we have used diphenylhydantoin only when the arrhythmia was suspected to be a result of digitalis intoxication. Published reports indicate that in severely failing hearts diphenylhydantoin may impair AV conduction. But experimental work indicates that diphenylhydantoin does not decrease AV conduction, (2, 24) and we have cautiously used diphenylhydantoin to successfully treat PAT with block that was suspected to be due to digitalis intoxication. If given intravenously, it should be administered slowly and cautiously (100 mg/5 min, and no more than 300 mg in 30 min).

PROPRANOLOL

Propranolol (Inderal) may also be used to control arrhythmias suspected to be due to digitalis intoxication. While it has been found to be effective in suppressing or preventing ventricular tachycardia and fibrillation in patients with acute myocardial infaction, we have not used it in patients with acute myocardial infarction because it also depresses myocardial contractility.

The drugs discussed above are contraindicated in patients with heart block and slow junctional or idioventricular rhythm, except when the rhythm has been controlled by electrically pacing the ventricles. Preexisting bundle branch block or intraventricular conduction defect (*e.g.* left bundle branch hemiblock) dictates caution (9).

DIGITALIS

Of the available digitalis glycosides we prefer digoxin (Lanoxin) because it is available for administration intravenously, intramuscularly or by mouth; it has a rapid onset of action and is excreted fairly promptly. Although no hard and fast dosage rule can be given, most patients can be effectively digitalized by the dosages given in Table 12–1. In general we give one-half the oral dose when the drug is given parenterally. Digitalis glycosides probably increase myocardial automaticity in patients who have an acute myocardial infarction. Consequently we seldom give full digitalizing doses to such patients. If the patient has not had previous digitalis medication, digoxin is given in an initial dose of 0.25 to 0.5 mg intramuscularly or intravenously and additional doses of 0.125–0.25 mg are given by the same route at 3 to 4 hour intervals until the desired digitalizing effect is obtained (usually control of the ventricular rate to less than 100/min) or ventricular automaticity appears. Often this is at half, or less, of the usual parenteral digitalizing dose.

Arrhythmias, particularly atrial arrhythmias, may be prevented or controlled by the effective treatment of congestive heart failure, if it is present. Digitalis glycosides are also useful in controlling the ventricular rate in patients who develop atrial flutter or atrial fibrillation.

ELECTROLYTES-POTASSIUM

Successful management of patients who are susceptible to arrhythmias requires knowledge of the serum electrolytes, particularly if digitalis medication is being given. Potassium salts may be effective in abolishing ventricular automaticity, especially if it is due to digitalis; but great caution is advised if there is any indication of AV block (29). In general if first degree, or greater, AV block exists, even though it may be considered due to digitalis, it is wise not to give potassium unless hypokalemia is known to exist. In this case potassium may be given cautiously, preferably by mouth and while the patient's rhythm is being monitored.

Prophylactic Measures

The question has been raised of administering antiarrhythmic agents prophylactically to all patients having an acute myocardial infarction (15). Because of the frequency with which patients having acute myocardial infarction develop arrhythmias which, by present criteria require suppression, it is difficult to resolve this question by a controlled trial. It has been shown that prophylactic administration of antiarrhythmic agents will decrease the incidence of ventricular arrhythmias, including ventricular fibrillation (3, 10, 15, 16). However the effective prophylactic agents, quinidine, lidocaine, and procaine amide, may have undesirable side effects, including pacemaker depression, impairment of AV and intraventricular conduction, and induction of ventricular tachycardia in sensitive individuals.

The cardiac rhythm of all patients who have an acute myocardial infarction should be monitored continuously during at least the first 5–7 days of their illness. The trend in the frequency of arrhythmias may be established from a routine hourly estimate of the number of ectopic beats. If arrhythmic activity is increasing, or if certain arbitrary limits are exceeded, then the patient should be treated with suppressive agents.

Electric Countershock

Arrhythmias with rapid ventricular rates may cause hemodynamic impairment manifested by heart failure, hypotension, decreased urinary output or loss of consciousness. Particularly in patients with acute myocardial infarction such an arrhythmia must be promptly reverted and the most effective means of doing this is electric countershock. Instruments which deliver a direct current (DC) shock programmed (synchronized) to discharge at a selected point in the cardiac cycle (usually right after the QRS) are used. The older alternating current (AC) instruments, although seldom used today, can be used effectively to treat ventricular fibrillation.

Electric countershock is the only effective way of dealing with ventricular fibrillation. It is also the most effective and rapid method of treating established ventricular tachycardia and should be used promptly to treat this arrhythmia if the patient develops hypotension or becomes unconscious.

Countershock, synchronized to be delivered immediately after the QRS, is indicated in the treatment of supraventricular arrhythmias with rapid ventricular response which cause circulatory impairment. Initial energy levels of 50–75 w-sec (joules) are tried and increased as necessary if no significant ventricular arrhythmia has occurred following the previous shock. Lower settings (10–25 w–sec) are used if the patient has received digitalis. Kimball and Killip (13) recommend positioning a pacing electrode in the right ventricle prior to electrically converting supraventricular arrhythmias thought to be caused by digitalis.

It may be necessary to give the patient sedation or analgesia, and for this purpose in the critically ill patient we prefer intravenous meperidine (Demerol) in a dosage (usually 25–50 mg) sufficient to make the patient sleepy and induce amnesia for the shock. This is usually sufficient for low energy shocks (less than 150 w-sec). Diazepam (Valium) has also been recommended for inducing amnesia for the shock. The dosage suggested is from 5–10 mg given intravenously. The safety of the procedure is enhanced by the presence of a person, usually an anesthetist, skilled in tracheal intubation and mechanical support of respiration.

Electric Pacing

AV block resulting from acute myocardial infarction can usually be successfully treated by using a pacing electrode placed in contact with the endocardium of the right ventricle. When endocardial pacing is used all electric equipment in contact with the patient should be well grounded to a common, isolated ground. Line current powered pacemakers should not be used because of the danger of inducing ventricular fibrillation; the patient should be paced with a battery-powered pacemaker. Demand (ventricular-inhibited) pacemakers, which respond to the appearance of a spontaneous QRS at the electrode tip by ceasing external pacemaker activity, have made the use of pacemakers less hazardous, because the possibility of a pacing stimulus being applied during the vulnerable period of the cardiac cycle has been materially diminished.

TECHNIQUES

We prefer to place the endocardial pacing electrode under direct fluoroscopic vision into the apex of the right ventricle. The electrode-catheter may be introduced into the right external jugular vein, but the left median antecubital vein is most often used because of the ease of passage of the catheter. Size 5F or 6F bipolar electrode-catheters with the electrodes at the tip are used.

When the pacing electrode is positioned in an area where pacing can be achieved at a relatively low amperage (4 milliampere (ma) or less), one should record the spontaneous endocardial QRS using lead 1 or 2 of the electrocardiograph and attaching the right arm lead to one pole and the left arm or leg lead to the other pole of the pacing catheter. It is necessary to manipulate the pacing electrode into an area where the spontaneous QRS voltage will exceed 2 millivolts (mV) when recorded in a bipolar fashion. This is the minimum voltage necessary to suppress most demand pacemakers.

By recording a unipolar or V lead from the pacing electrodes, endocardial contact can be identified by the inscription of a displaced ST segment (Fig. 12–2), usually from the distal electrode. Once successful pacing has been achieved subsequent failure to pace is usually due to dislocation of the pacing electrodes, often out into the pulmonary artery and occasionally into the right

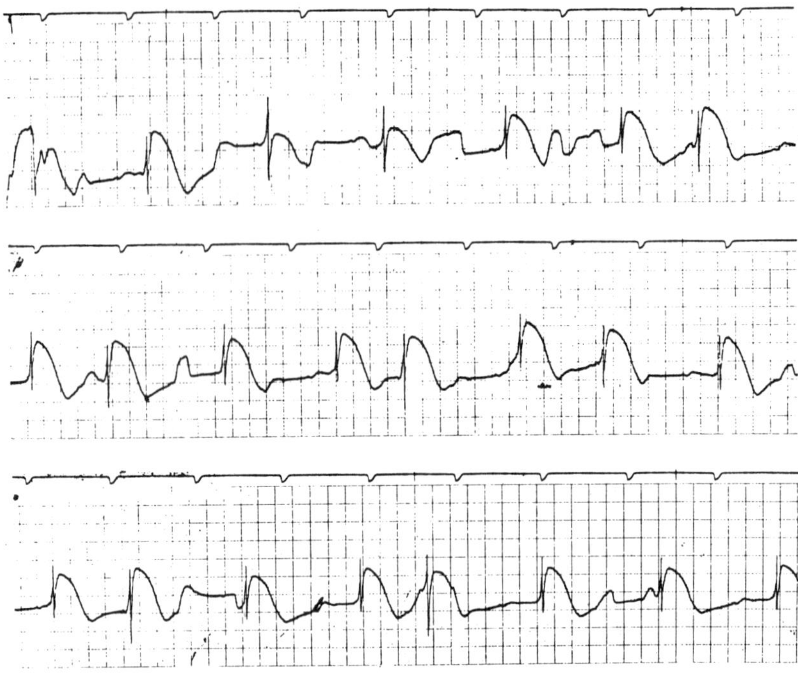

Fig. 12-2. From a patient with complete AV heart block, an idioventricular rhythm of about 45/min, and frequent PVCs. Recording was made from a pacing electrode in the right ventricle. Elevated ST segment indicates endocardial contact. Biphasic spikes represent the QRS complexes of the nonpaced ventricles. Their irregularity results from frequent premature ventricular contractions.

Fig. 12-3. Intraatrial and intraventricular recording from a 73-year-old man with complete AV block following an acute inferior myocardial infarction. Note the prominent atrial complexes recorded within the right atrium, which became very small when the electrode entered the right ventricle where large QRS complexes were recorded. Transient atrial tachycardia was caused by mechanical stimulation of the right atrium by the pacing electrode.

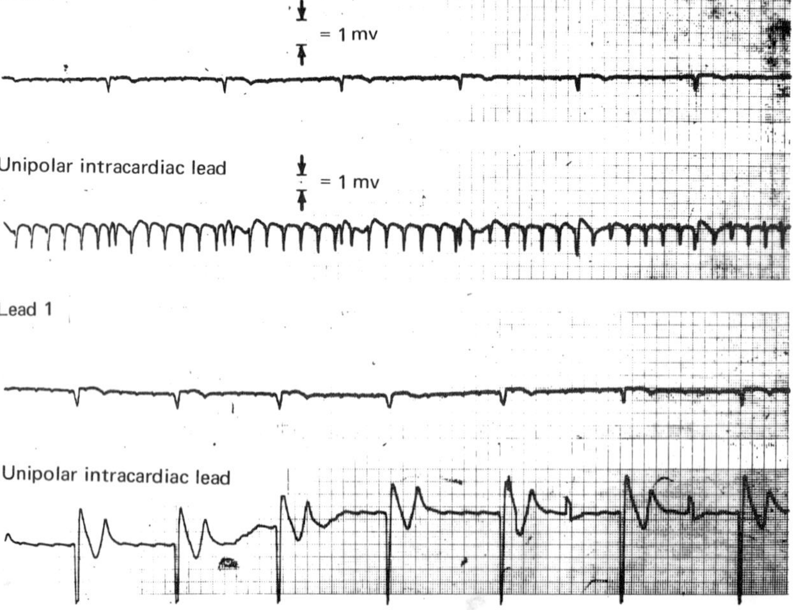

atrium. Rarely the catheter tip may penetrate the ventricular myocardium and lie free in the pericardial space. Once dislocation has occurred, successful pacing can be reestablished only by repositioning the electrode-catheter.

Frequently the pacing electrode can be manipulated blindly into the right ventricle after it has been introduced percutaneously and advanced while monitoring the unipolar electrocardiogram recorded from the electrode. The change in pattern of the P waves and QRS complexes as the electrode passes through the right atrium and into the right ventricle is used as a guide in positioning (Fig. 12–3). The floating, balloon-tipped electrode-catheters manufactured by Edwards Laboratories are useful for this purpose. These electrode-catheters are introduced into a large median antecubital vein or the femoral vein by use of a catheter introducer of proper size. (It may be necessary to cut down on the antecubital vein). The blind, percutaneous technique may be useful to establish pacing for the patient who is admitted with, or suddenly develops complete heart block before he is moved to the cardiac catheterization room. We have had a higher postpositioning failure rate with the blindly positioned catheters than the ones which we have positioned fluoroscopically. Ideally a portable image intensifier which can be brought to the patient's bedside should be used to position the pacing electrode without removing the patient from the CCU.

After positioning, the individual poles of the bipolar pacing electrode are connected to each pole of the pacemaker; however, the use of monopolar electrodes requires that the second pole of the pacemaker be placed in contact with the skin by passing a stainless steel suture through the skin. The positive pole of the pacemaker is then attached to the stainless steel suture and the negative pole to the pacing electrode.

INDICATIONS

The primary application of cardiac pacing is in patients who develop AV block, which must be distinguished from junctional rhythms causing AV dissociation by interference (Fig. 12–4). Both arrhythmias occur more often in inferior infarction. We believe that placement of a pacing electrode should be considered in any patient with an acute myocardial infarction who develops second degree AV block. Unless clearly due to administered medications such as digitalis or morphine, we view the Mobitz type I or Wenckebach phenomenon as an indication to place a pacing electrode. Statistically, mortality in patients exhibiting Mobitz I block has not been influenced by pacing. But complete block with slow idioventricular rhythms, ventricular arrhythmia or hypotension may develop in an occasional patient. Pacing may also be indicated in patients who have marked sinus bradycardia, particularly if escape beats or ventricular extrasystoles occur, or when the patient is hypotensive or shows other signs of circulatory failure. Pacing may be necessary in patients if the administration of antiarrhythmic agents for ventricular irritability causes sinus bradycardia or arrest (Fig. 12–1). In such cases if AV conduction is intact one may pace either the atrium or the ventricle.

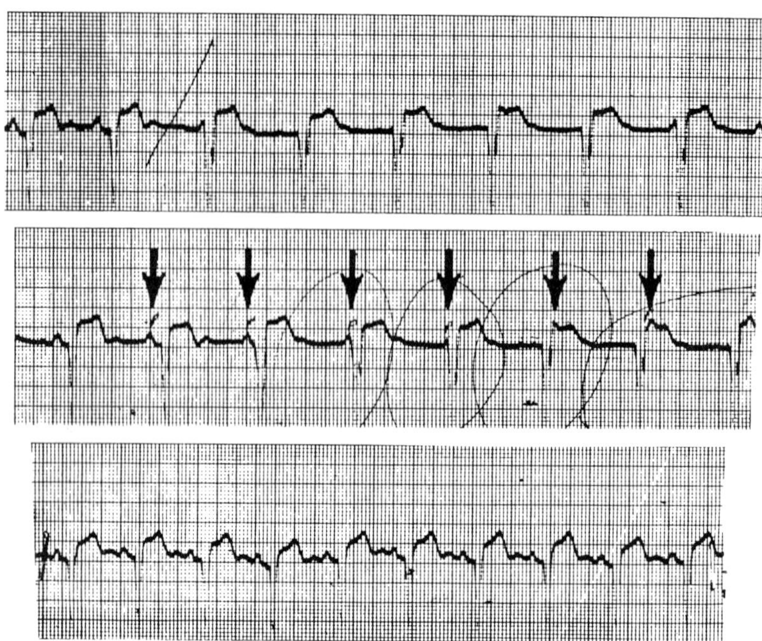

Fig. 12–4.   **From a 45-year-old man with an acute inferior myocardial infarction. Sinus rhythm at a rate of 63/min was interfered with by a slight faster junctional pacemaker. The P waves (indicated by ↓) can be seen entering the QRS complexes in second strip. After an intravenous injection of atropine, 0.3 mg the sinus rate increased to 86/min and again controlled the ventricles (bottom strip).**

Atrial or ventricular pacing may be used to suppress ventricular arrhythmias in patients when drug therapy has failed. Here pacing is usually done at a rate greater than the patients unpaced rate. If PVC's occur at a fixed interval from the preceding QRS, a pacing rate giving an RR interval equal to or less than the R-PVC interval should be tried, unless this results in an excessive heart rate.

VENTRICULAR ARRHYTHMIAS

Premature Ventricular Contractions

From 85–90% of all patients with acute myocardial infarction will have ventricular extrasystoles. Since many of these patients will require no treatment the problem becomes that of identifying the arrhythmia and deciding which patients should be treated. We use the generally accepted criteria of more than 6 PVCs/min, PVCs occurring in runs of 2–3 or more, or PVCs which occur on or near the T wave of the preceding systole as indications for suppressive treatment. The trend in the rate of occurrence of PVCs is also helpful in making decisions regarding treatment.

All patients who are admitted with the diagnosis of confirmed or suspected acute myocardial infarction should be started on intravenous infusion. This is useful should it become necessary to administer treatment for arrhythmias. Lidocaine is usually used to suppress PVCs and therapy is often started with intravenous boluses of 50–100 mg, which may be repeated until the arrhythmia is suppressed or a maximum of 5 mg/kg of body weight has been given during a 20–30 minute period. Following this, a continuous infusion of lidocaine (1–3 mg/min) is usually maintained, and the rate increased or decreased as is necessary to abolish the ventricular extrasystoles or at least to suppress the early PVCs, coupled or runs of PVCs. After 24 hours (or longer, depending on the seriousness of the arrhythmia and the time-course of convalescence from the acute infarct) the rate of infusion is gradually decreased and discontinued if the arrhythmia does not recur.

Quinidine and procaine amide are also useful agents for suppression of ventricular extrasystoles. Lidocaine, used as outlined, has great advantage in flexibility. Further, hypotension and impairment of AV or intraventricular conduction are less common.

Quinidine or procaine amide may be used to suppress PVCs in patients who do not have an acute infarct or in whom PVCs reappear as lidocaine is decreased. Procaine amide may also be added when an excessive dose (over 3 mg/min) of lidocaine alone is required to control ventricular automaticity.

Since there is evidence that the patients who develop ventricular arrhythmias are more likely to have higher levels of circulating catecholamines (14, 21, 26), it is worthwhile to attempt to control the patient's anxiety. During the first 3 or 4 days we prefer to sedate the patient so that he is drowsy and sleeps intermittently when not stimulated or disturbed. Phenobarbital (15–30 mg *q.i.d.*) hydroxyzine (Vistaril) (50–75 mg *t.i.d.*) or diazepoxide (Valium) (5–10 mg *q.i.d.*) are useful for sedation and are usually given by mouth.

Ventricular Tachycardia

Ventricular tachycardia (defined as runs of three or more consecutive PVCs usually at a rate of 150/min or greater) is of greater significance because it is frequently followed by sustained ventricular tachycardia or ventricular fibrillation. Therefore it must be suppressed promptly. This form of ventricular arrhythmia can usually be successfully handled by the methods used for PVCs.

Sustained ventricular tachycardia is a particularly ominous rhythm because of the resulting fall in cardiac output and also because it may degenerate into ventricular fibrillation. Therefore it requires prompt and effective treatment. Frequently a vigorous blow to the precordium will terminate ventricular tachycardia. Lidocaine, given as outlined above, is often effective; should the tachycardia persist, reversion by electric countershock is indicated. Should the arrhythmia present with serious hypotension or loss of consciousness, immediate electric reversion is indicated (Fig. 12–5).

The accurate diagnosis of ventricular tachycardia may be quite difficult. The staff of the CCU may have the advantage of seeing it develop from isolated, identifiable, premature ventricular contractions to runs of ectopic beats having a similar QRS configuration (Fig. 12–6). Supraventricular tachycardias with aberrant conduction or occurring in patients with preexistent bundle branch block, may be confused with ventricular tachycardia. In such instances the ventricular rate is often sufficiently rapid that prompt reversion of rhythm is indicated. In this case electric conversion is preferred to drug therapy, which might be hazardous in a patient with bundle branch block.

Quinidine or procaine amide, given as described above, may be used to terminate ventricular tachycardia. Because of the more frequent occurrence of side effects from these drugs we prefer lidocaine. Because of the serious nature of the arrhythmia, if full dosage of lidocaine does not revert the tachycardia (even though the patient may not be hypotensive) it is best to terminate the arrhythmia with DC countershock rather than to persist in further trials of drug therapy because of the delay and the problems resulting from the use of more than one such potent agent.

Ventricular Fibrillation

Ventricular fibrillation is tantamount to cardiac arrest and requires prompt and effective treatment if the patient is to survive (Fig. 12–7). Except in mortally damaged hearts ventricular fibrillation can usually be prevented by attention

Fig. 12–5.   **Continuous monitor strip showing the development of a rapid (> 200/min) ventricular tachycardia in a patient with recent anterior myocardial infarction. After about 20 seconds, reversion was accomplished by D.C. countershock (3rd strip) and was followed by sinus rhythm with runs of ventricular tachycardia which were controlled by injections of lidocaine. Elevated ST segment was present following the sustained ventricular tachycardia.**

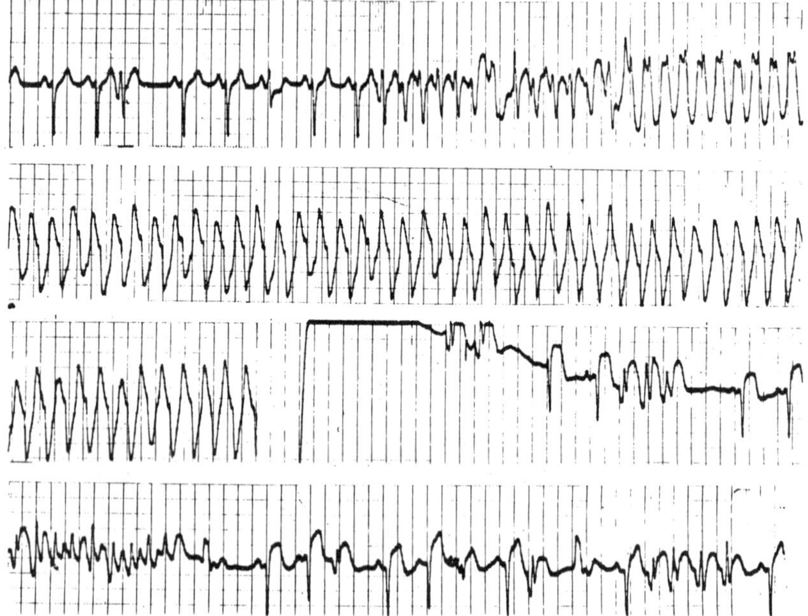

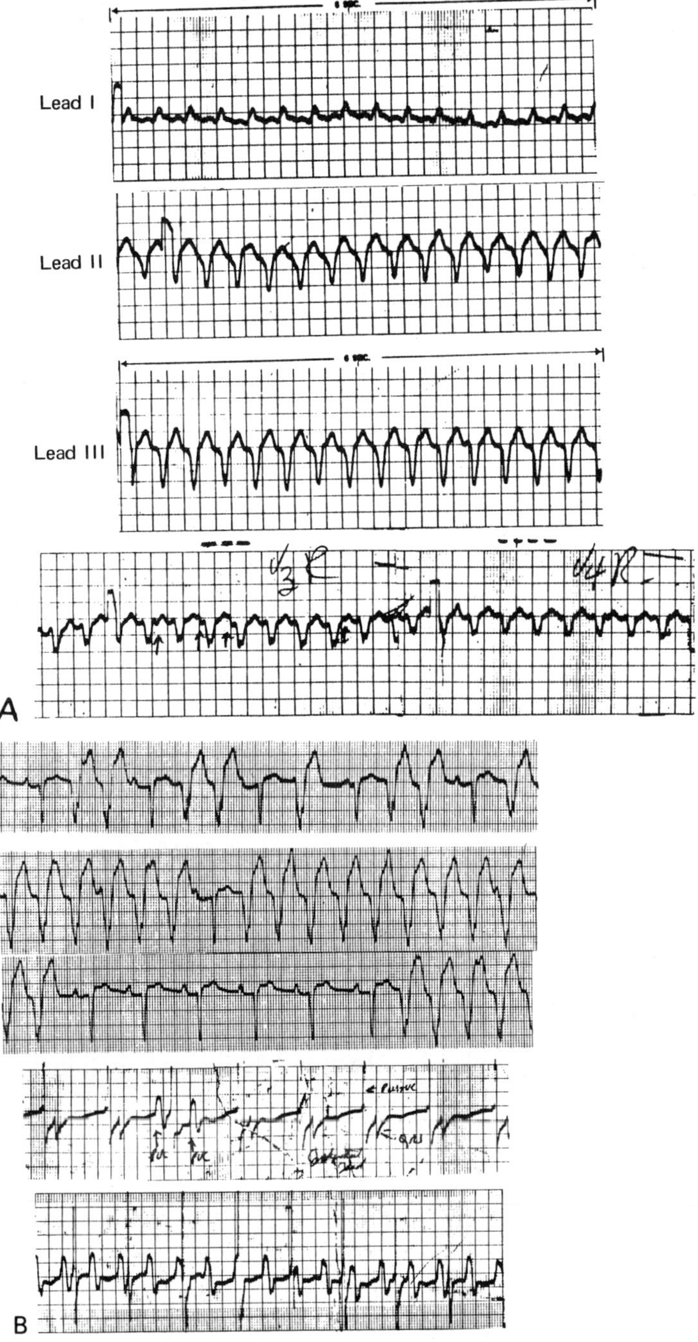

Fig. 12–6. **A. A 65-year-old man was admitted with a regular tachycardia (150/min) and heart failure. Dissociated P waves were thought to be visible in V_3R (arrows). The arrhythmia was reverted with lidocaine and the patient's EKG showed evidence of a recent anterior infarction. B. Same patient as Figure 6A, (monitor strips) Runs of tachycardia recurred (strips 1–3) and an electrode was positioned in the right atrium which recorded the P wave as a high amplitude, biphasic spike preceding the smaller biphasic QRS. In strip 4 the third and fourth QRS are PVCs independent of the P spikes. Strip 5 shows ventricular tachycardia at a rate of 140/min and the dissociated atrial rhythm (75/min).**

to premonitory arrhythmias (*e.g.*, PVCs), the prevention of anoxia, and the prompt treatment of heart failure. The only effective treatment is electric defibrillation, which should be done immediately once the arrhythmia is recognized. Our CCU personnel are instructed to carry out electric countershock as soon as the patient has lost consciousness, thus confirming the presence of cardiac arrest (and making analgesia unnecessary). To facilitate prompt defibrillation an electric defibrillator should be present at the bedside of each patient during the acute phase of myocardial infarction as well as those patients who manifest evidence of myocardial automaticity or are being electrically paced.

If for any reason it is impossible to promptly revert ventricular fibrillation, it becomes necessary to support the patient by effective cardiopulmonary resuscitation. Resuscitation procedures are detailed in another chapter in this book. It should be pointed out that most of our failures, other than those patients in whom ventricular fibrillation occurred as a terminal arrhythmia because of severe myocardial damage, have resulted from our inability to establish adequate support of respiration. CCU personnel should be proficient in the insertion of an endotracheal tube. But if there is no one present who is capable, it is best to use mouth-to-mouth resuscitation and to continue this mode of support until someone skilled in inserting endotracheal tubes is available. Attempts to use an Ambu bag attached to a face mask are frequently

Fig. 12–7.   **From an experimental animal. Ventricular fibrillation is present (EKG–top tracing) and lower tracings show fall of aortic pressure (Ao) to below 20 mm Hg and left ventricular pressure (lv) to 0. Following dc countershock (arrow), effective ventricular contractions promptly returned.**

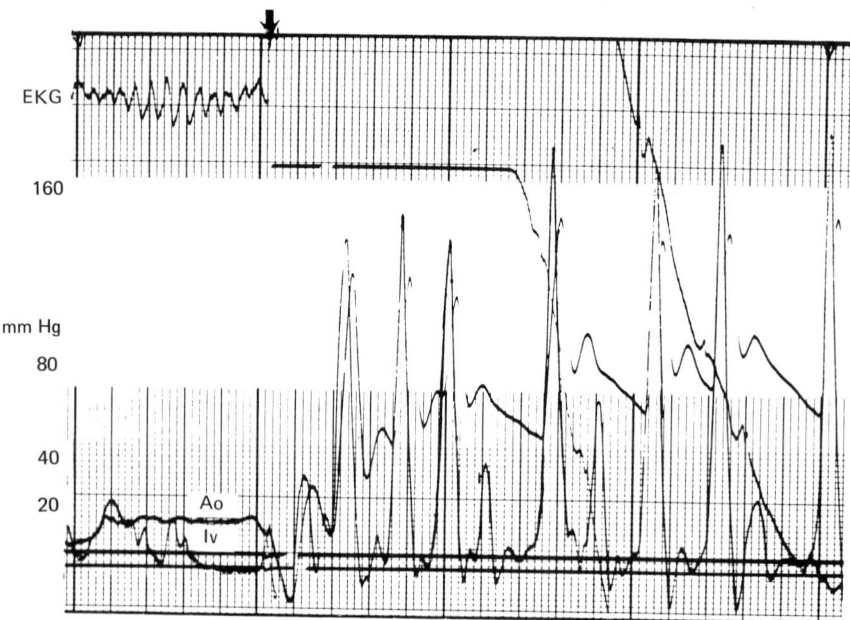

ineffective because of the difficulty in obtaining proper fit of the mask or failure to extend the neck properly.

Acidosis occurs promptly after cardiac arrest and continues to develop even with satisfactory resuscitation measures; this must be combatted by the prompt administration of sodium bicarbonate. Generally 2–3 ampules (40 mEq/ampule) are administered immediately to combat the acidosis and further bicarbonate is given, usually at a rate of 1 ampule/10 min that cardiac arrest persists.* Determinations of arterial blood pH are needed, as this is really the only satisfactory guide to further administration of alkali.

If the initial attempts to defibrillate the heart electrically are unsuccessful and the fibrillatory waves are of low amplitude, the intravenous administration of isoproterenol (Isuprel) 0.5–1 mg or 0.5 ml–1.0 ml of a 1:1000 dilution (0.5–1 mg) of epinephrine (Adrenalin), either intravenously or directly into the heart chambers, may make the fibrillatory waves coarser and more susceptible to electric defibrillation.

When considering equipment for the coronary care unit one should select defibrillators which do not have the option of synchronization, or instruments in which the synchronization switch must be deliberately set each time that it is desired to synchronize the shock. Otherwise defibrillators used for synchronized shock may be left with the synchronized mode set and fail to discharge when an attempt is made to convert ventricular fibrillation, since the fibrillatory waves usually are not of sufficient amplitude to activate the synchronizing circuit.

ATRIAL ARRHYTHMIAS

Premature Atrial Contractions

Atrial arrhythmias may occur in from 10–15% of patients with acute myocardial infarction. Premature atrial contractions (PACs) occur fairly often; when they are numerous and appear in runs and are multifocal, they often portend the appearance of either atrial fibrillation or less commonly atrial flutter or paroxysmal atrial tachycardia (PAT). However PACs are not actively treated except coincidentally, when they occur as a manifestation of heart failure.

Atrial Flutter and Fibrillation

About 10% of our patients with acute myocardial infarction have developed atrial fibrillation, and atrial flutter has occurred in 3% of patients. When atrial flutter or fibrillation develops, if the ventricular rate is not excessive (*i.e.*, 130/min or less), if the patient does not have severe heart failure (*e.g.*, pulmonary edema), and is not hypotensive, we generally prefer to control the ven-

*Editorial note: See Chapter 14 for precautions in the use of sodium bicarbonate.

tricular rate by the use of digitalis glycosides. Digoxin is used and is usually given parenterally as described above if the patient has not had previous digitalis medication. Often these arrhythmias appear in a paroxysmal fashion and may revert with no evident relationship to treatment. Usually they disappear after the ventricular rate is decreased by the administration of digoxin (Fig. 12–8).

If evidence of circulatory impairment is present the arrhythmia should be reverted by synchronized DC countershock. Because of the tendency for atrial flutter or fibrillation to recur during the acute phase of myocardial infarction even if quinidine is given, digoxin should also be given to control the ventricular rate in the event of recurrence.

Electric pacing of the right atrium can, in some cases, convert atrial flutter to sinus rhythm or to atrial fibrillation with a more readily controlled ventricular rate. A rapid pacing rate (120–180/min and often over 400/min) with a relatively high amperage is needed. It is necessary to verify that the electrode is not in the ventricle by recording intraatrial complexe. from both electrodes

Fig. 12–8.   A) A 62-year-old man with an acute anterior myocardial infarction developed atrial flutter (atrial rate 280/min) with 2:1 AV block. B) Conversion to sinus rhythm occurred after the intravenous administration of a total of 0.875 mg digoxin over a period of 2 hours (monitor leads).

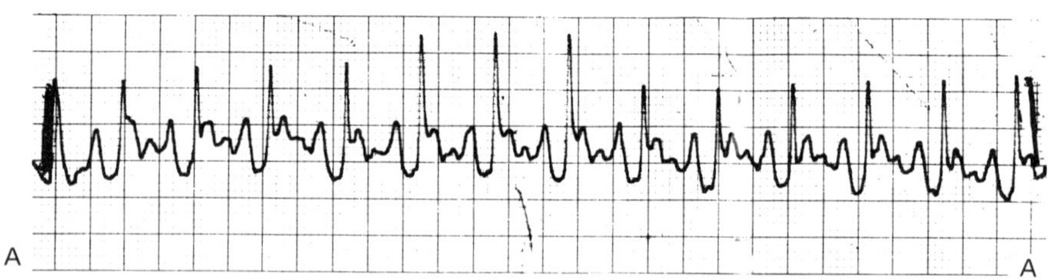

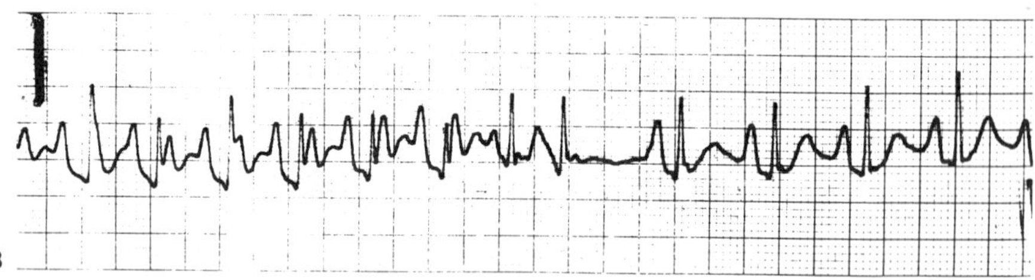

of a bipolar pacing catheter (Fig. 12–3). This method of treatment has the advantages of not requiring anesthesia and of not precipitating ventricular arrhythmias in patients who are receiving digitalis.

Paroxysmal Atrial Tachycardia

Paroxysmal atrial tachycardia (PAT), with or without block, is occasionally seen accompanying acute myocardial infarction (4% of our patients) and may be caused by digitalis. If the arrhythmia is present without block it may be necessary to resort to reversion by synchronized electric countershock because the ventricular rate is often rapid and poorly tolerated by the patient. If immediate reversion is not mandatory and the patient was not receiving digitalis glycosides, the arrhythmia may be treated with digoxin as outlined above. Attempts are usually made to convert the arrhythmia with carotid sinus pressure prior to electric reversion or digitalization. When block of sufficient degree is present it may not be necessary to treat the patient actively if the ventricular rate is slow enough to be well tolerated. Use of an α-adrenergic stimulating agent, such as phenylephrine (NeoSynephrine), to increase the blood pressure and reflexly inhibit the arrhythmia, may also provoke ventricular arrhythmias or angina and is not recommended.

In the absence of ventricular failure, propranolol or diphenylhydantoin (Dilantin) may be used for reversion of PAT; however, if significant AV block is present, these drugs should be given in smaller dosage increments and more slowly than usual. This is particularly so if digitalis intoxication or heart failure is suspected.

Sinus Bradycardia and Junctional Rhythms

Junctional rhythms are most commonly observed when the sinus rhythm is slow and the junctional pacemaker appears as an escape rhythm (Fig. 12–4). In such cases the problem is to identify whether or not heart block is present because as a general rule a junctional escape rhythm does not require electric pacing. This arrhythmia is seen more often with inferior myocardial infarctions. Morphine may contribute to the development of junctional rhythm.

Atropine or isoproterenol (Isuprel) may be used to show that the junctional rhythm is an escape rhythm and to establish that heart block is not present. If AV block is not present the patient seldom requires active treatment. Epstein and coworkers have questioned the advisability of using atropine to increase heart rate (6). They and others (18) cite the increased incidence of significant ventricular arrhythmias in atropine-treated dogs with experimental myocardial infarction. But if the heart rate is sufficiently slow that hemodynamic impairment or ventricular automaticity appears, increasing the sinus rate may overcome these problems (27). In some patients the repeated administration of atropine (from 0.3–1.0 mg) is sufficient to accomplish this (Fig. 12–9). It may be necessary to resort to electronic pacing, (atrial or ventricular) in an occasional case.

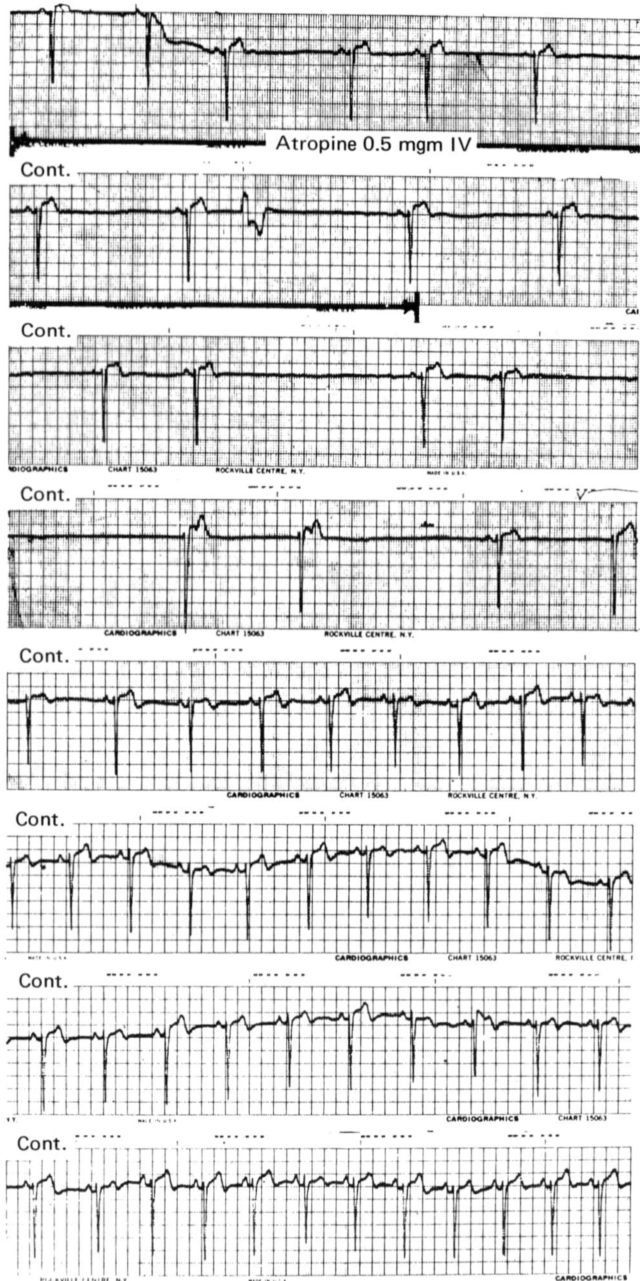

Fig. 12–9. **Marked sinus bradycardia in a patient with an acute myocardial infarction. Junctional escape beats appear in strip 4. After intravenous injection of atropine, the sinus rate increased to 80/min.**

We have experienced difficulty in maintaining continuous atrial pacing for long periods; but usually the sinus slowing is transitory, with normal rate reappearing after a few hours. Phrenic nerve stimulation may occur with pacing the right atrium and cause bothersome diaphragmatic contractions.

The development of a rapid junctional, or nodal tachycardia accompanying acute myocardial infarction is relatively rare in our experience, accounting for 2–3% of all arrhythmias. The ventricular rate is usually less than 130/minute and does not require aggressive treatment. If the patient has been receiving digitalis, then the possibility of the junctional rhythm being due to digitalis toxicity must be considered. In this instance, discontinuance of the drug usually suffices; if necessary, reversion may be accomplished by the cautious administration of diphenylhydantoin, propranolol or potassium. If the use of synchronized countershock becomes necessary, the energy level must be kept low (10–25 w-sec).

When junctional tachycardia (not due to digitalis) is present and is at a rate fast enough to cause hemodynamic impairment, synchronized countershock should be used to abolish the tachycardia. If the patient's cardiac function is adequate, digoxin may be used since in nondigitalis related cases it is usually effective in controlling or abolishing the arrhythmia.

COMPLETE HEART BLOCK

Complete AV block occurs in from 5–7% of patients with acute myocardial infarction. Particularly with inferior myocardial infarction, it may be transient and accompanied by a high idioventricular rhythm with narrow QRS complexes and a reasonable rate, (*i.e.*, 50/min or greater), thereby causing little difficulty to the patient. However if the block is established with broad QRS complexes and a slow ventricular rate the mortality is quite high. Even with prompt institution of effective electric pacing, it still exceeds 50% (19). When complete AV block complicates anterior myocardial infarction, it is more likely to be of the latter type.

Complete AV block occurs more commonly in patients who have inferior or diaphragmatic myocardial infarction. In some patients with inferior myocardial infarctions it may be induced by increased vagal tone, such as occurs after the administration of morphine sulfate, or with retching and vomiting. Consequently we feel it is important to give atropine (0.5 mg) with morphine. Meperidine (Demerol) seems to cause less nausea than morphine.

The appearance of complete AV block may be preceded by altered intraventricular conduction (left anterior hemiblock, right bundle branch block), increasing first degree block, the appearance of intermittent second degree heart block (Mobitz type II), and occasionally by the Wenkebach phenonmenon (Mobitz I). The Wenkebach phenomenon has been said to progress less often to complete heart block. But when it occurs in patients with infarctions of moderate or greater severity (as judged by pain, EKG changes, enzyme levels, hemodynamic stability), and is unrelated to medication, we believe it should be regarded with the same significance as Mobitz II (Fig. 12–10). Therefore when second degree heart block appears, we think it best to insert a pacing electrode. This is particularly true in patients with anterior myocardial infarction, because complete heart block may appear suddenly and be accompanied by hemodynamic collapse, cardiac arrest, or excessive myocardial irritability resulting in ventricular fibrillation. If this should occur and a pacing electrode is not in place, it may be difficult to establish pacemaking quickly enough to prevent the patient's death.

Should the patient present in difficulty from established complete heart block, a continuous intravenous infusion of isoproterenol from 1–4 μg/min may sustain the idioventricular pacemaker until an intracardiac pacing electrode can be placed.

ELECTRIC ARREST

Electric arrest (*i.e.*, absence of spontaneous electric activity) usually results from severe myocardial damage. Consequently, resuscitation is difficult and often unsuccessful. If no response is obtained from simply forcefully striking

Fig. 12–10.   **A 46-year-old man was admitted on 12–6–75 with an acute inferior myocardial infarction. He exhibited short runs of Mobitz I block during the first 24 hours, but was uncomplicated thereafter until 12–11–75 when he suddenly developed a short run of high degree AV block with junctional escape beats (A). Normal conduction returned (B), but was soon followed by an episode of complete AV block (C). A temporary pacing electrode was placed, but block did not recur and recovery was uncomplicated thereafter. No electrocardiographic or enzyme evidence was found to imply an extension of the infarction on 12–11–75 (monitor leads).**

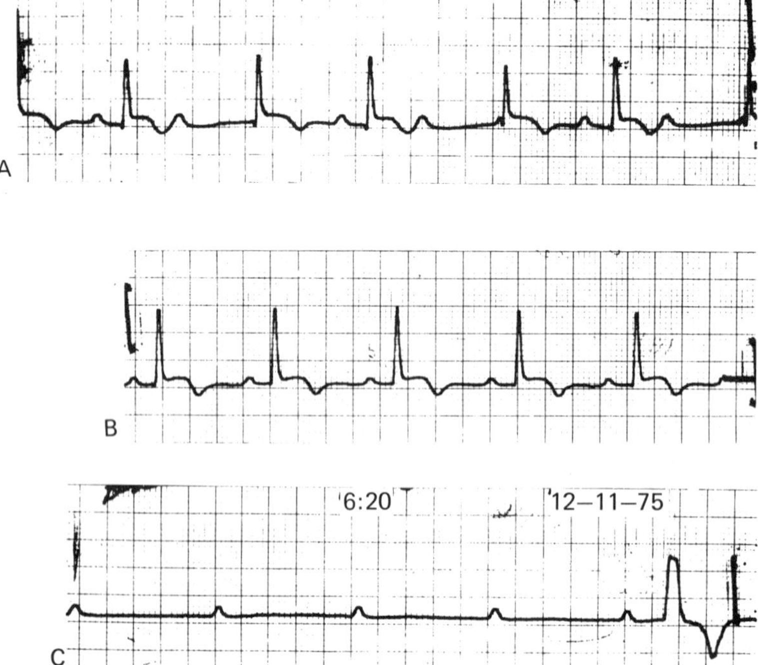

the chest, intracardiac administration of epinephrine should be quickly tried. If this is not successful a transthoracic pacing stylus should be inserted. Meanwhile, of course, effective cardiopulmonary resuscitation measures should be carried out.

The transthoracic pacing stylus is available from the Electro-Catheter Company. To place this stylus a thin-walled, 18-gauge needle is inserted at the cardiac apex and the tip passed toward the right shoulder. As soon as a free flow of blood is obtained the stylus is introduced and passed into the ventricle until the marker on the stylus is within the hub of the needle. The needle is then withdrawn, taking care to grasp the stylus at the point where it enters the chest, just as soon as the needle is withdrawn from the skin. The stylus is marked for connection by means of small "alligator" clips to both poles of the pacemaker.

REFERENCES

1. Austen WG, Moran JM: Cardiac and peripheral vascular effects of lidocaine and procaine amide. Am J Cardiol 16:701, 1965
2. Basset AL, Hoffman MF: Antiarrhythmic drugs; electrophysiological actions. Am Rev Pharmacol 11:143, 1971
3. Bloomfield SS, Romhilt DW, Chou TC, Fowler NO: Quinidine for prophylaxis of arrhythmias in acute myocardial infarction. N Engl J Med 285:979, 1971
4. Cote P, Harrison DC, Basile J, Schroeder JS: Hemodynamic interaction of procaine amide and lidocaine after experimental myocardial infarction. Am J Cardiol 32:939, 1973
5. Davis LD, Temte JW: Electrophysiological actions of lidocaine on canine ventricular muscle and Purkinje fibers. Circ Res 24:693, 1969
6. Epstein SE, Redwood DR, Smith ER: Atropine and acute myocardial infarction. Circulation 45:1273, 1972
7. Gianelly RE, vonder Groeben JO, Spivack AP, Harrison DC: Effect of lidocaine on ventricular arrhythmias in patients with coronary heart disease. N Engl J Med 277:1215, 1967
8. Grossman JI, Lubow LA, Frieden J, Rubin IA: Lidocaine in cardiac arrhythmias. Arch Intern Med 121:396, 1968
9. Gupta PK, Lichstein E, Chadda KD: Lidocaine-induced heart block in patients with bundle branch block. Am J Cardiol 33:487, 1974
10. Jones DT, Kostick WJ, Gunton RW: Prophylactic quinidine for the prevention of arrhythmias after acute myocardial infarction. Am J Cardiol 33:655, 1974
11. Julian DG, Valentine PA, Miller GG: Disturbances of rate, rhythm, and conduction in acute myocardial infarction. Am J Med 37:915, 1964
12. Kayden HJ: Current status of procaine amide in the management of cardiac arrhythmias. Prog Cardiovasc Dis 3:331, 1961
13. Kimball JT, Killip T: Aggressive treatment of arrhythmias in acute myocardial infarction: procedures and results. Prog Cardiovasc Dis 10:483, 1968
14. Klein RG, Troyer WG, Thompson HK, Bogdonoff MD, Wallace AG: Catecholamine excretion in myocardial infarction. Arch Intern Med 122:476, 1968
15. Koch–Weser J, Klein SW, Foo–Canto LL, Kastor JA, DeSanctis RW: Antiarrhythmic prophylaxis with procaine amide in acute myocardial infarction. N Engl J Med 281:1253, 1969
16. Lie KI, Wellens HJ, van Cappelle FJ, Durrer D: Lidocaine in the prevention of primary ventricular fibrillation. N Engl J Med 291:1324, 1975
17. Lown B, Fakhro AM, Hood WB Jr, Thorn GW: Coronary care unit. JAMA 199:188, 1967
18. Massumi RA, Mason DT, Amsterdam EA, Demaria A, Miller RR, Scheinman MM, Zelis R:

Ventricular fibrillation and tachycardia after intravenous atropine for treatment of bradycardia. N Engl J Med 287:336, 1972

19. McNally EM, Benchimol A: Medical and physiological considerations in the use of artificial cardiac pacing, Part 1. Am Heart J 75:380, 1968

20. Meltzer LE, Palmon F, Ferrigan M, Pekover J, Sauer H, Kitchell JR: Prothrombin levels and fatality rates in acute myocardial infarction. JAMA 187:986, 1964

21. Mixter CG, Moran JM, Austen WG: Cardiac and peripheral vascular effects of diphenylhydantoin sodium. Am J Cardiol 17:332, 1966

22. Robinson JS, Sloman G, McRae G: Continuous electrocardiographic monitoring in the early stages after acute myocardial infarction. Med J Aust 1:427, 1964

23. Romhilt DW, Bloomfield SS, Chou TC, Fowler NO: Unreliability of conventional electrocardiographic monitoring for arrhythmia detection in coronary care units. Am J Cardiol 31:457, 1973

24. Scherlag BJ, Helfant RH, Damato AN: Contrasting effects of diphenylhydantoin and procaine amide on A–V conduction in the digitalis-intoxicated and the normal heart. Am Heart J 75:200, 1968

25. Schumacher RR, Lieberson AD, Childress RH, Williams JF: Hemodynamic effects of lidocaine in patients with heart disease. Circulation 37:965, 1968

26. Valori C, Thomas M, Shillingford J: Free noradrenaline and adrenaline excretion in relation to clinical syndromes following myocardial infarction. Am J Cardiol 20:605, 1967

27. Webb SW, Adgey AL, Pantridge JF: Autonomic disturbance at onset of acute myocardial infarction. Br Med J 3:89, 1972

28. Wyman MG, Hammersmith L: Comprehensive treatment plan for the prevention of primary ventricular fibrillation in acute myocardial infarction. Am J Cardiol 3:661, 1974

29. Zimmerman HB, Gentsch KW, Gale AH: Action of potassium on the atrioventricular node in digitalized patients. Chest 43:377, 1963

Use of DC Shock in Cardiac Arrhythmias

JONATHAN D. SATINSKY
LEONARD S. DREIFUS

It is barely 15 years since precordial shock was first successfully utilized for the clinical conversion of cardiac arrhythmias. The method is rather simple and under most circumstances, extremely safe. The concept matured from precise electrophysiologic concepts and appears effective in the restoration of sinus rhythm in the presence of ventricular tachycardia and fibrillation, as well as in some of the supraventricular mechanisms. In fact the method is so simple that through the past decade nurse clinicians and paramedical personnel have successfully learned the indications and have carried out the method with the preservation of life in innumerable instances. A review by Driscol, *et. al.*, (7) reveals a most amazing history of electroshock restoring life in a number of unique experiments carried out by Peter Christian Abildgaard, an accomplished veterinarian (7). I believe that it is worthwhile to describe some of these experiments which were performed at least 124 years before Prevost and Battelli described defibrillating effects of weak and strong currents on the heart in 1899 (24).

Abildgaard succeeded in rendering hens lifeless by a shock to the head from electrostatic glass jars and then revived them by a second shock, which was to the chest, while a second shock to the head did not revive the birds. In another group of experiments Abildgaard shocked the hens once, allowed them to lie on the ground overnight, and was unable to revive them the next morning. These reports to the Medical Society of Copenhagen in 1775 can lead the reader to his own conclusions as to whether Abildgaard was, in truth, the inventor of therapeutic precordial electric shock.

It was not until 1956, however, that Zoll, *et. al.*, terminated ventricular fibrillation in man by externally applied countershock (36, 37). It was perhaps this innovation that contributed to the favorable survival rates following myocardial infarction now reported in the coronary care units throughout the world and will stand as one of the major medical advances of this century. Furthermore, Zoll reported the first use of externally applied alternating current countershock in the termination of ventricular tachycardia (35). By 1962 Lown had used this procedure on at least six patients (19). Subsequent publications by Zoll and Linenthal (35), and later by Lown and others, (15, 19, 20) led to the widespread use of precordial shock for the treatment of both supraventricular and ventricular arrhythmias. The theoretic principles and practical use of precordial shock have changed little during the past decade (6).

However certain specific issues deserve review and more precise indications have developed since that time.

Certain pertinent guidelines have evolved to aid clinicians in the use of this method (6, 12). Long-term studies by Hurst, *et. al.,* (11) and Morris, *et. al.,* (22) indicated that sinus rhythm was maintained in at least half of their patients for at least 6 months following electric shock treatment of atrial fibrillation. However Morris, *et. al.,* (22) had to employ repeated cardioversion to achieve similar results. Today such repeated cardioversion is seldom carried out. This is particularly true because the ventricular rate in atrial fibrillation is often easily controlled by pharmacologic techniques. Furthermore following electric reversion of atrial fibrillation, less than 30% of patients remain in sinus rhythm for more than 1 year unless quinidine is administered. Hence, it is unjustified to attempt to convert all patients to sinus rhythm merely because atrial fibrillation is present.

The initial enthusiasm for converting every patient with atrial flutter or atrial fibrillation to sinus rhythm has now subsided and the indications for elective precordial shock are now rather limited (6, 10). Patients now considered not to be candidates for elective DC precordial shock are listed in Table 13–1.

In patients with rheumatic mitral disease and a large left atrium, or with atrial fibrillation of more than 1 year's duration, sinus rhythm is infrequently maintained following DC shock (18). The longer the duration of atrial fibrillation, the higher the energy required for conversion to sinus rhythm and the lower the success rate for maintenance of sinus rhythm. Other contraindications for cardioversion are lone atrial fibrillation without significant hemodynamic derangements, and atrial fibrillation due to the so-called sick sinus syndrome, where precordial shock may be a hazard as the sinus node may not be able to pace the heart following conversion to sinus rhythm and cardiac arrest may ensue.

EMERGENCY CARDIOVERSION

Ventricular tachycardia and ventricular fibrillation are usually associated with an acute myocardial process or other significant cardiac disease. Ventricular

Table 13–1. CONTRAINDICATIONS FOR CARDIOVERSION OF ATRIAL FIBRILLATION

1. Elderly patients with slow ventricular response or the so-called sick sinus syndrome
2. Patients with advanced mitral valvular disease, especially with a giant left atrium
3. Certain patients with lone atrial fibrillation, especially those with a small heart and slow ventricular rate who would be little better if sinus rhythm were restored, or those in whom the ventricular rate is satisfactorily controlled with or without digitalis
4. Patients with the so-called sick sinus syndrome whose ventricular rate is more satisfactory during atrial fibrillation since there is an unstable sinus mechanism
5. Patients who can maintain sinus rhythm only for a short period of time after cardioversion in spite of antiarrhythmic drug therapy
6. Patients intolerant of antiarrhythmic agents, such as quinidine or procaine amide
7. Recent systemic or pulmonary embolism; cardioversion may be attempted after several weeks of anticoagulant therapy

fibrillation has the highest priority for electric conversion of any of the cardiac arrhythmias. The cardioverter must be set at a nonsynchronized mode, as consistent QRS complexes are not available for synchronization. The highest energy setting (400 w-sec) of the defibrillator should be utilized, as valuable time may be lost in delivering shocks of lesser intensity which may be ineffective in restoring a regular rhythm. Failure to restore a regular rhythm after the first shock requires additional measures. While the defibrillator is being recharged continuous external cardiac massage is carried out; an adequate airway is secured and respiration is maintained artifically. Correction of acid base balance is essential. Several ampules of intravenous sodium bicarbonate are often necessary to reverse acidosis. If the fibrillatory waves are of low amplitude an intracardiac injection of epinephrine, 1 ml, 1:1000, given before the next electric shock may be useful. Administration of a 50–100 mg intravenous bolus of lidocaine before the shock may help maintain sinus rhythm following DC shock. Multiple shocks delivered within a short period of time can be extremely useful, as the first shock may lower the skin resistance and allow a higher energy discharge to be delivered to the myocardium with subsequent shocks. Intravenous or intracardiac injection of bretylium, 300–600 mg, after several unsuccessful attempts at cardioversion has proved extremely useful in restoring sinus rhythm in refractory cases.

As with ventricular fibrillation, ventricular tachycardia is usually associated with advanced myocardial disease or an active myocardial process. An initial attempt to revert ventricular tachycardia to sinus rhythm should be made by a precordial thump. This procedure is usually accompanied by the intravenous administration of 50–100 mg of lidocaine. Failure to restore sinus rhythm indicates that precordial shock or other treatment should be carried out. Although ventricular tachycardia has been known to maintain an adequate cardiac output for long periods of time, the rapid heart rate without atrial contribution to ventricular filling usually compromises coronary flow and left ventricular function; furthermore, ventricular fibrillation often ensues. A 50–100 mg intravenous bolus injection of lidocaine can be helpful in maintaining sinus rhythm and probably should always be given before the electric shock.

Special attention should be directed to ventricular tachycardia associated with acute myocardial infarction. If the ventricular tachycardia is very rapid with a bizarre configuration that defies clear separation of the T wave from the QRS complex, synchronization could lead to impulse discharge on top of the T wave (the vulnerable period) rather than on the R wave. Theoretically, this could result in ventricular fibrillation 50% of the time. In such cases, the nonsynchronized mode should be used. The chances then of firing into the vulnerable period would be less than 10%.

Often one cannot distinguish sinus tachycardia with RBBB or LBBB or supraventricular tachycardia with aberrant ventricular conduction from ventricular tachycardia. This is especially true when the ventricular rate is rapid and the circulation is compromised. When sinus tachycardia is present carotid sinus pressure may temporarily slow the sinus rate and reveal the P waves hidden in the T wave in the preceding QRS complex and T wave of the electrocardiogram. However, carotid sinus pressure may not be helpful and cardioversion is utilized. If several shocks are unsuccessful in terminating the arrhythmia, particularly if the rate increases, a sinus mechanism is suggested.

Tachycardia accompanying the Wolff–Parkinson–White syndrome may simulate ventricular tachycardia when the QRS complexes are wide and bizarre. Reentry tachycardia, which enters the ventricles by the accessory pathways and returns to the atrium via the normal AV conducting system, is usually associated with a broad QRS complex. Precordial shock may be necessary to terminate the supraventricular arrhythmias of the Wolff–Parkinson–White syndrome.

Any tachyarrhythmia associated with lowered cardiac output or functional cardiac arrest must be managed by DC precordial shock regardless of the electrophysiologic mechanism. Recurrence of the dysrhythmia should be prevented by properly selected drugs.

ELECTIVE CARDIOVERSION

It is usually not essential to perform cardioversion in the operating room suite, but the anesthesiologist requires that facilities be available for suction, for administering anesthetic gases and for intratracheal intubation. While cardioversion can be done in outpatients, increasing medical-legal considerations require that maximum precautions be observed. Hence informed consent and a detailed discussion of the procedure, as well as psychological support of the patient are essential in preparing the patient. Special attention should be directed to the level of digitalis glycoside in the blood and to the withholding of digitalis preparations prior to conversion. In treating atrial fibrillation or atrial flutter, digitalis should usually be withheld for at least 48 hours. Digitalis toxicity may be evoked by electric conversion (6). Serious ventricular arrhythmias and standstill may ensue when precordial shock is attempted in the presence of digitalis glycosides and especially in the presence of digitalis and low serum potassium. If the patient cannot tolerate quinidine or procaine amide the desirability of cardioversion should be reconsidered. Most patients unable to tolerate one of these drugs will revert to atrial fibrillation within a short period of time. Quinidine, in a dose of 200 mg every 4 hours, initiated 24 hours prior to the procedure is useful. Occasionally the dysrhythmia may revert to sinus rhythm before precordial shock is instituted, saving the patient an unnecessary procedure.

Anticoagulant therapy should be used in all patients with a history of systemic or pulmonary embolization. In these instances anticoagulant therapy should be instituted 2–3 weeks before elective cardioversion and continued for 1 week afterwards or longer. Ordinarily anticoagulant therapy is not indicated in other patients, although Lown suggested anticoagulants in most patients prior to cardioversion (10).

Hemodynamic improvement is expected after reversion to sinus rhythm. Some, but not all, authors have been able to show hemodynamic improvement following successful cardioversion (5, 14, 21, 27, 31). Exercise tolerance is improved by conversion to sinus rhythm according to Resnekov (27). Phonocardiographic studies suggest that one or both atria may not contract well for hours to days after resumption of sinus rhythm.

Kinetocardiography (21) and echocardiography (5) showed evidence that reversion to sinus rhythm enhances the atrial transport mechanism, but this change does not always produce increases in systemic blood flow. Patients with depressed cardiac output tend to show improvement while those with normal cardiac output remain unchanged. Nonetheless almost all patients exhibited improved atrial mechanics, which must be taken as a beneficial change.

TECHNIQUE

When an arrhythmia necessitates emergency electrotherapy the electrode paddles are covered with electrode paste, placed in position, and the shock given. If time is available the patient may be lightly sedated with diazepam or a rapidly acting barbiturate. The electrode paddles must be clean and free from corrosion or dried electrode paste.

The following statements will outline the technique for cardioversion on an elective basis: The patient should fast for at least 6 hours prior to the procedure. Rapidly metabolized and excreted digitalis preparations such as digoxin should be stopped at least 24 hours prior to countershock, and digitoxin for a day or two longer. Serum electrolytes, especially potassium, should be within the normal range and diuretics should not be given on the day of cardioversion. In the case of elective cardioversion factors which predispose to atrial fibrillation should be abolished or stabilized before attempting the procedure. These factors include pulmonary infection, myocardial infarction and insufficiency, sepsis, uncontrolled thyrotoxicosis and heart failure. Patients who are to be cardioverted electively after cardiac surgery should wait at least 2–6 weeks for this procedure.

Many authorities suggest that patients receive quinidine prior to cardioversion and be maintained on this medication for as long as they remain in sinus rhythm. Three hundred mg of quinidine are administered orally every 6 hours for 24 hours prior to conversion. The last dose should be given approximately 3 hours before the procedure. This quinidine preparation reverts between 10–15% of the patients, thus making electric shock unnecessary in them. According to Rossi and Lown (30), postconversion arrhythmias occur less frequently and are of less severity in the quinidine-treated group. Furthermore the electric energy required to convert atrial fibrillation is 40% less. Certain patients will not tolerate quinidine. They may receive other antiarrhythmic prophylaxis, such as procaine amide or propranolol.

Prior to cardioversion the apparatus should be tested to be certain the synchronized mode is working correctly. This procedure varies with the machine but generally requires a direct writing mode to be absolutely certain that the impulse fires on, or just after, the upstroke of the R wave. The simplest method of doing this is to discharge the paddles through a saline-soaked towel not in contact with the patient or personnel.

Most patients undergoing elective cardioversion receive some form of sedation or anesthesia. Rapidly acting barbiturates may be administered intravenously. Diazepam is most commonly used. Generally the patient is given 100 mg of phenobarbital orally 1 or 2 hours before the procedure. Diazepam is administered in doses of 2–5 mg intravenously every 3–5 minutes until the patient is either somnolent or asleep. The patient is usually easily aroused but will have amnesia for the event. Older patients with congestive heart failure receive a smaller amount of diazepam while alcoholics may require the highest total dose with a range of 30–80 mg (9). The patient will often groan or cry out at the time of impulse discharge but will sleep for minutes to an hour afterwards. Someone must remain in attendance until the subject is at least partially awake. For all such procedures an intravenous needle should be well secured so that the convulsive movement at the time of discharge or some minor thrashing about while the diazepam becomes effective will not dislodge it. This site is used to administer lidocaine, atropine, or isoproterenol if necessary. The patient must have electrocardiographic monitoring prior to and for the first 60 minutes after cardioversion to detect arrhythmias.

Patients with atrial fibrillation may require anticoagulant therapy to prevent embolism, which follows the conversion to sinus rhythm in 1.5–3% of such reversion, whether it be effected by electric means or by quinidine (1, 17, 28).

The best position for the paddles is yet undecided. Nachlas reported that the vertical position of Kouwenhoven delivers greater energy to the heart than other positions (23). Here the electrodes are placed anteriorly, one on the upper right sternal edge and one at the lower left sternal edge. Another commonly used position is that of anterior-posterior paddle placement. The posterior paddle is flat and placed at the lower left scapular edge. The anterior paddle is placed over the right sternal border at the third intercostal space. Handheld electrodes must be pressed firmly to avoid burns secondary to gapping of the discharge.

It is difficult to determine the electric energy that will be required to terminate an arrhythmia. In emergencies high energy levels are used, 200–400 w-sec in the case of ventricular fibrillation and 100–200 w-sec in the case of ventricular tachycardia.

In elective cardioversion some investigators suggest starting at very low energies such as 1–10 w-sec and increasing the level progressively if the previous dose has failed to revert the arrhythmia. The rationale for using low energy levels initially stems from several facts. First, very low doses may revert a certain percentage of arrhythmias. Second, the higher the energy the more likely is the occurrence of postconversion arrhythmias and myocardial damage. Third, electric impulses have been shown repeatedly to accentuate digitalis effect and digitalis toxicity (10).

COMPLICATIONS AND HAZARDS

Cardioversion has proved to be of great therapeutic benefit, with a relatively low complication rate. Most of its complications are minor and do not prolong hospital stay or threaten life. Horn and Lown reported that in a series of 850 cardioversions for atrial fibrillation, there was approximately a 2% incidence of clinically significant complications, primarily systemic emboli (10). Most of these patients did not receive anticoagulants. There is rarely a late death reported. The majority of fatalities reported were in exceedingly ill patients and the deaths occurred at least several days after the procedure (28). Their relationship to cardioversion was often tenuous.

Most arrhythmias associated with cardioversion are due to abnormalities of impulse formation. Ventricular fibrillation is rare and develops immediately after impulse discharge. This complication may be fatal but usually can be reversed by switching the apparatus to the nonsynchronized mode and shocking the patient again (25, 28). Bjerkelund and Orning reported one young woman in whom ventricular fibrillation lasted 20 minutes despite all available medical therapy and then reverted spontaneously (1). By the next day she had completely recovered. It has long been thought by Lown and others that incorrect synchronization of the electric impulse, with discharge into or near the vulnerable period, leads to the rare case of ventricular fibrillation. The place of poor synchronization in the production of ventricular fibrillation has been disputed by Nachlas, *et. al.,* (23) and the incidence of this arrhythmia appears to be approximately the same whether synchronization is used or not (13, 16, 22, 25, 33).

Other ventricular arrhythmias may occur minutes to several hours after countershock (17). These range in severity from isolated PVCs to ventricular tachycardia. These complications are usually related to digitalis toxicity or the use of higher energy shocks, and may be treated with lidocaine (10, 23). Even isolated premature ventricular systoles should be treated with lidocaine bolus, followed by a continuous infusion of lidocaine for at least an hour after the procedure. When ventricular arrhythmias occur after unsuccessful counter-shock and lidocaine has effectively abolished the arrhythmia, another shock at the same or slightly higher energy may be used. If the arrhythmia is precipitated again, no further attempts should be made.

Arrhythmias which occur a day or more after cardioversion are often related to quinidine. Quinidine therapy may be complicated by as much as a 2.5% incidence of ventricular tachycardia or ventricular fibrillation (4, 29, 32). These arrhythmias are often accompanied by lightheadedness or syncope and usually terminate spontaneously. Quinidine must be stopped.

Cardioversion may be followed by failure of the sinus node to resume activity, often accompanied by multifocal atrial or junctional beats. This may be a feature of the sick sinus syndrome and may be followed by reversion to atrial fibrillation (17). Initial sinus bradycardia is usually transient and sinus rhythm remains. Intravenous atropine may hasten the process. AV junctional rhythms are common and are often replaced by sinus rhythm (17). If junctional rhythms last longer than several hours, the return to atrial fibrillation often occurs.

The problem of embolism has been discussed above. It is important to note that this complication, when present, usually occurs later than the first 24 hours after conversion. Any symptoms suggesting pulmonary or systemic embolism even several weeks after conversion require immediate attention.

Hypotension unrelated to anesthesia has been reported in approximately 3% of the patients. This complication usually lasts longer than an hour but is usually less than 4 hours. Although in some cases the low blood pressure has been associated with the pulmonary edema and/or ST and T wave electrocardiographic changes, its exact cause is not known; death has not been reported in any of these incidents (28).

Approximately 4% of subjects develop increasing heart size and pulmonary venous congestion on chest x ray within the first 24 hours after cardioversion. About one-third of these develop frank pulmonary edema. The exact cause of this complication is not known (17, 28). Although high levels of energy have been used in most instances: Budow, *et. al.,* reported three cases in which only 70 w-sec were delivered (2). In their one fatal case and in other autopsied cases, pulmonary emboli were not reported. Reale has shown that some patients undergoing cardioversion have significant increases in left ventricular diastolic pressure following the procedure (26). It has been suggested in the past that pulmonary edema was the result of a disproportionate increase in right atrial contractility over left atrial contractility. There appears to be little solid evidence for this. In an echocardiographic study failure of left atrial transport in two patients was associated with rapid return to atrial fibrillation (5). No mention was made of the development of increasing heart size or pulmonary edema. It is of interest that pulmonary edema has not been reported to follow quinidine reversion of atrial fibrillation so the change to sinus rhythm is probably not responsible.

In a 1970 review electrocardiographic ST and T wave changes following cardioversion were considered by one of the authors (LSD) to be innocent (6). Patients with these changes exhibit no increase in morbidity or mortality according to Resnekov and McDonald (28).

Warner, *et. al.,* (3, 34) found serum enzyme elevations following cardioversion; these have been attributed to skeletal muscle destruction in the chest wall. However myocardial necrosis was invariably produced in animal experiments when high energy shocks were delivered in rapid succession. In 54% of these animals the myocardial component of CPK (MB-CPK) appeared in the serum. In a group of patients subjected to countershock by the usual method, 30% had elevations of total CPK while in only 6% did the MB-CPK appear. Ehsani and his coworkers concluded that there is little evidence of myocardial necrosis following the clinical use of countershock (8).

SPECIAL CONSIDERATIONS

The use of precordial electric shock in patients with first degree or higher degrees of AV block may prove hazardous. When patients are receiving large doses of antiarrhythmic agents, such as propranolol, quinidine, and procaine amide, there may be a relative contraindication for the use of this method. Patients suspected of the so-called sick sinus syndrome should be carefully monitored before precordial shock; prophylactic insertion of a transvenous pacing electrode into the apex of the right ventricle may be necessary. Precise methods of electric isolation are necessary in order to prevent burns in and around the insertion site of the temporary cardiac pacing wires. Patients who have recently received β-adrenergic blocking agents for angina pectoris are particularly vulnerable to sudden sinus node arrest following attempted cardioversion. Postcardioversion bradycardia syndromes may be treated by the intravenous administration of 0.5–1.0 mg of atropine; hence, this drug should be available at all times in the postcardioversion state. If the patient has a permanent electronic cardiac pacemaker, cardioversion is not contraindicated. These units are usually protected by diodes that will prevent large discharge voltages from reaching the vital components of the pacemaker. However after the procedure the pacemaker should be evaluated for correct function in both demand and magnetic modes since a few units may be damaged by the shock. While it is generally agreed that cardioversion has proved to be a safe and extremely effective technique for the control of supraventricular and ventricular arrhythmias, the majority of patients must be eventually managed by carefully selected drugs. Finally it should be acknowledged that open heart surgery could never have been developed without this technique. More efficient wave forms and methods of delivery will undoubtedly emerge in the future, but the technique is extremely successful in its present form.

REFERENCES

1. Bjerkelund CJ, Orning OM: The efficacy of anticoagulant therapy in preventing embolism related to DC electrical conversion of atrial fibrillation. Am J Cardiol 23:208, 1969
2. Budow J, Ponnusway N, Kroop G: Pulmonary edema following DC cardioversion for atrial arrhythmias. JAMA 218:1803, 1971
3. Dahl CF, Ewy GA, Warner ED, Thomas ED: Myocardial necrosis from direct current countershock. Effect of paddle electrode size and time interval between discharges. Circulation 50.-956, 1974
4. Davies P, Leak D, Oram S: Quinidine-induced syncope. Br Med J 2:517, 1965
5. DeMaria AN, Lies JF, King FJ, Miller RR, Amsterdam EA, Mason DT: Echocardiographic assessment of atrial transport, mitral movement and ventricular performance following electroversion of supraventricular arrhythmias. Circulation 51:273, 1975
6. Dreifus LS: Use of DC shock in the treatment of cardiac arrhythmias. In Fowler NO (ed): Modern Treatment. New York, Harper & Row, 1970, p 176
7. Driscol TE, Ratnoff OD, Nygaard OF: The remarkable Dr. Abildgaard and countershock. The bicentennial of his electrical experiments on animals. Ann Intern Med 83:878, 1975
8. Ehsani AA, Ewy GA, Sobel BE: CPK isoenzyme elevations after electrical countershock (abstr). Circulation 48 (IV): 129, 1973
9. Forsell G, Hardlander R, Nyquist O, Orinius E: Diazepam in cardioversion. Acta Med Scand 197:255, 1975
10. Horn HR, Lown B: Cardioversion 1975: foremost therapy for tachyarrhythmias. Geriatrics 30:75, 1975

11. Hurst JW, Paulk EA Jr, Proctor HD, Schlant RC: Management of patients with atrial fibrillation. Am J Med 37:728, 1964

12. Jenser H, Lown B: Cardioversion of atrial fibrillation after valve replacement. Am Heart J 84:840, 1972

13. Kavanagh–Gray D: Non-synchronized direct-current countershock in cardiac arrhythmias. Can Med Assoc J 96:1460, 1967

14. Killip T, Baer RA: Hemodynamic effects after reversion from atrial fibrillation to sinus rhythm by precordial shock. J Clin Invest 45:658, 1966

15. Kouwenhoven WB, Milnor WR, Jude JR, Knickerbocker GG, Chestnut WR: Closed chest defibrillation of the heart. Surgery 42:550, 1957

16. Kreus KE, Salokannel SJ, Waris EK: Non-synchronized and synchronized direct current countershock in cardiac arrhythmias. Lancet 2:405, 1966

17. Lown B: Electrical reversion of cardiac arrhythmias. Br Heart J 29:469, 1967

18. Lown B, Amarasingham R, Newman J: New method for terminating cardiac arrhythmias: use of synchronized capacitor discharge. JAMA 182:548, 1962

19. Lown B, Newman J, Amarasingham R, Berkovits BV: Comparison of alternating current with direct current electroshock across closed chest. Am J Cardiol 10:223, 1962

20. Lown B, Perlroth MG, Kaidbey S, Tadaaki A: "Cardioversion" of atrial fibrillation. N Engl J Med 269:325, 1963

21. Mahlik J, Schweizer W, Burkart F: Atrial function after cardioversion for atrial fibrillation. Br Heart J 35:24, 1973

22. Morris JJ Jr, Peter RH, McIntosh HD: Electrical conversion of atrial fibrillation: immediate and long-term results and selection of patients. Ann Intern Med 65:216, 1966

23. Nachlas MM, Box HH, Mower MM, Sieland MP: Observations on defibrillators, defibrillation and synchronized countershock. Prog Cardiovasc Dis 9:64, 1966

24. Prevost JL, Batelli F: Sur quelques effects des descharges electriques sur le coeur des mammiferes. C R Acad Sci [D] (Paris) 129:267, 1899

25. Rabbino MD, Likoff W, Dreifus LS: Complications and limitations of direct current countershock. JAMA 190:417, 1964

26. Reale A: Acute effects of countershock conversion of atrial fibrillation upon right and left heart hemodynamics. Circulation 32:215, 1965

27. Resnekov L: Hemodynamic studies before and after electrical conversion of atrial fibrillation and flutter to sinus rhythm. Br Heart J 29:700, 1967

28. Resnekov L, McDonald L: Complications in 220 patients with cardiac dysrhythmias treated by phased direct current shock and indications for electroconversion. Br Heart J 29:926, 1967

29. Rokseth R, Storstein O: Quinidine therapy of chronic auricular fibrillation. The occurrence and mechanism of syncope. Arch Intern Med 111:184, 1963

30. Rossi M, Lown B: The use of quinidine in cardioversion. Am J Cardiol 19:234, 1967

31. Rowlands DJ, Logan WF, Howitt G: Atrial function after cardioversion. Am Heart J 74:149, 1967

32. Selzer A, Wray HW: Quinidine syncope. Paroxysmal ventricular fibrillation occurring during treatment of chronic atrial arrhythmias. Circulation 30:17, 1964

33. Waris EK, Scheinin TM, Kreus KE, Salokannel J, Scheinin BM: Non-synchronized direct current countershock. Acta Med Scand 178:309, 1965

34. Warner ED, Dahl C, Ewy GA: Myocardial injury from transthoracic defibrillation countershock. Arch Pathol 99:55, 1975

35. Zoll PM, Linenthal AJ: Termination of refractory tachycardia by external countershock. Circulation 25:596, 1962

36. Zoll PM, Linenthal AJ, Zarsky LRN: Termination of ventricular fibrillation in man by externally applied countershock. N Engl J Med 254:427, 1956

37. Zoll PM, Paul MH, Linenthal AJ, Norman LR, Gibson W: Effects of external electric currents on heart: control of cardiac rhythm and induction and termination of cardiac arrhythmia. Circulation 14:745, 1956

14 | Cardiac Resuscitation

JOHN C. HOLMES

Cardiac arrest may be defined as the sudden cessation of an effective heartbeat. It may result from ventricular fibrillation, from ventricular asystole, and occasionally from ventricular tachycardia. Cardiac resuscitation comprises those emergency measures taken to revive a patient following cardiopulmonary arrest. Cardiac arrest which occurs in patients with advanced congestive failure or cardiogenic shock, offers little hope for successful resuscitation. The outlook for successful resuscitation, however, is much more favorable when arrest occurs under other circumstances, such as during acute coronary insufficiency; following acute myocardial infarction in the absence of shock or heart failure; during anesthesia, intravenous medication, electrocution accidents, or coronary arteriography.

Although cardiac resuscitation was first described by Vesalius in the sixteenth century, it was not until 1901 that the first patient was resuscitated successfully (12). By the onset of World War I open-chest cardiac massage was accepted for the treatment of cardiac arrest. It was infrequently attempted outside an operating room. The first successful defibrillation of the human heart with electric current was reported by Beck in 1947. The real impetus to the modern treatment of cardiac arrest came in the early part of the present decade. In 1960 Kouwenhoven, Jude, and Knickerbocker first reported successful closed-chest cardiac massage (5). In 1962 Lown showed that direct current (DC) countershock was an effective and safe method of terminating cardiac arrhythmias including that variety of cardiac arrest produced by ventricular fibrillation (7). The use of direct current (DC) countershock has since gained wide acceptance. In 1963 Day introduced the concept of the coronary care unit, bringing together the resuscitation team and the acute myocardial infarction patient (4).

SOME GENERAL PRINCIPLES

The successful management of cardiac arrest is primarily dependent on the realization of the importance of the time factor. Because of irreversible cerebral damage, failure of the resuscitation attempt is almost inevitable unless proper resuscitative measures are instituted within 4–5 minutes after a cardiac arrest. Few medical emergencies challenge the speed and efficiency of the physician as does the problem of cardiac arrest.

Regardless of the cause of the cardiac arrest the initial resuscitative proce-

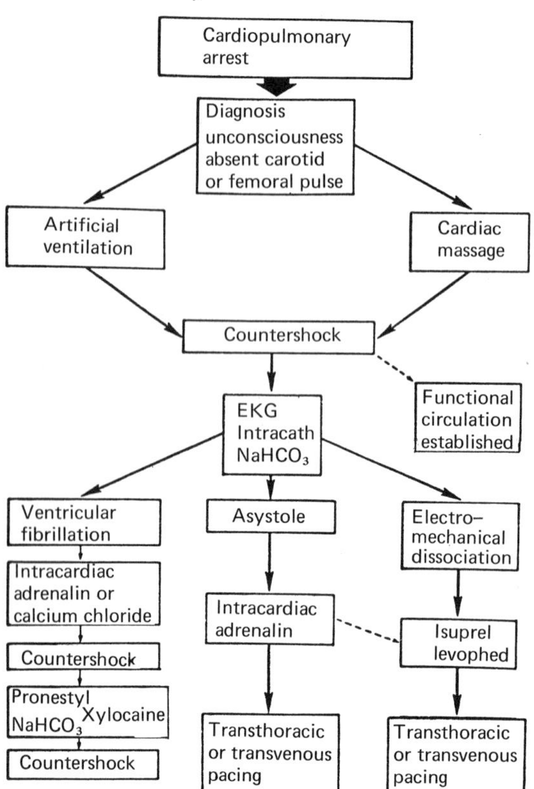

Fig. 14–1. **Flow diagram outlining treatment of cardiopulmonary arrest.**

dures are similar. The primary objective is to maintain a supply of oxygenated blood to the central nervous system. The chance of success will be greatly enhanced by carefully placing each aspect of the resuscitative procedure in its proper order (Fig. 14–1). This chapter will describe in detail the steps in resuscitation as well as the rationale for their use.

When cardiopulmonary arrest occurs a decision must be made whether or not to initiate resuscitation. If there is reasonable expectation that prompt treatment will restore the patient to a useful existence, then resuscitation should be attempted. In most instances the decision is not difficult. When one is dealing with an individual who sustains cardiopulmonary arrest during a surgical procedure there is no doubt that immediate efforts to resuscitate him are indicated. This is equally true in those cases in which cardiopulmonary arrest occurs following drowning, electrocution, or the administration of drugs or diagnostic agents. Resuscitation should be attempted in all such instances unless irreversible brain damage due to cerebral hypoxia has already occurred. Following cardiac arrest irreversible damage to the central nervous system occurs in approximately 4 minutes. In patients who are in the terminal stages of incurable disease, *e.g.,* advanced cancer, chronic cerebral vascular disease or terminal heart disease, resuscitation should not be attempted. Unfortunately cardiac resuscitation has become so commonplace in the past 15 years that frequently patients with terminal cancer or end-stage irreversible heart disease are successfully resuscitated only to continue to suffer without hope of recovery. Resuscitation in these circumstances may represent a violation of the patient's right to die with dignity.

There are other problems which are especially regrettable when a patient with no hope of a future useful life has been resuscitated, and then sustained by artificial respiration for days, weeks, or even longer. The relatives of such a patient are subjected to a prolonged period of suffering. The hospital intensive care facilities and personnel are being used ineffectively, and such care may be unavailable to a more hopeful case. Both relatives and hospital professional personnel may be faced with an eventual guilt-ridden decision to discontinue artificial support, with possible ethical and legal implications.

The physician should be alert to the possibility of cardiac arrest under certain circumstances; he should take certain measures to prevent arrest and must be prepared to deal with it promptly if it occurs.

Cardiac arrest may occur with any of the anesthetic agents. These agents may act directly on the myocardium or they may bring about their circulatory effects through the autonomic nervous system. Most instances of cardiac arrest associated with anesthesia can be prevented by preoperative sedation and atropine, as well as careful attention to the patient during induction and the operation to prevent hypoxia, hypercapnia, or hypotension.

The intravenous administration of any one of many different therapeutic and diagnostic agents, such as radiographic contrast media, may precipitate cardiac arrest. Although most instances cannot be prevented the prompt application of the proper resuscitative techniques will result in a successful outcome in most instances. Many catastrophes, such as drowning, electrocution, asphyxia, and massive pulmonary embolism may not directly damage the heart but may cause death by cardiac arrest. Cardiac arrest following acute myocardial infarction may occur in 12–13% of hospitalized patients.

The coronary care unit concept has been a major aid in the reduction of the mortality rate following acute myocardial infarction. The ready availability of the proper equipment and trained personnel in these units has brought about both preventive measures directed toward cardiac arrest, and its prompt treatment when it occurs.

DIAGNOSIS OF CARDIAC ARREST

Little time should be lost in the recognition of cardiac arrest. Time is a critical factor, not only for the preservation of cerebral function, but also for ease of resuscitation. Cardiopulmonary arrest is assumed to be present in an unconscious patient when breathing is absent and when one cannot feel a carotid or femoral pulse. Initial resuscitative measures should be instituted immediately.

Unnecessary diagnostic procedures, *e.g.,* auscultation of heart, obtaining an electrocardiogram, or visualization of the ocular fundi, must be postponed. The evaluation of the pupil size may be misleading as a guide to the degree of cerebral damage. Frequently the pupils are dilated following cardiopulmonary arrest, but in the presence of previous brain damage the pupils may be constricted. Auscultation of the heart for a faint or absent cardiac sound is unnecessary. Procurement of an electrocardiogram or the placement of an endotracheal tube should be delayed until after initial countershock (Fig. 14–1). The intravenous or intracardiac injection of drugs is usually of little value at this point. Occasionally a single firm blow to the lower third of the sternum with the closed fist, which requires only a few seconds, can restart the heart action and reestablish a functional circulation.

INITIAL PROCEDURE IN CARDIAC RESUSCITATION

Cardiopulmonary resuscitation has two principal objectives: 1) To establish immediately a flow of oxygenated blood to the central nervous system sufficient to maintain the viability of the brain cells, and 2) to reestablish a functional circulation so that the patient is able to sustain his own circulation and respiration. The first objective is accomplished by the initiation of artificial ventilation and closed-chest cardiac massage. Once artificial respiration and cardiac massage are begun they must be continued without interruption until a functional circulation returns spontaneously, or until it is determined that the resuscitative effort should be abandoned.

ARTIFICIAL RESPIRATION

Initially the lungs of the patient should be ventilated three to four times before beginning external cardiac massage. If one begins closed-chest cardiac massage without first oxygenating the pulmonary blood pool, one pumps systemic venous blood from the left ventricle to the central nervous system.

Mouth-to-mouth Breathing

The quickest and most efficient way to accomplish artificial ventilation is by mouth-to-mouth breathing (Fig. 14–2). Mouth-to-mouth artificial respiration has been used for many centuries and is, perhaps, the oldest of all methods of artificial respiration. The Bible, *II Kings,* 4:32–27, relates that Elisha used mouth-to-mouth respiration to revive the Shunammite boy. Before beginning artificial respiration one must be certain that the mouth and posterior pharynx are cleared of any mucus or foreign bodies. By placing several fingers into the mouth of the unconscious patient one can scoop out foreign material, mucus or vomit that may be present. After the oropharyngeal airway is cleared, the patient's neck is hyperextended by placing one hand behind his neck and elevating the chin with the other hand. One then places his mouth tightly over the open mouth of the patient and, while occluding the patient's nostrils with

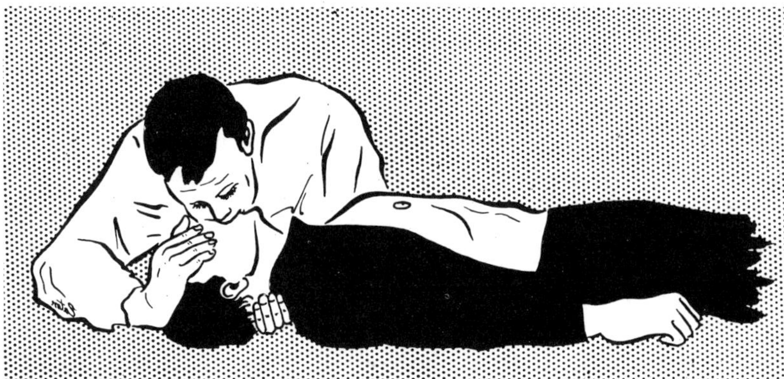

Fig. 14–2. **Technique of mouth-to-mouth artificial respiration. (see text.)**

the index finger and thumb, exhales, thus forcing air into the lungs. The resuscitator then removes his mouth from the patient's mouth, and exhalation occurs passively. This procedure is then repeated 12 times a minute. The patient's chest must visibly expand with each insufflation. If the chest cage fails to expand, either the head of the patient has not been extended sufficiently to prevent the tongue from blocking the posterior pharynx, or there is another variety of airway obstruction.

Variations of Mouth-to-mouth Technique

Variations of the mouth-to-mouth technique are equally successful in establishing adequate artificial ventilation. In particular the mouth-to-nose technique or the use of an airway adjunct, such as an S tube or Brook airway may be more appealing aesthetically. A distinct advantage of the S tube is that one may more readily observe expansion of the patient's thoracic cage and thus be more confident of adequate ventilation. This method also prevents direct contact with the patient which is particularly advisable when pulmonary infection or tuberculosis is suspected. It is possible to use an Ambu bag for artificial ventilation. The operator must make certain that the head is fully extended and the mask fits tightly to the patient's face. In my experience two people are usually needed to carry out adequate artificial respiration with an Ambu bag; one person maintains an adequate seal between the patient's face and the mask; the other compresses the bag.

An endotracheal tube should not be used in the initial management of cardiac arrest except when the endotracheal tube is already in place at the time the arrest occurs. This is likely only when arrest occurs during a surgical procedure. There are several reasons for postponing the use of an endotracheal tube. The passing of an endotracheal tube can delay more essential procedures. Frequently the endotracheal tube is placed in error in the esophagus and results in distension of the stomach. The endotracheal tube is often advanced too far and enters the right mainstem bronchus. Left lower lobe collapse and rupture of the right lower lobe with extensive pneumothorax may result from faulty and hasty placement of an endotracheal tube.

If during the course of the resuscitation it becomes evident that mechanical ventilation will be needed for a prolonged period, it may then be necessary to intubate the patient. This should be done by a thoroughly experienced operator with proper equipment.

MAINTENANCE OF EFFECTIVE CIRCULATION

Closed-chest cardiac massage is the method of choice for maintaining circulation in most patients with cardiac arrest. It requires no equipment and can be carried out by personnel who are relatively inexperienced or have minimal training.

EXTERNAL CARDIAC MASSAGE

Closed-chest cardiac massage compresses the heart between the sternum and the vertebral column. The vertebral column must be supported adequately. If the patient is in bed, one should place a firm board between the patient and the mattress. If the board is not available, the patient should be quickly moved to a hard table or onto the floor. One of the critical factors is the site of application of the external pressure to the sternum (Fig. 14–3). If pressure is applied too high it will be ineffective in propelling blood from the ventricles and may result in complications, particularly multiple rib fractures. If the pressure is applied too low over the sternum, it may be ineffective and may result in laceration of the liver or trauma to other abdominal viscera with consequent fatal intraperitoneal bleeding. The sternum should be compressed only over its lower one-third. The heel of one hand should be placed directly over the lower one-third of the sternum and the heel of the other hand placed on the dorsum of the first (Fig. 14–3).

Fig. 14–3. **Technique of closed-chest cardiac massage. (See text.)**

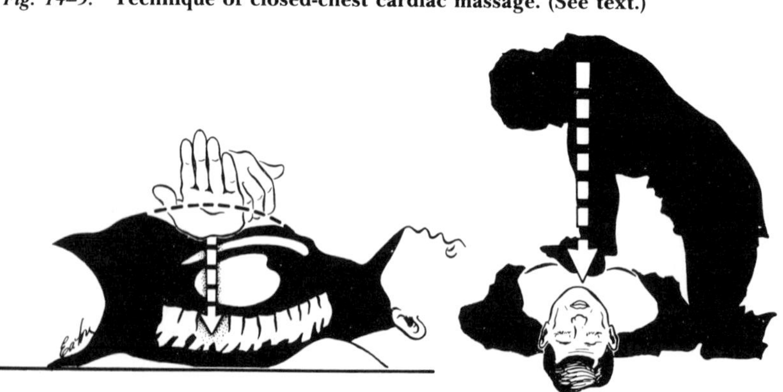

External cardiac massage may be a misleading term since it gives the impression that one should apply a slow milking action. To produce a good, vigorous pulse, palpable in the carotid or femoral arteries, one must quickly and forcefully depress the sternum 2–3 inches and then suddenly release the sternal pressure. In adults adequate depression of the sternum requires considerable pressure, but it is seldom necessary to cause rib fracture or sternocostal separation. Rapid release of pressure from the sternum following depression facilitates filling of the right heart from the great veins and the left heart from the pulmonary veins. Adequate cerebral circulation can be obtained by sternal compression at a rate of 60 times/min. More rapid rates may not allow sufficient time for adequate ventricular filling. Frequently it is necessary to carry out external cardiac massage for an extended period of time, hence one should be in a position so that he may employ not only the muscles of his upper extremities but those of his shoulders and back. This is best accomplished by kneeling beside the patient (Fig. 14–3).

If only one person is available to carry out the initial resuscitative effort, he may employ a sequence of ventilating the lungs twice, followed by external cardiac massage 10 times. This cycle is repeated until spontaneous breathing is resumed and an effective heartbeat is present, or until other facilities for artificial respiration become available. When two people are present to carry out the resuscitation, one can continually compress the sternum at a rate of 60/min, while the other effectively ventilates the lungs 12 times/min. Proper coordination of these two events is necessary and can be readily accomplished after a short period of practice.

DETERMINING EFFICACY OF RESUSCITATION

Once cardiopulmonary resuscitation has been initiated one must determine its efficacy. Effective cardiac compression should produce a palpable carotid or femoral pulse. If the pupils were initially dilated and then become constricted following initiation of resuscitative measures, effectiveness of the resuscitative procedure is probable. The onset of spontaneous respiration and an increase in the level of consciousness is evidence of effective resuscitation. One must continue artificial ventilation and artificial cardiac external massage until the patient has spontaneous respiration and an effective heartbeat, or until it is evident that the resuscitative effort is hopeless. When the patient with cardiac arrest is not in a hospital or a setting where more definitive treatment can be applied, then artificial ventilation and external cardiac massage must be continued as the patient is transported to a hospital.

DEFINITIVE TREATMENT OF CARDIOPULMONARY ARREST

Once effective artificial ventilation and cardiac massage are established and when sufficient personnel and equipment are at hand, one may proceed to the second stage of more definitive treatment.

ELECTRIC COUNTERSHOCK

The initial step in definitive treatment is the application of an electric counter-shock to the chest of the patient. I believe that this should be done before obtaining an electrocardiogram since there is frequently considerable time lost in obtaining the electrocardiogram and there is little or no advantage at this point in the definitive treatment. Most clinicians now prefer direct current (DC) to alternating current (AC) for this purpose. After extensive studies it was found that an underdamped impulse of 2.5 msec released from a 16 Faraday capacitor through a 100 mH inductance resulted in a low incidence of arr-hythmias (8). Lown showed that this form of modified capacitor DC discharge was safe and effective in termination of cardiac arrhythmias, and cardiac stand-still did not follow its use (6). Ventricular fibrillation is most readily reverted with 400 w/sec, the maximum energy level available in most or all DC equip-ment. In the treatment of cardiac arrest direct current (DC) countershock has become preferred; however, alternating current (AC) is also acceptable (13). In the treatment of cardiac arrest it is easiest and quickest to apply both electrode paddles to the anterior chest wall, one below the suprasternal notch and the other just below the left nipple. One must make certain that the equipment is adequately grounded so as to protect the operator and ancillary personnel (11). A single individual should be responsible for periodically checking the equipment and maintaining it in proper working condition with the synchronizing switch off. The skin surface between the two electrodes must be dry and clean. A low resistance bridge may be formed by ECG paste between the two paddles. This pathway can shunt considerable electric energy and thus inadequate current may reach the myocardium for successful defibril-lation. Inadequate use of electrode paste can cause severe skin burns. There is much to be said for using saline soaked 4 × 4″ gauze pads between each electrode and the skin. This is particularly true when closed-chest massage is to be done.

Following the initial countershock artificial ventilation and external cardiac massage are immediately resumed, unless adequate circulation and spontane-ous respiration return. If an adequate heartbeat does not follow the first countershock, it is our practice to apply a second countershock of 400 w-sec. If there is again no effect we resume artificial ventilation and external cardiac massage. At this time we obtain an electrocardiogram to determine the cardiac rhythm. In cardiopulmonary arrest one of four electrocardiographic patterns may be observed: 1) ventricular fibrillation, 2) electric asystole, 3) ventricular tachycardia, and 4) persisting spontaneous electric activity. In the last-named the QRS complex is rarely relatively normal. Usually slow and wide idioven-tricular complexes are present with ineffective ventricular contractions (elec-tromechanic dissociation) [Fig. 14–4].

Advantages of Procedure

We prefer to apply an electric countershock to the closed chest before obtain-ing an electrocardiogram. This order of procedure has several advantages. The

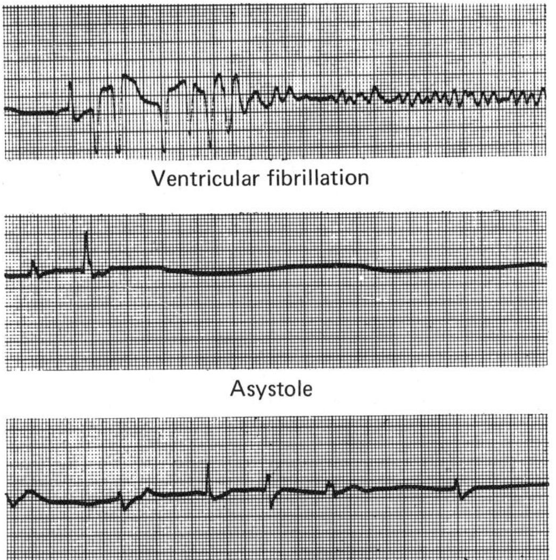

Fig. 14–4. **Electrocardiographic patterns observed in cardiopulmonary arrest.**

time lost in obtaining an electrocardiogram can militate against the success of the resuscitation. Countershock is not harmful with any of the four electrocardiographic patterns that can be observed in cardiac arrest. With ventricular fibrillation or tachycardia the initial countershock may immediately reestablish a functional circulation. In asystole, external countershock occasionally will be all that is necessary to reestablish a spontaneous rhythm. With electromechanic dissociation the countershock will probably have neither a beneficial nor a harmful effect. Synchronization of the countershock is not necessary in electromechanic dissociation. If the shock should cause ventricular fibrillation this complication can be readily treated by a repetitive countershock. Therefore there are no serious hazards in employing electric countershock before the cardiac rhythm is determined. If several rapid serial countershocks are not successful, we obtain an electrocardiogram while continuing artificial ventilation and external cardiac massage. In addition to the ECG, at this point an Intracath (a plastic catheter inserted through a large needle) should be placed in a suitable vein for a continuous infusion of 5% dextrose in water and sodium bicarbonate. Further treatment is guided by the ECG interpretation (Fig. 14–1).

Intracardiac Injection of Drugs

When the initial countershocks fail to convert ventricular fibrillation additional measures are required. When there are fine or poorly developed ventricular fibrillatory waves, repeated countershock is often unsuccessful. It may be helpful to change the fine fibrillatory waves to large or coarse fibrillatory waves by the injection of 0.5–1.0 ml of epinephrine (Adrenalin) 1:1000 solution, diluted to 10 ml with normal saline, directly into a cardiac chamber through the chest wall (Fig. 14–5). Although some prefer 1 ml of undiluted epinephrine 1:1000, the 10 ml volume is more easily and rapidly injected into a cardiac chamber. The needle can be inserted into the heart either by the subxyphoid approach or from the fourth or fifth intercostal space at the left midclavicular line. One would prefer to inject all intracardiac drugs into the left ventricle, since this facilitates rapid passage of the drug into the coronary circulation. This may not always be possible and one must settle for entering any cardiac chamber from which blood can be easily withdrawn. Following the injection of any drug into an arrested heart, one must externally massage the heart in order to deliver the drug to the coronary circulation. Not infrequently I have observed house officers, in the midst of a resuscitative attempt, inject a drug into a myocardial chamber and then step back from the bedside and wait impatiently for something to happen. Unless one massages the arrested heart following the intracardiac injection of any drug, little or no effect of the drug can be expected. Following the intracardiac injection of epinephrine (Adrenalin), one may see a change in the amplitude of the fibrillatory waves. If another electric countershock is then applied one is often successful in terminating the ventricular fibrillation. Failure to convert ventricular fibrillation may also be related to

Fig. 14–5. **Routes for intracardiac injection of drugs: the subxyphoid and the left fifth intercostal space approaches are shown.**

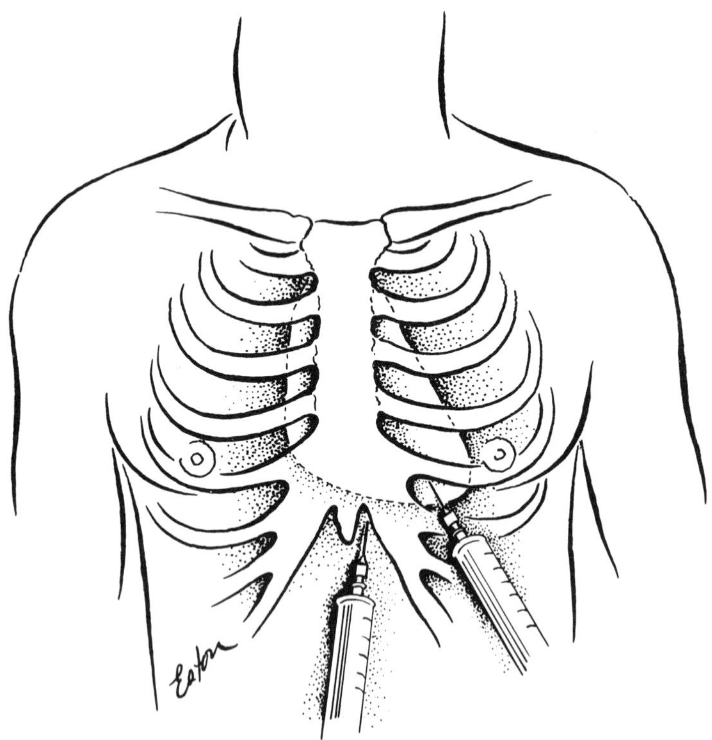

hypoxia resulting from inadequate artificial ventilation. If artificial ventilation is adequate and the ventricular fibrillation is not successfully treated with a countershock following the direct cardiac injection of epinephrine (Adrenalin), the intracardiac injection of 5 ml of a 1% solution of calcium chloride may facilitate conversion of ventricular fibrillation. If the above measures fail the intracardiac injection of procainamide hydrochloride (Pronestyl) 100 mg or lidocaine (Xylocaine) 100 mg followed by cardiac massage and then electric countershock may be successful. Successful treatment of ventricular fibrillation has been reported with propranolol (Inderal) 3–5 mg intravenously, followed by cardiac massage when other forms of therapy have failed (10).

Metabolic Acidosis

Failure to treat ventricular fibrillation successfully may be related to uncorrected metabolic acidosis. Metabolic acidosis is an inevitable complication of cardiac arrest and must be promptly and adequately treated. This is best accomplished by the intravenous administration of sodium bicarbonate, 44.6 mEq every 8–10 min from the onset of the cardiac arrest. One may give an initial bolus of two ampules followed by a continuous intravenous infusion (equal to one ampule every 8–10 minutes). Frequent determinations of arterial pH are desirable as a guide to the adequacy of this treatment.*

Not infrequently ventricular fibrillation or ventricular tachycardia recur soon after successful conversion. To prevent this event an intravenous drip of lidocaine (Xylocaine) 1–4 mg./min or a continuous intravenous infusion of procainamide hydrochloride (Pronestyl) 1–4 mg/min may be helpful in maintaining an adequate cardiac rhythm.

ASYSTOLE

If the electrocardiogram reveals asystole (Fig. 14–4) and the initial countershock prior to obtaining an electrocardiogram has failed to establish any electric activity, the treatment of choice is epinephrine (Adrenalin) 0.5–1.0 ml of a 1:1000 solution, diluted to 10 ml with normal saline, given directly into a cardiac chamber followed by external cardiac massage. Unfortunately this is rarely effective. Asystole is usually a difficult problem and successful resuscitation is unusual. Success or failure depends to a considerable extent on the underlying cause of the asystole which, at this point in the emergency treatment may not be readily apparent; and one must proceed with the empiric treatment of asystole. It may be necessary to repeat (at 2–3 minute intervals)

---

*Recently, this recommendation has been modified. Sodium bicarbonate, 1 mEq/kg body weight, is given intravenously initially. If arrest continues, this dose is repeated. Then further doses should be guided by determinations of arterial blood gases and pH. If these measurements are not available, one-half the initial dose is given at 10 minute intervals. Effective ventilation is needed to prevent CO_2 accumulation. Once there is an effective spontaneous circulation the sodium bicarbonate should be discontinued. (Standards for Cardiopulmonary Resuscitation (CPR) and Emergency Cardiac Care (ECC). JAMA 227 (Supp):837, 1974) the initial injection of epinephrine (Adrenalin) into a myocardial chamber several times before a sustained electric activity is again established.

Use of Artificial Pacing

If this fails one should then consider the use of artificial pacing of the heart. There are many disadvantages of external cardiac pacing, and this technique is rarely effective. However in many emergency situations on mobile units external artificial pacing is the form most readily available. External pacing is accomplished either through the electrodes used for obtaining an electrocardiogram, or by the addition of one or two other electrodes to the anterior chest wall. One sets the rate of the external pacemaker between 70–80 beats/min, and increases the amplitude of the electric energy level until effective pacing of the heart is obtained. Unfortunately the appearance of paced ORS complexes on the electrocardiogram is not necessarily indicative that an adequate myocardial contraction will follow. If artificial pacing is effective a strong carotid or femoral pulse is palpable. If successful, external cardiac pacing is continued until a more satisfactory variety of pacing can be established with a transvenous catheter and a battery-powered portable pacing unit.

A more effective emergency cardiac pacing may be accomplished transthoracically by passing a thin-walled 18 gauge needle through the anterior chest wall into the cavity of the right or left ventricle (Fig. 14–6). A unipolar or bipolar pacing wire is inserted through the needle into the ventricular cavity. The needle is then withdrawn over the wire allowing the wire to remain coiled in the heart through the anterior chest wall. The wire electrode is then attached to a battery-powered portable pacemaker and endocardial pacing is established (9). This application of cardiac pacing can be accomplished readily after one has practiced on a cadaver. The successful treatment of asystole is largely determined by the length of time asystole has been present.

Once circulation is restored the most effective and stable method of temporary pacing is by a transvenous catheter. A Swan–Ganz pacing catheter can be

Fig. 14–6. **Technique of transthoracic pacing using a wire electrode inserted through a thin-walled 18 gauge needle. [From Roe (9).]**

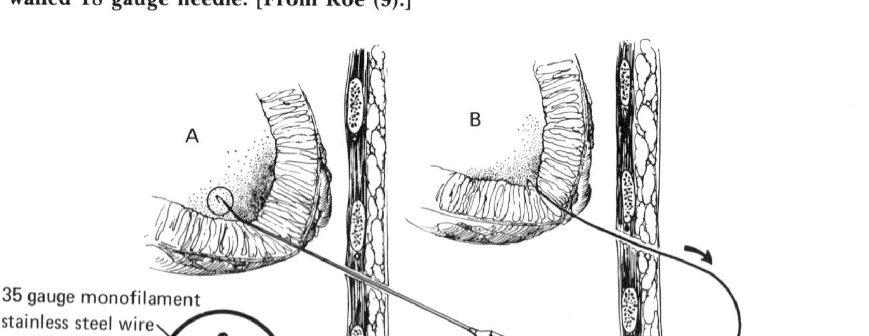

rapidly passed into the right ventricle with the aid of EKG monitoring. Image intensifier fluoroscopy, necessary for placement of the conventional bipolar pacing catheter, can thus be obviated. The catheter pacing systems are connected to a battery-powered portable pacing unit and may be used for days or weeks when necessary.

ELECTROMECHANIC DISSOCIATION

The treatment of electromechanic dissociation which is seen most commonly in advanced or terminal stages of chronic cardiac disease is nearly always unsuccessful. The successful treatment of this arrhythmia in association with an acute myocardial infarction may be a rare exception. The treatment of choice following the initial countershock is isoproterenol hydrochloride (Isuprel) 4 mg in 1000 ml 5% dextrose in water. The rate of administration is dependent upon the response of the myocardium to the isoproterenol (Isuprel). As the electrocardiogram is being obtained following the initial countershock, another member of the team establishes an intravenous infusion while external massage and artificial ventilation are going on. This is most readily accomplished by inserting an Intracath into either an arm vein or the subclavian vein. Dextrose (5% in water) is given continuously, and all drugs to be given intravenously can be readily administered by this route. The arrested heart must be massaged continuously in order for drugs to reach the coronary circulation and become effective. Occasionally pacing may be helpful in management of electromechanic dissociation.

USE OF PRESSOR AGENTS

In the course of treatment of a cardiopulmonary arrest it frequently is necessary to administer a pressor agent. Levarterenol bitartrate (Levophed) is given intravenously, 2 ampules (8 mg of base) in 500 ml of 5% dextrose in water, is the drug of first choice. Levophed is not only a potent α-sympathetic stimulator, but in addition has a marked positive inotropic effect on the myocardium. Metaraminol (Aramine), 200 mg in 500 ml 5% dextrose solution, may also be used as an effective pressor agent, but is less potent than levarterenol both as a pressor agent and in its inotropic effect on the myocardium. Dopamine HCL (Intropin), 200 mg in 500 ml 5% dextrose solution, may be useful in the shock syndrome frequently seen in cardiopulmonary arrest. When used in low to moderate doses (5–30 mcg/kg/min) it has little or no effect on total systemic vascular resistance, but may be useful alone or when used simultaneously with Levophed or Aramine because of its selective effect on increasing renal blood flow and its positive inotropic effect on the myocardium (3).

POST-ARREST THERAPY

Following cardiopulmonary arrest the products of anaerobic metabolism accumulate; the blood pH drops, and metabolic acidosis may become very severe and must be treated. This may be effectively treated by the administration of sodium bicarbonate 44.6 mEq intravenously/10 min from the onset of the resuscitative measures until the patient is completely resuscitated, and preferably the pH is within the normal range. If there is a delay in the administration of the bicarbonate, one must initially give a sufficient amount of bicarbonate to overcome the deficit which has accumulated. Occasionally a venous cut-down may be necessary for intravenous therapy when one fails to find a vein suitable for insertion of the Intracath plastic catheter.

Following successful resuscitation one may observe various cardiac arrhythmias even though a functional circulation has been established. Immediately following successful countershock there may be a brief period of AV dissociation or multiple ventricular contractions, which in both instances usually subside spontaneously. The brief periods of AV dissociation rarely require any specific therapy. Premature ventricular contractions which exceed 4/min can usually be suppressed by an intravenous loading dose of 100 mg lidocaine (Xylocaine) followed by 1–4 mg/min as a continuous intravenous infusion.

TERMINATING RESUSCITATION

When should efforts at resuscitation cease? It is difficult to state categorically the criteria for abandonment of the resuscitative effort. If one is fairly certain that the brain is not irreversibly damaged by anoxia then efforts at resuscitation should continue. One must maintain adequate cardiac massage as evidenced by a good carotid or femoral pulse. After prolonged periods of cardiac compression, one must question the advisability of continuing. When there is no sustained improvement after 30 minutes of intensive and adequate resuscitative efforts, success is unlikely and further efforts should probably be abandoned. Prolonged cardiac asystole which is refractory to drugs and artificial pacing precludes successful resuscitation. Definitive signs of central nervous system death may be more difficult to ascertain without an electroencephalogram. The size of the pupils may be misleading in certain patients and should be used with caution in evaluating the status of the central nervous system.

If external cardiac massage is carried out correctly one can expect little or no trauma to the heart, lungs, or abdominal viscera. However there is usually some separation of the costochrondral junction and some contusion of the anterior surface of the heart with closed-chest cardiac massage. Direct trauma to the heart is usually limited to contusion of the epicardium; contusion of the myocardium is unlikely except with acute myocardial infarction, in which case the infarcted area may rupture with cardiac tamponade.

In patients with chronic obstructive lung disease who have considerable increase in the anteroposterior diameter of the chest, it may be difficult to compress the heart adequately without fracture of one or more ribs. Not infrequently the increased force necessary to compress the heart damages the lungs and the abdominal viscera. Cardiac arrest in this setting may be an indication for internal cardiac massage. Internal cardiac massage should otherwise be reserved for patients with penetrating wounds of the chest, tension pneumothorax, chest or spinal deformities, or severe crush injuries of the thorax and instability of the thoracic cage. If cardiac arrest occurs in the operating room where the abdominal cavity is open, the surgeon may elect to enter the thoracic cage through the diaphragm and directly massage the heart. Internal cardiac massage should not be attempted outside of an operating room suite or emergency room with adequate facilities for mechanical ventilation and control of bleeding.

POST-RESUSCITATION CARE

Following successful resuscitation from cardiopulmonary arrest every patient should be observed closely for 24–48 hours with continous cardiac monitoring. This can best be accomplished in an intensive care unit. Not infrequently a patient will experience a second cardiac arrest following initial successful resuscitation. Continued support of blood pressure and assisted respiration may be needed for a variable period of time following successful resuscitation. Specific therapy for postresuscitation arrhythmias or hypothermia for cerebral edema in comatose patients may also be necessary. A careful evaluation of each patient for the underlying cause of his initial arrest should be made.

What can we expect from cardiopulmonary resuscitation? Successful resuscitation is most likely when cardiac arrest is treated promptly and occurs as the result of an accident involving a relatively healthy person. Several cities in the United States, including Miami and Seattle, have developed excellent out-of-hospital advanced mobile Life Support Units. These units have the ability to provide a trained team with the appropriate portable equipment to offer the basic and advanced treatment of a cardiopulmonary emergency and to stabilize the patient's condition prior to transfer to a continuing care facility. By providing central control, coordination, and a dispatching agency, these Mobile Life Support Units have reduced the early mortality associated with cardiopulmonary emergencies (1). Cardiac arrest as a complication of diagnostic procedures, anesthesia, drugs, accidental electrocution or drowning is an example of the foregoing. Patients with cardiac arrest in these settings have a better prognosis, since cardiac function was usually good before the arrest, and can in most instances be returned to normal. The outlook is best when the physician is in the room when the arrest occurs, since there will be minimal delay in initiating the resuscitation. In many hospitals the organization of emergency arrest teams, equipped with mobile defibrillation carts, who are on call at all times and available within 1 or 2 minutes, has increased the number of successful resuscitations. The continuous cardiac monitoring of high risk patients, *i.e.,* those with acute myocardial infarction, patients undergoing general anesthesia, and patients subjected to angiography and cardiac catheterization, enables emergency treatment to be promptly applied and increases the number of successful resuscitations. Nurses are often the only professional personnel immediately available to patients in coronary care units, intensive care units, or on general medical or surgical floors of hospitals. They are now routinely trained in the initial resuscitative procedures.